Psyche and Soul in America

Psyche and Soul in America

The Spiritual Odyssey of Rollo May

ROBERT H. ABZUG

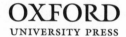

OXFORD
UNIVERSITY PRESS

OXFORD
UNIVERSITY PRESS

Oxford University Press is a department of the University of Oxford. It furthers
the University's objective of excellence in research, scholarship, and education
by publishing worldwide. Oxford is a registered trade mark of Oxford University
Press in the UK and certain other countries.

Published in the United States of America by Oxford University Press
198 Madison Avenue, New York, NY 10016, United States of America.

CIP data is on file at the Library of Congress
ISBN 978-0-19-975437-3

1 3 5 7 9 8 6 4 2

Printed by LSC Communications, United States of America

In memory of my parents, Seymour and Frances Wolff Abzug

Contents

Acknowledgments

It is a pleasure to recognize the many people who helped in the creation of this book. First and foremost was the late Rollo May, who in candid conversation and by granting access to his manuscripts enabled me to capture the extraordinary breadth of his life. Georgia Johnson May was extremely helpful in adding to this picture both before and after May's death. The Mays showed me the warmest hospitality at their home in Tiburon, California, where I did virtually all of the work in his papers, and in Holderness, New Hampshire, where we engaged in wide-ranging and illuminating discussions of his life and life in general. Rollo's niece, the late Barbara May, added a touching dimension to my understanding of his last years. May's half-brother, the late Gerald May, in his own right an author and therapist, met with me over two long lunches in Maryland and provided insight into the father they shared. Of course, I would not have had the opportunity to commence this work without the aid of the late John Vasconcellos, a friend for forty years, who introduced me to May and shared anecdotes concerning his own interactions with the humanistic psychology community.

May's colleagues and friends aided the project as well. Irv Yalom commented on parts of the manuscript and discussed May's impact on his own work and personal life. I gained special insight into May's New York years from the late Bob Akeret of the William Alanson White Institute. In emails and conversations long and short, I learned much from therapists who knew Rollo or who were connected to the White Institute in New York and various Bay Area institutions, had written about major figures in the story, or were in private therapeutic practice: the late Sabert Basescu, Sandra Buechler, the late Jim Bugental, the late Leo Caligor, Steven Diamond, Jackie Doyle, Sibel Golden, Tom Greening, Ed Hoffman, Peter Koestenbaum, Ed Mendelowitz, the late Don Michael, Maureen O'Hara, Barbara Rosen, Kirk Schneider, and the late Miltiades Zaphiropoulos. A special thanks to Shirley Kessler, who enabled my use of her interview transcripts for an unproduced film about Rollo May.

As for the world of Esalen, Michael Murphy and Walt Anderson helped me get the big picture, while chats with my friend Jeff Kripal as well as his scholarship helped supply the fine grain. Among others who shared their personal impressions of May were Ingrid Kepler May, the late Diane Middlebrook, and the late Harold Taylor. I owe a special debt to George Cotkin, cultural historian of so many things and most especially Existentialism, for his scholarship and for the times we have been able to discuss ideas related to this book. The same can be said of fellow biographer and friend Larry Friedman, who graciously let me look at some of the material he had collected for his biography of Erich Fromm and with whom I compared notes on the Fromm-May relationship and the profession in general.

Friends, colleagues, and students in Austin shared ideas, editorial advice, and support over many years. I am especially grateful to Alyssa Ramirez, whose detailed comments on virtually the entire manuscript improved its structure, style, and clarity. My friend of almost forty years, Mary Cook, read most of the manuscript and blessed it with acute observations. Joe Holley took time from his own writing to give the manuscript a final once over and helped shore up some important points. The work of three of my doctoral students and now peers—Chris Babits, Jess Grogan, and Matt Hedstrom—deepened my understanding of ideas and movements directly related to May's life. Friends and colleagues who provided research aid and insight, read chapters, and in other ways lent support include Daniel Coonan, Carol Dawson Randy Diehl, Betty Sue Flowers, Kathleen Higgins, Steve Hoelscher, Jim Magnuson, Mark Micale, Elizabeth Moore, Rachel Ozanne, Frank Richardson, Mike Stoff, Jennifer Westrom, and Hannah Wojciehowski. In addition, members of the University of Texas's Humanities Institute Seminar of Fall 2017 provided a warm and supportive environment in which to test ideas that proved important to shaping the final manuscript.

I would also like to recognize the archivists without whose aid much of this story could not have been told. Early on, the archives and staff at Michigan State University and Oberlin College, along with Oberlin's award of a Frederick Binkard Artz Summer Research Grant, eased the collection of unique material that illuminated May's college years. In New York, I had the privilege of utilizing the archives of Union Theological Seminary, the William Alanson White Institute, and Columbia University. In Cambridge I spent profitable days at Harvard's Houghton Library and Divinity School Archives. Jess Grogan shared material she had gathered at the University of Akron for her own research. Steps away from my office at the University of Texas, the Harry Ransom Center's manuscript collections provided me not only with archival material but also with a delightful environment within which to work. In addition, the Phi Beta Kappa papers at the Library of Congress proved enlightening on the subject of the Ralph Waldo Emerson Award. Finally, while I utilized May's manuscripts in his home office, they have found a more orderly and secure home as the Rollo May Papers at the Humanistic Psychology Archive, Special Research Collections, the Davidson Library, University of California, Santa Barbara. I owe a special debt of gratitude to David C. Gartrell at Special Research Collections, who oversees the Rollo May Papers and went above and beyond the call of duty by providing quality scans of most of the photographs in this book on short notice.

This study would not have been possible without generous funding for research travel and leave from my on-campus responsibilities. A Guggenheim Fellowship as well as yearlong and summer fellowship support from the National Endowment for the Humanities head the list. The Guggenheim and NEH Fellowships were matched by the University of Texas, whose University Research Institute also provided a semester's leave as well a number of travel grants. After 2001, I held the Oliver H. Radkey Professorship in History and the Audre and Bernard Rapoport Regents Chair in Jewish Studies, which gave me full freedom to travel on research missions and to present parts of this book to various audiences. In these and many other ways, the University of Texas has been a wonderfully supportive academic home for over four decades.

Very special thanks go to Susan Ferber, longtime friend and peerless editor at Oxford University Press. She embraced this project at a liminal moment and displayed an ideal mix of encouragement, patience, and editorial advice as I proceeded to finish it. Joellyn Ausanka, who worked with me on my first book for Oxford many years ago, oversaw copyediting and various other production tasks and guided me through the everchanging editorial procedures of the digital age with expertise and good humor. I very much appreciated the wise comments and careful copyediting provided by Ben Sadock.

There are more deeply personal debts to recognize. Thanks go to Dan Horowitz, who for fifty-six years has been the warmest and most supportive of friends at every stage of my academic and personal life and a shining model of humane scholarship. Steve Maizlish and Clarence Walker have offered sustaining friendship since our first years of graduate school at Berkeley.

As for family, I will repeat with only slight changes what I wrote in another book twenty-five years ago. I thank my wife, Penne Restad, who offered expert editorial advice and historical wisdom matched only by the love and patience with which she watched this project grow. Ben and Johanna have made it all worthwhile by simply becoming their uniquely wonderful selves. And now I can add Johanna's daughter, Wren, our first grandchild, born as this book was going to press and who arrived just in time to make these recent months ones of joy and inspiration despite the dark clouds of pandemic and more.

Austin, Texas
August 2020

Preface

Rollo May once joked that in his World War I–era youth, folks around him "thought Homer was something Babe Ruth knocked out" and that, aside from the Bible, the only book his parents owned was John Bunyan's tale of salvation, *Pilgrim's Progress*. May meant the quip to mark his own progress from modest roots in small-town Michigan to international fame as one of the most influential psychologists and public intellectuals in post–World War II America. His books—*The Meaning of Anxiety, Man's Search for Himself, Existence, Love and Will, Power and Innocence, The Discovery of Being*, and *The Courage to Create*, among others—reached millions of readers in America and abroad, illuminating a search for meaning in a modern world May viewed as increasingly disenchanted and unsure of its higher truths and common values. *Psyche and Soul in America* reveals May's inner and public life and the ways they intersected with those forces of modernity that corroded tradition and bred new definitions of selfhood, healing, and spiritual life.

May focused most of all on the consequences of modernity on everyday consciousness. He argued that the overvaluation of technology and science, as well as the regimentation of modern life and mass culture, had ensnared men and women in false choices, engendering in them a deep sense of powerlessness, loneliness, and apathy. He did not seek a return to "old values" or traditional religion but instead sought to promote individual and social regeneration through the courageous embrace of personal freedom and responsibility not only for oneself but also for the community at large.

May shared these concerns with many public intellectuals of the postwar years. During the 1940s and 1950s, Erich Fromm, David Riesman, David Potter, William H. Whyte, Vance Packard, and John Kenneth Galbraith, among others, focused on signs of alienation evident amid the seductions of prosperity. For the most part, their interpretations relied on political, psychological, sociological, as well as historical visions and methodologies. Collectively they shed a kaleidoscopic light on the era, one expressed in such evocative book titles as *Escape From Freedom, The Lonely Crowd, People of Plenty, The Organization Man, The Status Seekers*, and *The Affluent Society*.

May's contribution borrowed much from these interpretations but aimed more squarely at spiritual anxiety, depression, and feelings of emptiness that seemed endemic to the period. He enriched a basic psychoanalytic framework derived from Freud, Alfred Adler, and Otto Rank with meditations on the philosophies of the ancient Greeks, Kierkegaard, Nietzsche, and the neo-orthodox Protestant theology of Paul Tillich.

May's success at attracting a broad readership came as much from the power of his prose as it did from the psychological, philosophical, and religious ideas he merged into meaningful form. He displayed a peculiarly democratic and American sensibility, writing less to elucidate the finer points of one or another theory or belief system than to inspire a sense of intellectual and emotional engagement, one that would be both educational and therapeutic. He wrote in a style befitting his origins in the Protestant heartland, that of the plainspoken ministerial sermon. May mixed ideas and insights, quotations from Euripides, Kant, and Camus, with examples and applications literally clipped from daily newspapers. In doing so, he sought to demonstrate the relevance to their own lives of thinkers with whom most might be unfamiliar or know only by name. Some critics pointed out the sermonic nature of his prose, and not always as a compliment. However, at their best May's lectures and books were sophisticated, compelling, and spiritually inflected sermons for their times, ones that many continue to find relevant to this day.[1]

May came by that voice honestly. His father was a YMCA field secretary, his mother a devout Methodist, and his aspirations as a young man were to embrace the calling of as yet unspecified "religious work." He chose to study at Union Theological Seminary, graduated in 1938, and for several years pastored his own church. At Union he studied homiletics with the legendary preacher Harry Emerson Fosdick and forged a lifelong friendship with the great émigré theologian Paul Tillich. Even after he renounced his commitment to Christianity, pursued a career in psychoanalysis, and championed existentialism, he continued to emphasize the human capacities for love, transcendence, courage, and creativity that most men and women felt to be the very essence of the human condition. He spent the better part of his professional life helping to make more room for these dimensions in the worlds of psychological theory and psychotherapy.

May's life, fascinating in its own right, takes on much greater significance when seen as part of a central drama in modern American culture—the simultaneous decline of liberal Protestantism as a cultural arbiter and rise of a "therapeutic" vision that transformed the ways in which many Americans understood the emotional and spiritual issues of life. Critics have been fascinated and sometimes appalled by what the late Philip Rieff called "the triumph of the therapeutic," some seeing in its manifestations the maturing of American culture and others the ooze of a quiet cultural apocalypse. May himself worried about such developments and late in life wrote about the dangers of individualism untethered to a common mythos.[2]

It was not by accident, then, that May chose *Pilgrim's Progress* to symbolize his upbringing, for even as it marked his modest beginnings, it continued to resonate with the central concerns of his life. May used psychology and a broad philosophical framework to answer new, if less religious, forms of the Pilgrim's agonized question, "What shall I do to be saved?" In his first book, May equated successful therapy with religious experience, comparing "the transformation from neurosis to personality health" to "what it mean[t] ... to experience religion."[3] In his second book, he equated "the fulfilled personality" with "the 'saved' personality."[4] Much later, in "The Delphic Oracle as Therapist," an essay written at the height of his involvement in existentialism, he noted that the insights of myth came as much from "revelation" as psychological analysis, that "Aeschylus and Sophocles and the other dramatists could write great tragedies because of the religious dimensions of myth."[5] For May, "What shall I do to be saved?" was but a variation on that basic question "What does it mean to be human?" In his mature work, the fullness of creative encounter with the world and other human beings became May's yardstick for the meaningful life.

* * *

The evolution of May's career raises a complicated but important question: What was the relationship between the philosophy of life May came to espouse and his own most intimate choices, thoughts, and actions? This exploration is particularly appropriate for someone who grappled directly with issues that cut to the core of existence. I have assumed that no one obsessed by the meaning of love or life or meaning itself could have had a painless time of it. May himself once began an autobiography that he planned to call "The Wounded Healer." Wounds there were many, both suffered and inflicted. Nor did loving come easily. Fortunately, in a great act of courage, he put at my disposal, without prior censorship or restrictions, his extraordinarily large and intimate set of personal and professional manuscripts—letters, diaries, dream analyses, draft manuscripts, and sermons, as well as the often revealing ephemera of a long life. I have felt privileged to reach deeply into May's consciousness and life experience over virtually his entire adult life. This intimate vantage has allowed me to write about May from the inside out, so to speak, rather than attempt to fit his life neatly into existing narratives or controversies within the histories of psychology, religion, or philosophy.

The reader may wonder why there is only passing reference to his three children—Bob, Allegra, and Carolyn. Early on in this project, they collectively expressed the desire not to be interviewed or to have their lives play a substantive role in my account of May's life. I have honored their wishes as completely as possible, knowing that writing a biography involving living persons has an ethical dimension of paramount importance. At no point have they attempted to impede progress on my work, and all of our contact, largely through Carolyn May, has been one born of trust and encouragement.

The book owes its life to a serendipitous conversation. In the mid-1980s my friend the late John Vasconcellos, a humane and powerful member of the California legislature, came to Austin on state business. We invited him to our house for dinner, and somewhere around dessert he raised a heart-felt concern. Carl Rogers, the eminent psychologist whom John revered as both mentor and friend, was not well. John wondered whether anyone would write a biography of Rogers that did justice to his importance. I expressed sympathy and assured him that *someone* would write about him. I didn't expect John's next words to be "Bob, you ought to write about Carl." To which I replied with a simple "No."

I could have left it at that or added: too many projects, too much committee work, or the time-honored academic response—not my field. Instead, I told him that a biographer had to feel some gut connection to the subject and that Rogers didn't move me. I added that if I ever were to write about a psychologist, it would be someone who displayed his emotions, someone like Rollo May. Even as I spoke those words I wondered where they had come from. I had read only one of May's books (*The Courage to Create*), which did have a significant impact on my writing. I had heard him give exactly one public lecture. Suffice it to say I knew nothing of his inner life.

Nor did I have time to figure out why I had invoked May as a better subject for biography. John's almost instant response was, "Let's get together with Rollo the next time you are in the Bay Area." A year later, the three of us met in a Sausalito café. Being with Rollo was a treat, but I wondered if I really had an interest in his telling his life story. Nor was he necessarily eager to have a stranger write about what he considered a somewhat messy life. So we talked about everything but the biography while John sat impatiently, a matchmaker at the first date, waiting to broker a deal and faintly amused by the coyness all around. Rollo and I exchanged addresses and phone numbers. I sent him copies of my books and plunged into his work and to basic accounts of his life.

The courtship lasted for more than three years and involved numerous visits to May's home in Tiburon and summer place in Holderness, New Hampshire. We talked about each other's work, his transition from minister to therapist, the Vietnam War, Watergate, sex, love, and the fate of America under Ronald Reagan. We took walks along Tiburon's precipice overlooking Angel Island and along beaver-dammed streams in the New Hampshire woods. We grew to trust each other, and in 1991 May granted me permission to have unrestricted use of his papers. I agreed to do the biography. Rollo and I developed a respectful relationship, one that at times sparked a warm encounter in which each of us learned something about ourselves and the other. He urged me to present his life in full—his ideas, accomplishments, shortcomings, obsessions, and fragilities. Decades later, I have finally completed the task. I came to understand the power of May's appeal even now and its relevance to life in the twenty-first century. I am still perplexed as to the origins of my dinner table declaration but not sorry it took me down this long and enlivening path.

Psyche and Soul in America

1

"Epitome of America"

In late August 1987, after a troubled morning of writing, Rollo May emerged from the tiny work cabin at his summer home in New Hampshire to receive word from the American Psychological Association that it had awarded him a Gold Medal for Lifetime Achievement. At age seventy-eight, having been in the public and professional limelight for almost four decades, May was plagued by the fear that he and his work would soon be forgotten. "I was deeply moved," he wrote in his diary the next day. "My colleagues think well of me—I felt like crying." The honor came at a crucial time, for May was writing what he knew might be his last book, *The Cry for Myth*.[1]

The Cry for Myth summarized themes May had grappled with before but did so with new piquancy and focus: the disintegration of myth in modernity and yet the need for cultures and individuals to frame meaning, memory, and community in these overarching narratives. Pulsing beneath his elucidation of myth and the quest for meaning—stretching from the Greeks to Alex Haley's *Roots*—lay the contemporary individual's task, to discover a compelling narrative for one's life in a world without a shared sense of meaning. May, who had devoted his mature professional life to psychoanalysis, now defined therapy as "the search for one's own myth."[2] He warned of the power of unconscious personal narratives to imprison but also the possibilities of freedom inherent in making the chains visible and reclaiming liberating memory through a new story. And he quoted the foreboding lines of Canadian feminist poet Susan Musgrave: "You are locked / in a life / you have chosen / to remember."[3]

May wrote for his readers but also for himself. As he labored on *The Cry for Myth*, he was reworking his deepest understandings of his life story. Just a few weeks after receiving notice of his APA award, he recorded a startling dream:

> I living at home, with Mother and Dad. He not coming home mornings. I know something was wrong, I did not know what—no one would tell me. . . . Then I heard Dad in mother's room. I realize it was family trouble again. I felt empty, like old time feelings—I without any mooring—as

though world is unknown. I look to a bleak life, to the biting feeling of loneliness, emptiness—anything would be better than that. . . . Everything was
lonely . . . with me wandering through it.

"This my childhood neurosis," he wrote in his diary. "That world sad, lonely,
empty. At last, at 78, I have a clear dream about my childhood!!" It was "the
root," he claimed, of a lifelong "melancholia."[4]

Yet all was not so simple. May had been disturbed and intrigued by similar
dreams throughout most of his adult life, and as a psychoanalyst sought in
them the sources of an endemic sadness and anger. What is known of his early
life—a mix of facts and his own highly subjective and evolving memories—
hardly adds up to a balanced or objective sense of May's childhood. However,
he crafted from the memories, dreams, and nightmares about his youth an
explicit personal myth. These encapsulated snapshots became the basis of
his most profound public meditations on courage, love, and creativity. Even
as he sought meaning in the great cultural currents from antiquity through
modernity, he translated them for himself and his public through the conscious and unconscious shape of personal experience. To understand Rollo
May and his significance, then, one must begin in the murky memories of a
lonely youth.

* * *

"I am an American to the core," Rollo May declared in 1972, "indeed
middle western." The culture of his native region, he noted, mixed "generosity, friendliness, courage to risk and to experiment" with "violence and
money-mindedness" and a fear of "thinking too much." It was the "epitome
of America."[5] Born in 1909 in the village of Ada, Ohio, and raised in a dozen
small Michigan cities and towns, May experienced a world that bore the
marks of dynamic transformation. In those days, new mill, farming, and factory communities punctuated the dominant landscape of fields and woods,
where young boys searched for Indian relics and ministers preached piety
and good works in churches knit together by gossip and prayer. At family
dinners, aging veterans' memories of Civil War battles competed with excited reports of the latest automobiles and stunt flyers in biplanes. Three of
the four great American metropolises—Chicago, Detroit, and Cleveland—
connected the towns in Illinois, Ohio, and Michigan to food processing and
heavy industry and, by railroad and Great Lakes shipping, to the rest of the
world. From family farms to Detroit's assembly lines, from small-town seats

of self-proclaimed white Protestant virtue to new immigrant and African American communities, the Midwest conjured for Rollo and many others not only the epitome of America but also the epitome of American aspiration.

This romantic view warred with sordid realities. While Rollo navigated grammar school, midwestern writers were building literary monuments to the suffocating narrowness and hypocrisy of small-town life. A voice of the dead in Edgar Lee Masters's *Spoon River Anthology* pleaded for rebirth with the town "rooted out of [his] soul," while the inhabitants of Sherwood Anderson's *Winesburg, Ohio* betrayed a poignant universe of blunted spirits, secret passions, and family madness.[6] One might escape to the city, but there, depravity and injustices of an urban sort engaged crusading writers as varied as Theodore Dreiser and Upton Sinclair.

May's Midwest was of a piece with Winesburg or Spoon River but with its own virtues and darkness. His father, Earl Tuttle May, worked as a YMCA field secretary and earned a salary that allowed the Mays only a marginally middle-class existence. As important, his job involved founding and supporting YMCA chapters across the state of Michigan, which meant a constant uprooting that created predictable problems for the family. Rollo spent his youth in a dozen towns. Making friends was difficult, and all too often other kids bullied or teased the gawky new boy in town. These moves prevented sustained connection to any one place and lent intensity to a household awash in the lofty purpose of practical Methodist piety.

No one felt the church's call more strongly than Rollo's father. E. T., as he was known by all, was a trim, handsome, even dashing man—five foot six, a natural storyteller and gifted teacher, one quick to make friends and extremely successful at recruiting supporters of the Y. Earl's grandfather, Milton May, had been a wealthy slaveholder in Virginia who, before the Civil War, emancipated his slaves and took them with his family to Ohio. Milton and his wife had a daughter, who died in infancy, and two sons. The eldest, Lewis, taught school, served as justice of the peace, ran a general store, voted Republican, and by some accounts drank to excess. He married Emma Tuttle, who, at least by family tradition, was artistic, temperamental, beautiful if sickly, and a Democrat. After her first child died in infancy in January 1880, she gave birth to Rollo's father.

What little is known about E. T.'s early life comes through the prism of family lore. His parents instilled in him a heady spirit of rectitude and service, yet the boy graduated high school with little sense of direction. He taught grammar school for a few years and enrolled at Indiana's Valparaiso

University in 1902. Valparaiso had recently expanded from a normal (teacher training) school into a regional college and early on garnered a reputation for academic excellence. Nonetheless Earl took little advantage of its new curriculum. He felt smothered by the endless routine of classes and study. Only friendships, activities at the Y, and the passion of a tumultuous if disastrous love affair sustained him.

He needed to escape and decided to make a pilgrimage to the Holy Land. Such wanderlust was hardly novel for a young man, and the destination not exotic for a serious Christian. He spent the summer selling maps to finance his voyage and embarked from New York in December 1903. On the way he stopped in Cairo, observed daily prayers at a mosque, toured the pyramids in the company of tip-hungry touts, and visited a spot his tour guide assured him was where Pharaoh's daughter had rescued the baby Moses. In Jerusalem, he visited the Western Wall of the old temple and a Jewish synagogue but mainly concentrated on Christian sacred sites.

Earl's trip bore the outward signs of a religious quest, but his diary and letters home reported not one moment of awe, inspiration, or renewed faith— not in the shadows of Europe's cathedrals, nor in Bethlehem or Jerusalem. The ground trod by Jesus elicited no more excitement in his diary than an brand-new Ottoman railway station. Indeed, he seemed more concerned about propriety than religious experience. When visiting the Vatican and ancient Christian ruins, he shunned the beauties of the Catholic mass and, on a Sunday, expressed condescending surprise that Italians went about their business "as on week days." He seemed truly agitated only by sexual longing, noting in his diary that "fast women" on his ship to Alexandria had rekindled an "old trouble" and provoked "an odd dream."[7]

By mid-March, Earl had happily returned to the comforts of his Ohio home. He attended prayer meetings, judged local debate competitions, and assisted his father at the general store. In September, he attempted a fresh start at Valparaiso, but the break had improved neither his study habits nor his devotion to the university's "scientific" curriculum. In his diary, day after day he simply noted the word "college," except for once, when he wrote "depressed." Bible rallies and prayer meetings were the highlights of his campus life. The YMCA became a second home.

It was perhaps at the Y that Earl met the intense and attractive Mary Martha Washington Boughton. Matie (as she was called) descended from a mix of Methodists, Quakers, and Catholics from French and English roots (including, the family assured all, a line that descended from the family of George Washington). Her mother had one child and then lost her husband in the Civil War. Eight years later, she remarried to William Eric Boughton, settled on a farm in Michigan, and had six more children. Matie was her last. Her mother died while Matie was still young, and Matie's father arranged for his daughter to be raised by relatives. An orphan among family, Matie became virtually a live-in maid even as she struggled through school. Rollo remembered one story his mother repeatedly told her children: She had failed the seventh grade because of her home responsibilities but pleaded with the principal to promote her. Her wish granted, Matie applied herself and improved her performance, crediting her will to a renewed Christian faith.

Such commitment and a small inheritance allowed her to attend Valparaiso. The Matie Boughton that Earl May met was a bright-eyed redhead, a "new woman" of the twentieth century who sought an education and career. She took courses in a number of fields but majored in education. She and Earl married in 1905. That same year, Valparaiso granted Matie a "normal" diploma with a specialization in kindergarten. Her new husband left without graduating. The newlyweds moved to Ada, Ohio, where Earl finished college at Ohio Northern University. Matie volunteered at church, kept a small general store to make ends meet, and fashioned a modest home. E. T., as friends and family began to call him, took various jobs before finding a niche as an organizer for the YMCA.

We will never know the satisfactions or disappointments of the Mays' year of marriage before Matie's first pregnancy, but once the children started coming, their family became an emotional battleground. Matie gave birth to a tempestuous daughter, Ruth, in May 1907, whose erratic behavior helped to snuff out the joys of her birth and added to her parents' marital stress. Perhaps they were also disappointed, as Ruth later contended, that she had not been a boy. Matie became pregnant again little more than a year after Ruth's birth and on April 21, 1909, bore Rollo Reece May. E. T. had left on Y business the afternoon before and returned three or four days later. Matie was sure he was with a lover at the time, and sixty years later Rollo and his sister argued over their mother's suspicions that at the very moment of his birth his father was, as Ruth put it, "screwing another woman."[8] However, the birth of a son inspired Matie's fantasies and moved her to give him a special name. "Rollo" was the hero of Jacob Abbott's fabulously successful series of mid-nineteenth-century Christian children's books. Generations of American children had followed the boy's growth from *Rollo Learning to Talk* (1835) to

Rollo in Rome (1858), all reprinted many times through the early years of the twentieth century.[9]

Abbott's Rollo was the exemplary product of a Christian upbringing, trained in Protestant virtue and guided by the example of high-minded adults. Matie's Rollo certainly received a version of Christian nurture, though one colored by the more harrowing dimensions of his mother's love. She indulged him and cast him as her special child—the first-born son destined for great things. Rollo became the object of her intimacy in love and anger, her desperation and suspicions about E. T.'s affairs overburdening the child. "Mother needed me—father gallivanting—other women—she hugged me to her bosom—I owned her milk, caressing," he scribbled in his diary when in his seventies.[10] She proved unpredictable and often unhinged, snuggling him one minute and screaming at him the next.

Corporal punishment complemented desperate psychological manipulation. Physical discipline was the norm of the culture, but Matie's state of mind inspired extreme and frequent penalties. Rollo remembered more than once being whipped on the behind and many times clubbed on the backs of his legs. He recalled listening at an open window or door every day after school, trying to discern his mother's mood. He began wetting his bed, which further inspired parental wrath.[11] When Rollo was old enough, he built a treehouse to remove himself from the fray, a pattern he later recognized in a lifelong habit of retiring to heights, physical and mental—safe places from which to "give to others" but "at the price of figuring it out alone, being alone, going off on my own, inhabiting a mountain-top."[12]

As the family grew, so did Matie's despondency. She gave birth to another son, Don, in 1911. The following year, she bore a second daughter, Dorothea. In 1915 came a third daughter, Yona, whose birth triggered in Matie what Ruth later termed "a big *psychological break* (2 and a half hours)." Her depression persisted and deepened. Rollo remembered bringing a friend home, only to find his "mother in a soiled dress sitting in the middle of the room nursing the baby. . . . Brown feces on the dirty diddies strewn about the floor, a toy or two and books." His sister once questioned Rollo's sentimental regret that his father was mostly absent. "If Dad had been home oftener those childhood years," Ruth wrote to him, "there would have been *more* fights and *scenes* and probably more children." In fact, Matie bore one more child, Louis "Pat" May in 1922.[13]

Rollo did remember "happy times," such as when his mother exclaimed one Sunday morning, "Let's have a picnic!" and turned the entire family to the task of making sandwiches while she baked a cake. On such occasions, his father might demonstrate how to swing on a birch tree or perform some other amusing feat. Rollo recalled that when relatives came to visit, E. T. sometimes donned a fez, red silk bloomers, and sash he had brought home from the Holy Land and brandished a glinting scimitar before the amazed throng.

More ingrained in memory were nights the children heard threats and cries echo through the heat vents. E. T. once invited a colleague from the Y office in Detroit to counsel the couple and to lead them in prayer, but it didn't help. Soon after, Matie flew screaming from the bedroom wielding a pair of scissors and threatening suicide. Her husband wrestled the scissors away from her but then stormed out of the house and announced he was leaving for good. Rollo remembered Matie gathering the children around the kitchen stove and bewailing their lonely future. She got up after an hour, cranked up the wall phone, and finally located Earl at a hotel. "Earl," she said simply, "the children want you to come home." And, at least as May recalled, home he came.[14]

Such was the drama of the domestic scene, more humorous versions of which he would relate to intimate friends and occasionally allude to in public settings. In particular, his experience with his mother and sister tinged his life with sadness and distorted his deepest yearnings toward women. He feared their power but could feel powerful by helping to save them. The pattern constantly appeared in his own periodic seeking of therapeutic understanding at difficult moments in love or marriage. In the wake of a particularly difficult session with his psychoanalyst, Rollo recorded a haunting image that resonated with guilt: "Mother—sad-faced, walking with her stockings half down . . . hunched over for no reason . . . Mother sitting looking out, dazed, no reason to get breakfast . . . Ruth is there sour faced, mouth turning down, eyes like a mad Indian, resentful, a wolf or mad dog ready to jump . . ."[15]

Matie and Ruth's sad fates seemed particularly dark compared to that of E. T.'s blossoming YMCA career. Rollo's father embraced Y work with a booster's ebullience and the passion of a saint. He preached, raised funds, ran athletic programs, befriended troubled youth, and established new branches across the state. E. T. envisioned his efforts in each town and village of Michigan as part of a worldwide endeavor to preserve and extend Christian values amidst the tumult of modernity. Founded in England and established in the United States in the 1850s, the early Y sought to aid youth far from home, especially those surrounded by the temptations of the city. After the Civil War, its American branch broadened its mission by channeling the energies of young men—the group at highest risk of abandoning traditional values—into reforming and solidifying both body and body politic.[16] Across towns, cities, counties, states, and nations, the Y built an interlocking web of activities that would "Christianize community life" by strengthening "the Home, the Church, the School, and the Municipality in their relations to the social, recreational, educational, moral, and spiritual life of the community."[17]

The American Y translated these general commitments into a progressive reform program. It supported educational and moral uplift projects for African Americans, abolition of child labor, and protection of workers from "dangerous machinery, occupational diseases, and mortality." It endorsed the right of employees to organize and worked toward the eradication of poverty. It also campaigned for the prohibition of alcoholic beverages. YMCA activists imagined themselves to be on the front line of a global struggle for spiritual and material progress, "a 'world power' . . . laying the foundations of a new social and religious order . . . not only in North America, but in the Orient, the Levant, Latin America, and Europe."[18]

E. T.'s commitment to the Y crusade brought him respect and even adoration in the community but only conflicted feelings at home. Ruth's memories probably stood for Matie's as well. "The Business and Professional men whom he organized in each County esteemed him," she noted fifty years later, "the women fairly doted on him," and his fellow Y activists "worshipped" him. However, Ruth noted with bitter irony that E. T. gave "heady" sermons on humility and the imitation of "our *common* Lord" while mostly shunning familial responsibilities. "Never," she remembered, "did his wife or children share in this reflected glory." The Mays felt "shut out" as E. T. showered love upon his favorite Y "*boys*," who were privileged to call him "Earl." Yet, at least in one area, Ruth came to her father's defense. She, like Matie, took his infidelities as a given. She imagined him caught in a struggle between his "*baser instincts*" and the Christian life but was sure that he eventually experienced a "tremulous religious experience, conversion, and saw the light." If E. T. refrained from womanizing after his conversion, though, she was just as certain that it brought little peace to the family circle.[19]

E. T.'s impact on Rollo was especially complex. The son found in the father a model of Christian calling that he had already begun to make his own. Yet he also internalized Matie's rage at E. T.'s neglect and took on the role of his mother's helper. He yearned for his father's respect and attention but also sought to surpass his accomplishment and avoid his alleged hypocrisies. Nothing is ever simple in the love between father and son, and some of

Rollo's conflicts were those a psychoanalyst would term Oedipal. However, for Rollo, rivalry with and estrangement from E. T. had more complicated roots and remained with him his entire life.

The family seemed calmer for a while as Rollo entered his teens and E. T. moved the Mays to Marine City, Michigan, in 1921, where they would stay for almost five years. Marine City was a town of about 3,700 inhabitants, just across the St. Clair River from Canada and fifty miles northeast of Detroit. Its inhabitants worked in agriculture, shipbuilding, and the refining of sugar and salt. Almost 90 percent of were white and native-born. Its 462 "foreigners" were either Canadians or Germans, except for six "Asians." No African Americans lived in Marine City.

That was in stark contrast to neighboring Detroit, then America's fourth-largest city with a population of almost one million. Germans, Poles, Greeks, and other immigrants made up 29 percent of the population, and another 4 percent were African American migrants from the South. Twenty-nine different automobile manufacturers employed close to 150,000 workers, and autos were just the largest of several heavy industries centered in the area. Detroit's grit, variety, dynamism, and poverty sat as a challenge, seduction, and object of fear almost within sight of the wheat and corn fields of surrounding Marine City. Young Rollo shared those fears and developed a particular repugnance to the noise and stench of Detroit's industry. He preferred the quiet of his small town and its space for solitude.

Not coincidentally, it was in Marine City that Rollo and his father spent more time together and found an array of common interests. The two would read aloud to each other and chat in the meadow near their home. At Y camp in the summers, they would fish in Lake Superior or silently contemplate the beauty around them. Rollo later attributed his love of nature to these moments with his father. Most of all, he remembered that E. T. helped to give him a sense of competence in the world. He would allow Rollo to try out new activities and make mistakes. Once, building a porch on the back of their house, he asked his son to pick out the perfect board for a certain spot and waited patiently until, by trial and error, Rollo found the right one. Competence, self-reliance, confidence in one's skills—all of these the father carefully instilled in his son.[20]

E. T. also welcomed Rollo's own initiatives, as when he listened to the boy's homemade crystal radio, which pulled in WJZ in Detroit and, on clear evenings, a station from Atlanta that featured Wendell Hall, the "red-headed music man." "He would hold the earphone to his ear and I am quite sure that he grasped some idea of the miraculous," Rollo recalled. In fact, E. T. even preached a sermon on the miracle of radio.[21]

Still, Rollo experienced a typical teenage sense of isolation as he sought to find his place in the world, a loneliness heightened by being caught in the crossfire of often hostile and unreliable parents. While E. T. had many lessons to teach the young Rollo and delighted in his son's accomplishments, Rollo's enduring feeling was that he was in the world alone and crippled by the insecurities of a marginal social and emotional environment. One story that he later told to intimates bordered on self-pity. Deciding to enter a model airplane contest, Rollo carefully fashioned balsa side struts and a propeller as well as three-foot wings from silk-covered, varnished pruning wire. He cut a large rubber band from an inner tube to power the propeller. After a month's hard work, Rollo tested his model in the backyard only to watch it collapse into "a ruined heap." He attended the judging alone and without an airplane and saw dozens of beautiful models made from prefabricated sets of parts bought by "rich kids," who also brought their mothers and fathers to watch them. Rollo envied these children and later connected such feelings with a sense that he would never accomplish much despite his dreams and talents. The advantages they enjoyed were a slap in the face. "I knew these things were never for me," he wrote late in life; "a strange 'poor boy' experience, should I say myth, stayed with me and was never quieted."

Rollo thus appeared in high school as a mild paradox—a handsome, willowy teenager, six feet tall, but with a hesitant awkwardness that mirrored an inner turmoil. The swirl of guilt, anger, high purpose, fear, and resistance whipped up at home cramped his presence in the world. He completed his academic work like a drone, doing the normal four-year course in three years but earning mostly Bs and barely making the high school's own standard for college—despite an exemplary intelligence confirmed by IQ tests the high school administered.[22] He played football but remained a "second-stringer." In an emblematic story of self-definition, he remembered a game in which he was the only player on the team who could block an opponent's touchdown. He purposely stumbled and the other team won. "I was afraid of something— afraid of succeeding physically?" he wondered years later, worrying that he lacked courage. He did excel in public speaking, won countywide oratory competitions, and led the debate team to victory. Perhaps the shield of the rostrum helped him create a charismatic persona.[23]

Such sparkle often dimmed when others, especially women, sought his company. Rollo felt overwhelming desire but fierce inhibition. Like many youths, he had first learned about sex through rumor, humor, and chance. He cherished memories of his first-grade crush on a girl with curly golden tresses and his innocent backyard experiments with both girls and boys. He experienced the normal awkwardness of puberty, later still recalling school parties where dancing brought on unbearable arousal and embarrassment. It was all very titillating, but Rollo grew up in a household where sex was viewed with an extra helping of guilt and suspicion. One memory summed it up. He remembered that when he was nine or so, as he and a girl "played" in the backyard, Matie bounded out of the house singing "Onward Christian Soldiers" and gave him a brutal whipping. E. T. took a less violent but no less pointed approach, once hiring a Y speaker to educate his boys and girls separately about "reproduction" and urge abstinence upon them. For Rollo, the equation of virtue with abstinence as well as nagging suspicions about his father's adulterous proclivities complicated an already sensitive subject.

Hemmed in by school, home, and his own conflicts about assertion and success, Rollo found fulfillment and peace where he could. A paper route, clerking in a grocery store, and, in summer, a horse-and-wagon ice cream route earned him some spending money and whetted his appetite for independence. He felt most free on long walks, especially by the banks of the St. Clair River. The river became his companion and its past loomed large in his imagination. He knew of the great raft that in 1875 had transported two million board feet of oak from Bay City to Buffalo, and the replicas of the Niña, Pinta, and Santa Maria sailing to Chicago for the World's Fair of 1893.[24] However, for Rollo the river represented most of all the timeless, sublime, and sometimes brutal force of Nature. He delighted in the quiet beauty of flatboats towing houses in and out of the fog, but also in the gale force winds that ripped at docks and houses and in colossal waves that crashed boat against boat and washed the splintered remains onto the shore. In summer, he swam from an abandoned coal dock. In winter, he streaked across the ice-bound St. Clair in a homemade iceboat. In spring, he watched in awe as the annual thaw loosed great frozen blocks of ice, "transparent like the glass agates we used to shoot in marble games," battering anything that stood in their way. "It was a solace in my loneliness and occasional despondency," he later wrote of the river, "and it shared my joys."

The river gave young Rollo a place to ponder the troubling but inescapable question: What would he do with his life? The question blended invisibly with the anxious query of John Bunyan's Christian in Pilgrim's Progress: "What shall I do to be saved?" Whatever the drama of his family life, the Methodist and YMCA culture that shaped him gave a singular answer: service to humankind. His father's devotion to the Y provided a prime model. Given a special name, should Rollo not also possess a special future? Destiny became a craving, not only because of his parents' expectations but also because of his marginal place in school and among his peers. Fulfilling a great destiny might lift him out of family misery and loneliness. It might make him somebody in the world.[25]

The wounds of childhood, no matter how tentative, distant, and "strange" they made him feel, shaped the agenda for his concerns as a writer and psychologist. He replayed early pain and failure, in diaries and dreams, as a goad to accomplishment. If he had been cowardly on the football field, he would work out the meaning of "courage" for a new, psychological era. If the powerfully mixed messages of affection and hostility from his mother and Ruth made him wary of commitment to women and yet achingly crave their love, he searched for ways to unblock love and intimacy in modern society. Nowhere was this more evident than in Rollo's troubled religious life. The cacophony of faith, high ideals, and family madness would lead him toward a lifelong spiritual odyssey, one that subverted tradition even as it affirmed the centrality of the quest.

On the cusp of young adulthood, Rollo's dreams of destiny found voice in a poem that he discovered in an anthology he had received for his high school graduation in 1926, Sam Walter Foss's "The House by the Side of the Road." The first stanza proclaimed his imagined future:

> There are hermit souls that live withdrawn
>   In the peace of their self-content;
> There are souls, like stars, that dwell apart,
>   In a fellowless firmament;
> There are pioneer souls that blaze their paths
>   Where highways never ran;—
> But let me live by the side of the road
>   And be a friend to man.[26]

Rollo took its Christian altruism to heart. He would seek greatness through humility. He might find friendship by being a friend to "man," because he had yet to forge many such bonds with actual men and women. He did not yet have any sense of what that house by the side of the road might look like.

Would it be the simple cottage of a small town minister or one attached to the local YMCA? Or would it involve some grander, as-yet unknown mission?

Foss's poem never survived as literature, yet the power of its challenge stuck with May. He remembered every word well past his eightieth birthday. And a yellowing typescript of it remained tacked to the corkboard in his study on the day he died.

2

"A Deep Craving, a Keen Urge"

Rollo May entered college in 1926 with a lively sense of mission but only a vague of idea of direction. The example his father had set in working for the YMCA and the special honor his mother bestowed upon him as her "helper" pointed him to a career in "religious work." The rest was unsettled, even May's own spiritual life. He hoped to find himself and some compelling shape for his scattered emotions and ambitions. The task was made more difficult by the fact that college offered little escape from the embattled May household. E. T. had the YMCA transfer him to East Lansing so that Ruth and Rollo could attend Michigan State College while living at home "within the family finances." As a college administrator later noted on a scholarship form: "Family . . . more wealthy in children than money."[1]

East Lansing potentially offered Rollo the variety and ferment associated with academic life. Michigan State, with its faculty and more than three thousand students, was a community of its own but merged seamlessly with Lansing proper, the capital of Michigan. Campus culture exposed him to new kinds of people, new dress styles, more liberal sexual mores, and an open atmosphere for exploring ideas, literature, and the arts. A small number of wealthier students indulged in the mythic life of the 1920s—jazz, flappers, fast cars, wild parties, and bootleg gin. Rollo and the majority of students only gawked at such hijinks. They were serious-minded, preparing for work in the cities of industrializing America and on increasingly mechanized and commercialized farms or, as in May's case, finding a calling to match his nascent ideals.[2]

Launched in 1855 as the Agricultural College of the State of Michigan, the school sought to advance scientific agriculture and to keep the health and wealth of the state's economy at a peak. By the turn of the century, however, its narrow curriculum left Michigan Agricultural College vulnerable in an increasingly urban world where public higher education thrived on pre-professional training and the humanities. Worrisome symptoms abounded: declining enrollments, rapid faculty turnover, and the stranglehold of the State Board of Agriculture. In the 1920s, soldiers returning from

World War I crowded institutions with programs in business and liberal arts but avoided agriculture and veterinary medicine. Overcoming the resistance of the Agriculture Board and its legislative allies, Michigan Agricultural College responded with a new arts and sciences curriculum in 1921. Enough had changed by 1925 for it to adopt a new name: Michigan State College of Agriculture and Applied Science (this last part brought the farm lobby on board).[3] It was onto this newly named campus that Rollo first walked in the fall of 1926. He took the basics of Michigan State's new liberal arts curriculum— English composition, literature, Spanish, European history, basic zoology, and public speaking. He enriched his schedule with ornithology, drawing, decoration, and design, as well as religious education. His grades were respectable— a string of Bs punctuated by Cs and As. Still, freshman year threw him into turmoil. Among strangers but living with family, he missed out on the excitement of leaving home experienced by thousands of young men and women from Michigan's farms and small towns. He was also younger than most of his classmates and a gawky, self-conscious "townie" deprived of the camaraderie of dorm or boarding house life. Classes, assignments, and the extracurricular opportunities of campus life competed with his parents' expectation that he would help raise his brother Pat even as increasingly rancorous arguments between E. T. and Matie shook the household.

As a small-town "good" boy with little money and no social standing, he felt assaulted by the freewheeling horseplay and class snobbery that pervaded college life. "Of the fellowship of the college campus I felt I was left out," he reflected a few years later. Living at home and not having the "social punch," he perceived himself as invisible and insignificant. The "B.M.O.C.'s" on campus snubbed him as a "nothing."[4] Of course, he feared he was just that—a nothing—and searched for ways to distinguish himself.

He found little inspiration except in English classes. Professor W. W. Johnston, chair of the department, sparked his love of the literary imagination. Literature and loneliness helped Rollo to see himself as a sensitive rebel lost among farm boys, engineers, and spoiled snobs. The poet became his ideal and poetry a source of inspiration. Eventually, he found friends among like-minded souls, those he termed "the minority, 'reforming' group" on campus—young men and women who delighted in each other's company and flaunted a moral superiority compared to those they considered the dullard majority.

Still, Rollo often distanced himself even from his fellow reformers. Much as the camaraderie appealed to him, he had little experience of intimacy with peers in his earlier life. He had never lived in one place long enough and felt too embarrassed by his family life to invite friends home. Now within a group that accepted him, he still felt apart, opening up only when called upon for support or advice, to be a "friend to man." However, too often he offered a sweet but condescending brand of Christian "help" rather than the fuller embrace of friendship. One chum gave Rollo this piece of advice: "I am griped by your continual chatter, 'Pollyanna-ness.' Always 'over-nice.' Can't you be hard once in a while?"[5]

While intimacy remained a problem, literature and the freer intellectual life of campus unleashed in May an explosive exploration of ideas and meaning as he sought a place in the world. He banded with Roscoe Bloss and four others of his rebellious group to launch a five-cent biweekly newspaper, *The Student*, "dedicated to the Quest for Truth on the Campus of Michigan State College."[6] While Bloss concentrated on specific free speech issues, student elections, and university politics, May wrote about the "big" themes: morality, martyrdom, will, and rebellion.

Rollo searched especially for models of manhood, admiring action itself as much as any particular cause. His values echoed those of his father and the YMCA, albeit with a rebellious, autobiographical edge and little intellectual consistency. In the very first issue, he focused on Theodore Roosevelt's college years as a saga of the weakling transformed into a mighty leader. May depicted Roosevelt as "no different from the rest of young college men" except for "that invincible determination to make his life into something worthwhile." Perhaps thinking of his own cowardice on the gridiron in high school, May highlighted Roosevelt's immortal advice to young men: "In life as in football, the principle to follow is: Hit the line hard, don't foul and don't shirk, but hit the line hard."[7]

May also raised the question of courage and manhood in an excerpt, printed in bold type, from Elbert Hubbard's legendary Spanish-American War pamphlet "A Message to Garcia," which told the story of a "fellow by the name of Rowan" who, against all odds, delivered a secret letter from President McKinley to the leader of the Cuban rebellion. May plucked its lesson from the opening: "It is not book-learning young men need, nor instruction about this or that, but a stiffening of the vertebrae which will cause them to be loyal to a trust, to act promptly, concentrate on their energies; do the thing—'carry a message to Garcia'!" Yet for May's generation there were as yet no battlefield messages to deliver, no combat in which to suffer or die.[8]

Rollo did find one battle worthy of his soul, the defense of individuality in a world of leveling democracy and industrial society. "The iron bands of conformity," he thundered in "Are We Slaves?," "have in their deadly grasp the majority of American people!" Education no longer fostered "character and individuality," but rather taught skills that "fit" students "into the vast industrial system." Only the courageous individual could solve the problems of a "storm-swept world!" "The path of the strongest individuals is lonely," he declared, and constructed an American pantheon of courage: Lincoln, Whitman, Emerson, and Thoreau. Above all stood Jesus: "Society called Him a radical, a fanatic, and heaped abuses on His back. Had He not had the power to be an individual, you and I would not be here today!" May identified with these extraordinary figures as loners, indicating the shape of his own first feelings about what it might mean to "be somebody." This concern for individual autonomy in a world of conformity would remain a central theme of May's writing throughout his life. [9]

As it turned out, a less heroic piece in the same issue of *The Student* guaranteed the paper's downfall. In April 1928, May's fellow editor, Roscoe Bloss, fired a nasty salvo at Michigan's Board of Agriculture (which had sought to fire Michigan State's president), calling MSC "not a college at all, but a political playground, where the college presidency is a bait for party electioneers, a state institution for governors to practice economy upon, to cover up graft elsewhere in the machine." The college suspended Bloss and reprimanded May, who took over as managing editor of *The Student* under the watchful eye of the administration. May avoided directly contentious editorializing but found other means to raise embarrassing issues. In an Open Forum feature, for instance, he printed the "opinion" of a student who compared Bloss's controversial story—a mere "journalistic blunder"—to one local paper's bolder suggestion "that accepting the chair of the president at Michigan State College was about equivalent to committing professional hari-kari."[10] By the end of the term, despite attempts to keep the issue of Bloss's censure alive and perhaps win his own glory with a suspension, Rollo had managed only another reprimand. The unheroic whimper no doubt disappointed him. Yet editing *The Student* helped him define his commitments and make his mark on the world.

Less evident but far more profound were Rollo's struggles with religious faith, which reached a crescendo over precisely the same months as his involvement with the "reforming group" and *The Student*. "I suddenly came into the realization," he recalled a few years later, "that the views of

God . . . the beliefs I had absorbed from my parents—the belief that God was a great father always watching personally over his children—had become empty and without meaning to my life." Gaining some solace from eternal ideals like Beauty, Truth, and Goodness, he nonetheless felt that these were too abstract to allay "a deep craving, a keen urge to feel myself at home in the universe." All too often he found himself "bitterly lonely" and caught in "spells of despondency." He finally declared himself an atheist but at the same time sought spiritual counsel.[11]

He turned to Bennett "Buck" Weaver, a charismatic young poet and as-sistant professor of English. Born in 1892, Weaver had grown up on a farm in Wisconsin and in 1916, while pursuing a doctorate at the University of Michigan, joined the faculty at Michigan Agricultural College as a specialist in Victorian literature. He was also an active, progressive, and ecumenical Christian. In 1922, Weaver's spiritual proclivities moved him to accept the intertwined posts of director of religious work and religious education at the Peoples Church of East Lansing and YMCA secretary for the college commu-nity. Weaver, along with pastor Reverend Newell McCune, helped to launch what McCune called a "Great Experiment" by reconfiguring the church as a vibrant, nondenominational hub of ecumenical education, social action, and ministry to the students and faculty at Michigan Agricultural College. Weaver also launched "The College Christian Conclave," a lecture series at which national religious leaders discussed current affairs.[12]

The Mays joined the Peoples Church upon arriving in East Lansing, and Weaver soon got to know the whole family. Rollo was drawn to the young poet, who impressed upon him the stakes of spiritual life. He moved Rollo by speaking frankly about his strengths and weaknesses and the need to find his own religious truth. Weaver viewed faith as the product of a search for inner and individual wisdom and mystical experience. He placed little emphasis on theological exactitude or behavioral imperatives and instead focused on the growth of "personality," reflecting a liberal Christian view on the meaning and conduct of life in keeping with E. T.'s YMCA precepts and attitudes—at least the ones he promulgated in his public life.

Buck Weaver was the first of a number of new spiritual fathers Rollo would adopt in his life, and he came along at the right moment. Early in their rela-tionship, he helped May through a particularly harsh and lonely depression, the heart of which in Christian tradition would have been seen as a deepening "conviction of sin." Weaver coaxed him into a more ameliorative mood, one in which May somehow could remind himself that "hosts of persons through the age had found complete comfort in prayer" and had lost their loneliness by "finding a personal, loving God." Indeed, Weaver led May to his first "conversion experience." At one point, in the solitude of his room, he suddenly heard familiar phrases: "Come unto me" and "I will send you a comforter." He fell on his knees and tried to pray: "As I knelt there I suddenly seemed to see a light through my closed eyes; I felt a warmth permeating where my loneliness had been—at last the real lasting comfort of a personal God!"[13]

Buck Weaver's influence on Rollo extended far beyond this first of a number of religious experiences. In fact, May soon crystallized his approach to religious healing as an example of the most genuine and caring of relationships, an ideal for both counseling and life. He treasured Weaver's ability to "love me and believe in me," to take special interest in someone like himself from "personal liking" rather than as an object of missionary impulse. Buck Weaver defined what being "a friend to man" was all about.

Rollo spent the summer of 1928 working with his father at a YMCA camp near Lake Geneva, Wisconsin. There he immersed himself in nature, fellowship, and meditations on his religious state. He also pondered what to do the following fall. Weaver had already suggested that he might think about transferring to a college friendlier to his passions and nature, and Rollo returned to East Lansing in early September to seek Weaver's further counsel as well as that of his beloved English professor, W. W. Johnston. His religious experience, friendship with Weaver, and renewed engagement in his father's Y world pointed him toward a future in religion. He felt that Michigan State offered him little in this regard.

Weaver recommended that May apply to Oberlin College. He saw Oberlin as the perfect choice for Rollo because of its excellence in the humanities and its long tradition of Christian activism. Founded in the 1830s, Oberlin had been a hotbed of abolitionism, pioneered the education of Blacks and women, and bred in its students a fervor for all varieties of reform. After the Civil War, Oberlin exemplified the most progressive denominational colleges by seeding its faculty with new, university-trained specialists committed to combining a broad liberal arts education with Christianity. The presidency of Henry Churchill King (1902–27) saw a merger of a fervent liberal Christian faith with belief in the virtues of critical scholarship in all fields, including biblical studies. As one of Oberlin's historians put it, "The old evangelical faith, with its emphasis on individual salvation and personal moral codes, was giving way to a new faith combining reverence for the worth of the individual with social redemption."[14]

These values were hardly strange to Rollo. He had experienced them in action under Weaver's caring counsel. May knew Oberlin by reputation and had already read one of King's inspirational books, but not until the fall of 1928 did he conceive of the possibility of enrolling there. Attending a private school like Oberlin, with the expenses of tuition, room, and board, never seemed an option. Now, however, whatever the cost, it had become a spiritual imperative.[15]

Rollo decided to apply in person. Just before the term began, he hitchhiked 210 miles to Oberlin and, if we are to believe his usually accurate memory, pulled into town with suitcase in hand and five dollars in his pocket and walked the half block to campus to seek his educational fortune. He immediately confronted the Memorial Arch, which commemorated the Oberlin missionaries massacred during the Boxer Rebellion. The noble neoclassical design of the structure and one of its inscriptions left him awestruck: "The blood of the martyrs is the seed of the church." As he surveyed the list of names on the memorial, he suddenly felt "completely at home." This was not a "cow college," as he called Michigan Agricultural College, but a place that honored mission, destiny, even martyrdom—all that May dreamed about for his own life.[16]

At Peters Hall, he met with E. L. Bosworth, professor of theology and dean of men. The dean had already read letters about him from Weaver and Johnston, as well as Rollo's hastily thrown-together application. Weaver had emphasized "his unselfed thoughtfulness . . . his fearlessness of conviction and 'going on' quality." He felt that Oberlin would provide "the right environment" to deepen him. Johnston characterized him as "a high-grade, clean-minded, young man of fine integrity, high ideals and much independence of thought and judgment."[17] May's own essay expressed the desire for "the development and education which will come through studying under learned and Christian professors and associating with sincere and purposive students." May and the dean chatted for an hour about the YMCA, Christian commitment, and May's aspirations, after which Bosworth declared, "Okay, you're in."[18]

Paying for tuition and living expenses was another matter entirely. May's parents loaned him $350 at 6 percent interest, which he agreed to pay back by 1932.[19] He had earned $90 at the Y camp and planned to continue work there each summer. He put together the rest taking on jobs, loans from the college, and small scholarships and immediately began a search for affordable lodging. He investigated a boarding co-op that students dubbed "The

Poor House," but it had no vacancies. Rollo finally secured a room on East College Street in the home of a schoolteacher and traded kitchen work for rent. He traded similar duties for meals at a women's rooming house nicknamed "The Vatican" because it was in sight of Peters Hall (a joking reference to Saint Peter's Basilica in Rome). The following year he moved to the Men's Building as a resident adviser, though he continued to eat with the women.

Living within the college environs proved an adventure all its own, and the tight-knit Oberlin community seemed more like an extended family than an institution. At his boarding house and across campus, Rollo found an acceptance, friendship, and intimacy mostly absent at Michigan State. "The students at the Vatican took me in completely," he remembered. "Everybody loved me. I thought I loved everybody else." No one passed another acquaintance on campus without saying hello. He once knocked on the wrong door in his search for a room and, instead of meeting a student boarder, was greeted by the recently retired Henry Churchill King himself. King chatted amiably with the young man and sent him to the right address. Rollo was charmed by Oberlin's aura of genteel innocence. At the Vatican, this "country boy" learned that a man helped a woman with her chair and other "rites of politeness." He had "made it," being accepted by those who, he had always assumed, considered themselves his betters.

Such friendliness, grace, and the indefinable sense of finding a spiritual home helped open him to a new and joyful intellectual seriousness. One memory in particular encapsulated the meaning of Oberlin in his life. At the center of the seminar table of his first Greek class, he gazed at a beautiful reproduction of a Greek vase. "I used to look at that and wonder," he recalled, "how can human beings make something so beautiful? And I looked at that hour after hour." The study of ancient Greek culture became a portal through which art, philosophy, and literature came to acquire central meaning to his life, even as other courses awakened him to later foundations of the Western tradition. His classes that semester—Shakespeare and the Drama of the Sixteenth and Seventeenth Centuries, an introduction to Bible as history and literature, as well as Renaissance Architecture, the English novel, American literature, and an introduction to philosophy—kept his mind spinning with new and illuminating ideas.

He also found new models of manhood among the faculty, exemplary souls unafraid to live by their ideals and honor their emotions. His political science professor, Oscar Jászi, an exiled Hungarian patriot and member of a short-lived post–World War I government, enthralled him. Jászi brought to the classroom a sense of politics tempered by tragic experience. Most of all, Rollo came under the sway of Charles Wager, a legendary professor of English. Wager had come to Oberlin more than twenty-five years earlier and personified the college's spiritually charged embrace of the humanities. He taught classics and English literature and urged upon his students a quest for intellectual as well as moral excellence.

May especially remembered the last lecture of Wager's two-semester Victorian prose course, in which he spoke of "eternal verities" and the importance of rest, solitude, and a belief in personal destiny. Wager recited a poem that would become one of Rollo's lifelong favorites, George Eliot's "Oh May I Join the Choir Invisible." Eliot expressed, with greater elegance and cosmic dimension, the yearning for noble achievement to which Rollo was first drawn in Sam Walter Foss's "The House by the Side of the Road": "Oh may I join the choir invisible / Of those immortal dead who live again / In minds made better by their presence."[20]

As Rollo's advisor, Wager guided the young man in questions of life and character as well as curriculum. This was the Oberlin way. Students routinely conversed with professors outside of class, at the dorms or boarding houses or in the faculty's nearby homes. They would invite themselves to their professors' homes for Sunday evening chats. Such conversations ranged from the intellectual to the moral to the personal, imbuing a spirit of familiarity that reinforced the notion of the professor as humane authority.

Oberlin offered Rollo a special kind of intellectual nourishment. Assigning original texts and plain-spoken syntheses, professors presented the entire Western tradition of art, philosophy, and literature in single-semester or year-long courses. They considered it their mission to bring meaning and beauty to life and encouraged students to assess a text or piece of art for both its practical value and its theoretical truth. For one assignment, May's philosophy professor asked students to judge for themselves the various systems presented in Will Durant's recently published *The Story of Philosophy*.[21] Rollo's ingenious response was to pluck a "minute modicum" of truth from each of an array of thinkers from Plato to Nietzsche. He then assembled "a philosophy of philosophies" (as he called the paper), "almost the perfect philosophy." In six and a half pages, he boiled down the great ideas of the West since the Greeks to a few categories:

> Old Socrates seems to say to us, "Seek true wisdom", and he was right. Plato says, "Dream beautiful Utopias"; let us do that. Aristotle's message is, "Be

scholarly", and we surely ought to follow this precept. Bacon begs us, "Be scientific"; Spinoza says, "See the Unity of the universe"; Voltaire says, "Don't take life too seriously;" Rousseau advised us, "Follow your nature"; Kant says, "Listen to the small voice of duty"; Schopenhauer tells us, "There is a great Will behind all"; Spencer says, "The universe is a colossal evolution", and so on. Can we stretch our minds and observe the hidden unity in all these philosophies: If we can, then we have the combined truth of the ages, the philosophy of philosophies.[22]

The paper revealed a very early version of May's later urge toward synthesis and his propensity to marshal great minds across centuries to analyze present-day questions. It also marked May's first grappling with the puzzle of Nietzsche, whom he would later celebrate as an important influence in his turn toward existentialism. At the time, May noted that his "thought does not fit well with the others, for Nietzsche is alone in his world." However, rather than ignoring this loner, he devoted almost a whole page to him, more space than he gave to any other thinker. The tone reflected May's identification with the philosopher, as well as a striking juxtaposition of biblical phraseology and psychological description. "He was a voice crying in the wilderness," he wrote, bestowing on Nietzsche a John the Baptist role, "abnormal and psychologically-maladjusted, warped and unhealthy in outlook, but a philosopher of deep sincerity and backed by much suffering." In Rollo's reading, Nietzsche's call for *Übermenschen* was in reality a "demand for strong, courageous living" comparable to the "message of him who said, 'I have come that ye might have life abundant.'" Rollo saw in Nietzsche's persona the paradox of an anti-Christian Christ. And he revealed early on how the popular vocabulary of psychology had begun to mix with that of religion.[23]

May garnered a B-plus for his efforts, a better grade than most he made at Oberlin. Despite his intellectual and spiritual awakening, by the usual standards he remained a mildly indifferent student. Generally he scored Bs, though he received a C-plus in a philosophy course and a C in one of his favorite classes, Wager's Victorian prose. He made As only in Bible and Greek. His professors, who noted his class comments and other signs of creativity, puzzled over his performance. One psychology professor made a point of telling him that, according to the school records, his IQ was as high as or higher than 97 percent of the students. Why, then, had he compiled such a mediocre record?[24]

Years later, May explained it mainly as a conflict between his father's booster vision of the world, a world of clubs and committees, and his new intellectual passions. Often intellect lost out. Indeed, in addition to his jobs and classes, he seemed to be involved in everything on campus. In his first semester, he joined the YMCA cabinet and other student groups; that spring, he worked on the staff of the *Oberlin Review*. He filled his senior year with more intense activity: he continued on the *Review*, chaired the meetings committee of the YMCA, served on the executive committee of the Student Chest, joined the Oberlin Outing Club, played in the Oberlin concert band, and presided as chaplain at the Vatican (which meant leading prayer at each meal). The academic costs were significant, though not crippling. May forfeited two credits in one semester for excessive absences from class. Having observed his love of Greek, Rollo's professor urged him to continue with the sequence during his senior year, yet, as he remembered it, May "got control" of himself and "became more a Middle Westerner" again and dropped Greek so that he could concentrate on extracurricular activities.

Oberlin's liberal Christian commitments did direct Rollo's activities through its tradition of service. His sense of the school's sacred purpose deepened as he learned of the college's history of leadership in such reforms as abolitionism, women's rights, the social gospel, and foreign missions. All around him, students and professors debated the great issues of the day— socialism, war, domestic politics, and, after October 1929, the stock market crash. May summed up his outlook in those years: "I was very much a social gospelite. I was very liberal. I would have voted socialist."[25]

The positive side of Rollo's whirlwind engagement in non-academic activities did not escape the notice of others, especially the aid he gave to other students. Oberlin's much-loved Congregational minister, the Reverend James Austin Richards, and others were particularly impressed with Rollo's abilities as an informal counselor and confidant, a role in keeping with his avowed future in "religious work" and imbued with Weaver's example. Writing in support of his financial aid application for senior year, Richards observed that in "a group of young men, talking over some of the perplexities of the Christian view of life, he showed himself the most mature and positive of them all." The minister noted that May already seemed "to have in tow some of the lads who have come to me in spiritual perplexities, and to be trying to help them." There was not "any man on the campus," Richards added, "more useful for the things in which I am most interested."[26]

Rollo, the sensitive counselor who effectively aided those in need, however, still felt somewhat ill at ease with his peers as simple friends. His outward confidence in well-defined situations veiled deep shyness, insecurity, and awkwardness. Though he had traveled some distance from the depths of alienation he felt at Michigan State, Oberlin made his reserve in some ways more unbearable. He could no longer blame the institution. He had to face himself. He sought the counsel of the Reverend Richards, to whom he confessed self-doubt, hypocrisy, and utter frustration in trying to "let go." Richards told him, "Let's get one thing straight. You're very unfair to yourself." He reassured him that he was "one of the outstanding people on the campus" and that he simply suffered from an "inferiority complex." And so, perhaps for the first time, May heard his malaise analyzed in a merger of religious and psychotherapeutic terminology.[27]

Hearing that term—inferiority complex—used by a minister of the gospel might well have startled May. He recalled that his only exposure in college to psychology as a discipline was a boring class that dwelled upon statistics, and that he was mostly ignorant of something called psychoanalysis. It was liberal Christianity that opened May to the realm of psychotherapy, albeit as a variant of ministerial pastoral work. By the 1920s, the penetration of the psychoanalytic theories and therapeutic techniques of Sigmund Freud, Karl Jung, and especially Alfred Adler, duly filtered through American needs and sensitivities, became central to the most progressive corners of liberal Christianity. Many in the church and the Y found that psychoanalytic ideas illuminated age-old religious questions and that clinical approaches promised exciting innovations in the special world of the pastoral study.

Such interest in psychology and religious experience had been building among Protestants since the middle of the nineteenth century and reached a watershed with the publication of William James's *The Varieties of Religious Experience* in 1902. The first major experiment in merging psychotherapy and religion came in 1906, when three doctors and two ministers from Boston's Emmanuel Episcopal Church inaugurated a lecture series at the church on mind-body connections and the moral life. Later, they opened a clinic to do emotional counseling from both medical and spiritual perspectives. However, it was James's first doctoral student in psychology at Harvard, G. Stanley Hall, who most directly brought psychology to the churches. In 1909, as president of Clark University, Hall sponsored Jung's first and Freud's only speaking engagement in America. Later, he championed Adler's work in America. His own scholarship concentrated on bringing together the sciences, morality, and religion. Best known for his massive work on adolescence, he also devoted two lengthy volumes to a reinterpretation of Christian faith, *Jesus, the Christ, in the Light of Psychology*.[28]

May's own exposure to the possibilities of a dialog between psychology and spirituality began at Oberlin in a course called Types of Religious Experience, for which James's *Varieties of Religious Experience* was the central reading. His sessions with Richards exposed him to psychologically informed pastoral counseling. Then, in the summer of 1929, he participated in counseling workshops sponsored by the YMCA College at Lake Geneva. Rollo attended lay seminars and lectures on new psychological insights into religion, marriage, sexuality, and the counseling of adolescents. This little-remembered aspect of the Y's agenda helped to shape May's receptivity to therapy.[29]

The workshops at the Y College featured some of the most respected names in the movement. The first speaker in the counseling sessions was Harrison Elliott, author of such books as *The Bearing of Psychology on Religion* (1927) and *How Jesus Met Life Questions* (1920). Elliott neatly applied G. Stanley Hall's concerns to specific life situations. As May noted after Elliott's first lecture, "New psychological and psychiatrist research enables one to much more effectively interpret power of religion in aiding one's personal development." Subsequent talks highlighted Alfred Adler's "individual psychology" and suggested that human needs might best be looked at as a set of Adlerian progressions from bad to good:

> ignored ➡ looked up to
> physical distress ➡ physical well-being
> failure ➡ mastery
> non-loved ➡ loved
> worry ➡ peace of spirit
> routine ➡ adventure

Elliott noted that Jesus emphasized "goals" and that he looked upon sins as inadequacies not to be condemned but rather to be worked on. The modern counselor would imitate Christ by setting the counselee on the road to a productive life. Of course, such wisdom struck Rollo as good advice for others as well as himself.

As germane to Rollo's concerns were lectures given by "Mrs. Elliott" (Harrison Elliott's wife and future YWCA president Grace Loucks Elliott), who sought to clarify misconceptions about the opposite sex and place sexuality in proper perspective. She addressed misunderstandings between the sexes, especially the tendency for boys and men to idealize women as innocent (because women were taught to hide their true feelings and desires). She explained that women felt sexual urges as strongly as men, though certainly in a different way. As Rollo recorded: "Girls have more emotion connected with sex, since their organs are invisible. Men localize, women feel, not knowing where from."

Prefacing her discussion of sex in Christian marriage with the remark that "no one would embark on a business enterprise with as little knowledge as he enters marriage," Mrs. Elliott declared that marital sex, far from being something to stigmatize or "overcome," was in fact "a fundamental giver of power, zest—abundant living, dynamism. Sex can weld man and woman into complete unity." It was "the most glorious element in life," especially when both husband and wife achieved orgasm together. She left the job of explaining just how to achieve that sexual state of grace to John Quincy Ames, president of the YMCA College. He detailed the stages of intercourse, methods of sexual stimulation, examples of infantile sexuality, and such "unsatisfactory" sexual forms as adultery, prostitution, and homosexuality. In each of these cases, sexual pleasure came without true union, especially when measured against the ideal of perfect mutual orgasm in marriage. Such mutuality brought "spiritual impetus—better relation to God." "Petting" and "heavy petting" (each partner to orgasm) did not.

Nor did masturbation. In a certain sense, Ames offered a more stinging critique of solitary sex than simply calling it a serious sin. As May noted concerning Ames's lecture, "Masturbators do so because they are failures in life." Such assertions left him uneasy, since he spent much time chastising himself over what he viewed as his own obsessive indulgence in self-pleasure. He thus listened closely as Ames argued that there was "nothing so opposed to development of our Christian personality" as "depreciating ourselves." Invoking Adler, Ames blamed feelings of social or physical "inadequacy" on childhood suggestions from parents. He recommended speaking frankly with a counselor and letting the counselor be blunt in his analysis and advice. Ames's charge to these would-be counselors: "In sex, etc. *Talk* with person concerned, giving facts, letting him realize that same problems trouble all other people."

Rollo was so agitated that he asked Ames for a private consultation, where he confessed extreme worry over his habits. "My self consciousness," as Rollo recorded Ames's diagnosis, "is due 1) primarily to my sex problem. i.e. believe I am different from others because I have masturbated, and I assume they have not." Contributing to this feeling was the fact that he had been "teased" about his genitals when he was young and that his parents never discussed sex. Ames assured him that "99 out of 100" boys masturbated, which Rollo could confirm by talking with a trusted friend. He would then realize that he is in the "same boat as they."

The immediate impact of these and other workshops on May can only be indirectly gleaned. He did not adopt psychological terminology as his everyday language, despite the clear benefit of his meeting with Ames. Rather, his vocabulary remained primarily etched by Christianity and, notably, by the discovery of literature, especially spiritualized Victorian poetry and prose. Even as May was learning the rudiments of psychotherapy at YMCA College, he experienced a renewal of faith lacking Christian particulars but imbued with Victorian awe. "What I remember is that I was walking down some path at this camp," he recalled sixty years later, "and there was nothing very special about it, but I had a sense then of communion with God. . . . Well, the verse I like very much is from Wordsworth: 'We sense a being beyond thee whose dwelling is the light of setting suns and the round ocean and the living air . . . ' My religion was very much like those Victorian or Romantic poets like Shelley and Keats and Wordsworth."[30]

May's post-graduation plans displayed an idealism common among Oberlin graduates. He saw his future in "Christian religious work" and planned to serve as a missionary before attending Union Theological Seminary in New York. He had hoped to go to China as part of Oberlin's famed Shansi Project but was not selected. Oberlin had nominated him for a Rhodes Scholarship, but he was eliminated early on in the competition. However, he met with a recruiter from Anatolia College, a missionary school in Salonica, Greece, who convinced him to sign up as a teacher. When he graduated in June 1930, he was sad to leave Oberlin but thrilled by dreams of Greece's majestic ruins and the beginning of a new life.[31]

3

"I Must Change My Life"

In September 1930, Rollo May traveled by train from Lansing to New York and boarded a freighter for Greece. He was one of a group of teachers sent to the lands of the old Ottoman Empire by the American Board of Commissioners for Foreign Missions. The ABCFM took care of every travel arrangement, issuing Rollo a clergy pass for his rail trip to New York and booking him on a retrofitted World War I cargo ship it had leased from the American Export Line. At no time between Lansing and Salonica did Rollo leave the watchful presence of the mission board.

No matter how closely monitored, Rollo experienced the journey as a great liberation. He had lived only in the small towns of Michigan and Ohio, amid the culture of midwestern Protestantism. At age twenty-one, he looked forward to walking among the iconic ruins of the culture with which he had fallen in love at Oberlin. Rollo spent hours alone in his cramped room or on deck gawking at the ocean, dreamily lost in thought or writing in his diary. He continued to frame his feelings with lines from the romantic poets. Early on, he quoted Matthew Arnold's "Self-Dependence":

> Still, still let me, as I gaze upon you,
> Feel myself becoming vast like you!

Perhaps he also had in mind other lines from the same poem:

> Resolve to be thyself; and know that he,
> Who finds himself, loses his misery![1]

He wasn't always alone. Rollo found himself attracted to a young woman, Elizabeth Weaver, who had volunteered to teach at Anatolia College's school for girls. The two missionary teachers passed endless hours chatting and watching flying fish and porpoises. He shared with Elizabeth a warm friendship and, as he made clear in numerous diary entries, had fallen in love. He cursed his shyness and never mustered the courage to reveal his true feelings, nor even to elicit a kiss.

Delight overwhelmed frustration as Rollo caught sight of the coasts of Portugal and Spain and cruised so close to the African shore he thought he could smell the lemon and orange trees of Morocco.[2] One day, as the mist cleared, Rollo gasped at the sight of the Parthenon and the Acropolis and loudly declaimed the dramatic lines of Byron's hymn:

> The Isles of Greece, the Isles of Greece!
> Where burning Sappho loved and sung,
> Where grew the arts of war and peace,
> Where Delos rose, and Phoebus sprung![3]

At Piraeus, the port of Athens, representatives from Anatolia met May and his fellow teachers and led them to a refitted yacht. The next morning they sailed into Salonica. As Rollo stepped off the boat, he entered a city of deep significance for Christianity. In the days of the Apostles, Paul preached and established a Christian community there. His letters to its converts became immortalized in the New Testament as the Epistles to the Thessalonians (Salonica being Thessaloniki in Greek). The city itself was founded by King Cassander of Macedon in 315 BCE and named after his wife.

Over hundreds of years, Salonica experienced alternating periods of prosperity and conflict under Greek, Roman, Byzantine, and Latin Christian control, each culture leaving a mark on its art, architecture, and ethnic communities. Muslim rule began in 1430. Over the next four and a half centuries, the Turks built Salonica into a prosperous, cosmopolitan western gate to the Ottoman Empire. They were aided in no small degree by the city's large Sephardic Jewish community, whom the Muslims welcomed after Spain had expelled its Jews in 1492. Nineteenth-century European entrepreneurs linked Salonica by rail to western Europe and modernized the city's harbor. Salonica's Jewish majority set the cultural tone but also lived in reasonable harmony with Turks, Greeks, Bulgarians, and western Europeans. It was a thriving entrepôt, second only to Constantinople as a jewel of the realm.[4]

In 1930, however, May and his fellow teachers encountered a blackened and bleeding city, a victim of accident and awful historical circumstance. By the turn of the century, the city's prosperity had begun to crumble under the pressure of competing Balkan nationalisms and the growing precariousness of Ottoman rule. Corruption and confusion undermined the social order and inspired a burgeoning nationalist movement under Kemal Atatürk, the father of the Turkish nation. Salonica was Atatürk's birthplace and, later, the headquarters of the "Young Turks" revolt that established a constitution and parliament and toppled the sultan in 1909. Yet Turkey soon became embroiled in the Balkan Wars of 1912–13, losing Macedonia and with it Salonica. The city became part of Greece in 1912. After the outbreak of World War I in 1914, it became a major headquarters for Allied operations against Turkey, which the Central Powers had pressured into active alliance.

Salonica increasingly became the destination for thousands of Greek and Armenian refugees. With the outbreak of war, the Turks saw already suspect Armenian and Greek populations—foreigners and Christians in a time of nationalist upheaval—as dangerous subversives. Xenophobia soon grew into a concerted effort to destroy the Greek and Armenian communities of Asia Minor. Beginning in late 1914 and continuing through the mid-1920s, millions were killed or deported, as peoples who had lived for centuries among their Turkish neighbors now found themselves unwilling exiles. Salonica's location near the border with Turkey made it a favored destination for refugees. The Greeks settled them in a ring of shantytowns surrounding the city proper. For decades after, the Greeks called Salonica "The Refugee Capital" or "Poor Mother." Meanwhile, in 1917, an apparently accidental fire gutted a third of the city's central district, destroying many of its ancient labyrinthine neighborhoods. At least seventy thousand were left homeless, over two-thirds of them Jews.

Anatolia College had itself found refuge from the Turks in Salonica. Established by American missionaries in 1886 on the site of a seminary in the Ottoman city of Merzifon, the school had quickly become an important outpost of Protestant and Western culture in Asia Minor. However, its missionary goals and the large Armenian student contingent made it suspect in the eyes of the authorities, and even official approval from the government could not immunize it from occasional attack.

The college became a virtual hostage in World War I and the Turkish campaign against the Armenians. In 1915, Turkish soldiers methodically rounded up Merzifon's Armenian population (half of the city of thirty thousand) and took them to the mountains for execution and burial in mass graves. Over the protests of college president George White, Turkish soldiers broke through the gates of the school and dragged away all the Armenians they could find—teachers, families, and students. Turkish authorities closed the school in May 1916. The nationalist campaigns under Atatürk after 1919, as well as a renewal of hostilities with Greece, destroyed any hope of Anatolia College continuing in Turkey. President White finally found a new home for the institution in Salonica, where its most immediate mission became the education of refugee children. By the late 1920s, Anatolia and its sister school, the American Boarding School for Girls, had acquired buildings in the suburb of Charilaou and began educating hundreds of Greek and Armenian teenagers.[5]

As May and his comrades proceeded to campus on the outer edges of the city, hard roads turned into muddy paths. Hastily constructed tents and shacks made of tin, scrap wood, or oil drums dotted the flatlands and hillsides. Refugee families clothed in tatters foraged among the garbage of slightly more affluent neighbors, staring silently at the neatly dressed newcomers, even as the Americans encountered scenes of poverty and despair unknown to them at home.

Rollo's whirlwind journey into living history soon settled into routine. He lived with the rest of the faculty and many administrators at the Personnel House. His classes included English, (Protestant) Christianity, and Bible. He awoke each morning at seven, ate breakfast with his fellow teachers, and rushed off to the "quadrangle" to meet an 8:15 class. He then led his students to chapel, taught more classes until 12:30, broke for lunch, and headed back for classes and study hall until 4:15. In the YMCA tradition of sound mind and body, May ran the Athletic Council and often spent the rest of the day coaching handball, football, and basketball.[6] Some afternoons he would walk in the foothills of Mount Hortiati to the east beyond the city. From these modest heights, he often watched the sun set behind Mount Olympus across the bay. Yet it was hardly a comfortable life. Salonica's beautiful fall soon gave way to the short and often bitterly cold days of winter. Driving rainstorms turned the streets to mud, while overnight freezes glazed the ruts and puddles with an icy scum.

Rollo's duties and routines as well as the physical discomforts he experienced characterized the life of the missionary teacher, a role for which his upbringing had prepared him. At the same time, as sometimes happened to missionaries, the alien culture and people he came to transform into good Christians seduced and unhinged him. He sought textbook understanding at first, studying modern Greek and Greece's recent history. However, the beauty and mystery all around soon engulfed his imagination. He was struck especially by the demeanor of his students, who seemed so steeped in tragic knowledge of a world beyond May's own experience. They also appeared relaxed, unencumbered by Protestant catechisms of virtue, hard work, and missionary innocence. The boys' names—Platon, Aristoteles, Socraton, Agamemnonos—charmed him with echoes of classical antiquity. The missionary in him saw them as souls to be enlightened, but he also felt drawn to their dark sensuality.

Nor was it only the boys that began, at first imperceptibly, to crack May's brittle façade of wisdom and authority. Rollo encountered aesthetic allure everywhere. The Ottoman architecture, Byzantine churches, Greek and Roman ruins dotting primitive pastures, the color, the faces, strange languages and laughter, dramatic gesticulations, the very glint of the sunlight— all awakened excited yearnings. He sometimes simply wandered through the hubbub of Salonica's busy port to experience its sounds, colors, and aromas. Years later, he could still picture in his mind "the barques sailing in from Asia Minor, their decks loaded high with oranges."[7]

Rollo journeyed far and wide on school holidays and shaped his diary entries and letters home into romantic adventures. His first major trip was at Easter in 1931, when he boarded a small Italian ship to visit the city once known as Constantinople but recently officially renamed Istanbul by the Turks.[8] He sent home a five-page, single-spaced typed letter, and when words failed him he filled the margins with sketches of boats and minarets. From the full moon "rising as a great orange ball behind the hills of Salonica" as he commenced his trip to his return on a "spasmodic" train that traversed the battlefields of Thrace and Macedonia, he delighted in visual beauty and sensuous surprise. He savored the courses of his "dandy supper," watched "the thousands of far, twinkling, golden lights of the city of Salonica grow dimmer and dimmer," and found other boats sailing by in the moonlight so bewitching he needed to draw one. He pored over guidebooks at breakfast or sat entranced as a fellow passenger recounted the history of Istanbul and the Great War. They passed through the straits of the Dardanelles and to the fortress of Dardanellia, its twelve huge cannons standing guard. Rollo awoke before daybreak and stood freezing on deck to catch a first glimpse of "the dim lines of minarets sticking up into the heavens."

Rollo devoured Istanbul like a feast. The city walls—"high, thick, strong"— inspired a kind of fear, as did a deep hole into which the bodies of executed prisoners were dropped and allowed to float out to sea. A steamboat trip up the Bosporus revealed beauty "beyond description," as did the deposed sultan's palace with its swords, jewels, and golden mirrors. Then came the anarchy of the bazaar—"all is color! Red, yellow, orange, brilliant blankets, bright clothes, polished brass candlesticks and trays, smelly spices, fantastic perfume, fruits, foods, everything!"

May's feelings were more mixed about Islam. He visited mosque after mosque and admired their vast, dome-capped interiors, the "bright red, gorgeous rugs over the floor, the high place where the Mohammedan priest climbs to lead the service." He attended a Muslim service and was gripped by the preparatory washing and rhythmic kneeling of "three hundred Mohammed worshippers bowing and praying in unison." Yet he felt the need to dismiss what he saw, comparing those in prayer to "a bunch of soldiers taking setting-up exercises" and emphasizing that he "could not approve of their religion. It is not an intelligent religion." His words became more strident after he toured Istanbul with acquaintances from the city's Mission Board offices: "History shows unmistakably that the Turk is a killer. . . . The modern Turk still holds himself untouchable to Christianity." He reiterated his rejection of the Turks through romantic identification with Greece. "Until the Greeks achieve their dream and get [Istanbul] back from the Turks," he declared with conscious echoes of Lord Byron, "the city will be nothing more than a pageant of history. But—I'm a Greek—and some day we will have our ancient city back again!"

During the summer of 1931, May ventured to the safer cultural soil of Italy. He made a tourist's pilgrimage to Naples and Rome—took in the art museums, stood in awe of the ancient ruins, saw the pope in a group audience, gorged himself in the trattorias—and felt sickeningly lonely. His luck changed when he traveled north to Florence. As he descended the stairs of the Palazzo Pitti, spied he Charles Wager from Oberlin and gleefully cried out his name. Flattered that Wager remembered his face, he was only faintly disappointed when the professor asked to see pictures of his family in order to catch a glance at May's name in his wallet. Nonetheless, he was struck by the professor's kindness. Wager gave him an expert's tour of Florence, took him to tea, and, when May told him about his ramshackle room in a pension, offered to share his more luxurious accommodations. Rollo accepted. They toured and discussed literature and life.

The encounter inspired an intimate correspondence with Wager as he continued his journey. Rollo rhapsodized over the beauty of the French Alps but complained that he was "weary of himself." Wager protested that May seemed the "last person in the world" to fit that description. The professor noted some new companions, a young American high school teacher and a twenty-one-year-old German student, whom he had shown around, and described with special delight the view from his window of young men and boys bathing in the Arno. He also betrayed a special affection for Rollo, noting in response to May's expression of "growing loneliness" that "we Florentines like to be missed." And, in a second letter: "I can see no reason why my letter should be preserved among the May archives. Letters of friendship and affection cannot be rare in your experience. You attract them." Wager volunteered that May had been a "godsend" to him and regretted only that he could not stay longer. "Why do you suppose it is that the people one really wishes to have about," he asked wistfully, "are nearly always somewhere else?"[9]

They made a curious pair, the energetic young idealist and the worldly sixty-four-year-old professor-aesthete. Each basked in the light of the other. May relished the attention lavished upon him by his favorite professor. Wager was smitten with Rollo. Wager praised him not only for his vigor and good looks but also for his appreciation of beauty in literature and art. "You are a poet yourself, *Rollo mio*," he noted a few years later as they corresponded about Byron, "a poet in action."[10]

Many years later, after May heard that Wager was a homosexual, he wondered about the professor's attentions to him. Yet such same-sex attractions were common for the time, often filled with erotic intensity but only at times leading to sexual intimacy. May savored an uncomplicated affection for his professor, something shared by many of Wager's students. Indeed, if young Rollo was awkward in his intimacies with women and his peers, he gave himself over to mentors like Buck Weaver and Charles Wager.

Returning to Greece for his second year at Anatolia, Rollo began to slide toward crisis. His first year in Europe had been revelatory, but it had also knocked him off balance. Shaken by the loneliness of his months in Italy only relieved by his encounter with Wager, he faced the drudgery of a new term. His colleagues bored him, and he felt jealous of the attention "his" boys lavished on two new teachers. These were the first symptoms of much deeper trouble. Quite simply, his religious faith and sense of self had begun to fail him in the face of his new experiences. "As the year went on," he remembered, "I found that my habits and principles, coming from a typical small-town, mid-western childhood, such as hard work, fidelity, honesty and so on, stood by me less and less as the year progressed."[11]

Four months into the school year, May began a grappling with his soul of the sort time-honored by religious ascetics, a self-possessed self-critique he recorded in his diary as "new thoughts for living."[12] He explored every aspect of his being and bearing in the world, what others thought of him, and his relation to God. First came a strategy for renewing his faith. The answer to bad faith was more faith, the answer to loneliness was resignation, and the cure for self-concern was losing oneself in God. "Steadily and increasingly, through God's good grace," he wrote, "I am learning to forget myself in Him." He sought to "matter not at all, except as God's son, as one loved of Jesus," and to live by the command "Be Ye Perfect." "I shall trust that God is leading me day by day," May declared, "into the capacity to serve Him better—nothing else matters."

May attributed his problems mostly to "natural" causes—the difficulties of a new job, homesickness, everyday adjustments to a foreign culture, and, last but not least, the "uneasiness" caused by his "affection for Betty," the object of his shipboard infatuation and his inability to muster the courage to contact her at Anatolia's Girls School. He vowed that in the coming months he would be "less impatient and have more energy" for his work. He would learn to love his "associates and boys." From God he asked for the simple virtues— patience, industry, courage, trust, and love. "The worry is not mine," he declared. "I am not the general; I am merely His soldier."

With each declaration, Rollo seemed more lost. He grew a mustache in order to appear more serious, but his face displayed only growing despair. He worked to exhaustion each day, and each day he felt more isolated. Soon, he had trouble getting out of bed. In early March, he simply stopped. Others covered his classes, and the dean and his wife invited him to live with them in the hills overlooking the campus. They counseled him and nursed him back to health. It took Rollo a few weeks to regain his physical strength, but he remained deeply troubled, the comforts of the dean's house almost an affront to his unsettled emotions.

Unable to contain himself any longer, he made an extraordinary ritual pil-grimage as venerable in religious tradition as his project of self-scrutiny. On March 23, 1932, at about ten in the evening, after a profound talk with the dean—one that cut to the heart of his despair—he decided to climb Mount Hortiati. Right then. No matter that it was teeming a freezing rain, no matter that the base of the mountain was miles away or that its peak stood high above the city. Rollo plodded along shepherds' paths swamped in mud. Rain turned to snow as he reached the mountain's first plateau at about four in the morning. But his body pushed on without stopping as one thought led the way: "I must change my life."

At daybreak he reached a little village below the peak. The villagers were just rising as they saw a large young man in frost-caked clothing stumble into the *kafenio*. In rough Greek and sign language, Rollo rented a room upstairs and slept until the early afternoon. He arose and walked downstairs to see a dozen or more men huddled around the charcoal-burning iron stove. Dressed in lambskin and tasseled black shoes, they drank coffee and ouzo and roasted tiny fish on the flat top of the stove as snow fell outside. The men nodded and smiled in acknowledgement of this strange-looking fellow who had joined them around the glowing charcoal.

May took a small pad out of his pocket and began to write in a silent fury. Soon one of the men inquired, "Ti graphíte?" (What are you writing?) Rollo responded in his broken Greek, "Ti ine Zoeis." (What is Life?) They all had a hearty laugh, and one said: "That's very easy. If you have bread you eat, if you don't have bread, you die."[13] Rollo's question was really two: Why had his sense of life and meaning crumbled? Where did his true calling lie? These were modern versions of Bunyan's immortal question, "What shall I do to be saved?" He spent the better part of three days filling page after page with minute jottings that effectively began to redraw the boundaries of his life and faith. He set goals of "genuineness" and "spontaneity" for a new "personality," an agenda that came directly from the world of psychologized Christianity he had encountered at YMCA College. The extraordinary characteristic of these meditations, however, was their stark revelation of what was at stake—spiritual life or death.

Rollo began with "Situation I am in Now," in which he confessed that "conscientiousness and zeal" gave his teaching the false appearance of excellence. He did the "little jobs" well and "follow[ed] instructions." He seemed the "prototype of man who is a dependable cog in machine, but not much else." With horror, he saw himself in twenty years "sliding along road of conscientious conventionality" as "a moderately successful preacher preaching 'his best,' taking pains to make contacts and call on congregants." The problem became especially acute in his interactions with Anatolia's students. He seemed more interested in doing a "good job" as a missionary than truly engaging the "boys." The few times that spontaneous contact with his students had given him "keen, genuine pleasure" only underlined the "forced ungenuine feeling" of most other encounters. It was not simply that the missionary outlook, which emphasized "contact" for the ulterior purpose of conversion, seemed false to him. He also painfully recognized more of E. T.—God's salesman—in himself than he liked. "I enjoy, subconsciously, being seen in these contacts [presumably by those in charge at Anatolia]," he scribbled. "If I were to meet one of the boys in Rome, I should not go out of my way to converse and to

[go] places with him. . . . Therefore my main reason for 'making contacts' is the doing of my job well."

Rollo meant two things in his contrast of person as "contact" and as "personality." He recoiled at the idea of individuals being used to further personal or religious causes without recognition of their unique qualities. Indeed, he had come to doubt that his own specialness had been recognized. From the time he had returned to Anatolia that fall, his sense was that any "deference and kindness" shown to him by his colleagues was what they would have done and did do "exactly same to any other—the fact that I was Rollo May made no difference." He even resented the dean and his wife's nurture after his breakdown, "without regard to my being myself and also for the ulterior motive of putting stars in [their] own crowns."

Rollo defined "personality" as a person's individual and unique genius. He had come to believe, along with many other liberal Christians, that its recognition was at the heart of Christianity. The preservation of that respect for one's own uniqueness and that of others expressed itself religiously in a variety of ways: by avoiding anger or lusty thoughts of others, by turning the other cheek, and "by giving your coat also to him who asks your shirt, show[ing] your personality is worth more than material things." Interestingly, despite the deeply Christian attributes described, May identified modern models of authentic personality types that were in essence hardly Christian or even "religious" at all: the "artist" and the "philosopher." "The philosopher, the artist, are happy," he asserted, "because their personalities are kept as sovereigns of their lives." He made a further distinction: "Artists have best recognition of individual personality—men of literature best of personalities of other people."

Perhaps Rollo wondered unconsciously whether he was straying too far from the fold. He titled the next section of his notes "What was Jesus' idea?" (At a later date he notated this passage: "Still took my main cue from Xianity—had to rationalize that.") He assumed that God the Father had created a consciousness for human beings that encouraged them to believe that "life is good" and "men are brothers in the very nature of things." May drew a natural conclusion: "The way to live is simply to allow one's natural, good instincts expression. Simply remove cramping influences, let one's self free to love."

He saw resistance to freeing oneself as both a national and a personal flaw. What had prevented Americans in general and Rollo in particular from "simply" unchaining themselves for love? It was, he argued, the "Puritan idea . . . that God is a stern task-master; that life and man are not good, but [that] we must fight—fight ourselves, our instincts, and each other to arrive at salvation." In the American soul, a "mostly Puritan" heritage warred with "natural instincts, to love spontaneously, etc." However, those instincts could win out and were a potential source of "salvation." "Then," he noted, "a conversion to true, genuine religion is always possible."

"True" religion involved recognizing the uniqueness of individuals rather than focusing on the collective "saving of souls." The examples of Buck Weaver, Professor Wager, and Dr. Richards at Oberlin, who had been "interested in me as Rollo May," held out hope for change. Their actions illustrated a "primary law" of "genuineness": "Personality is one thing in us really of worth—it was put in us originally by God. It is our self. Everything done contrary to it, or not promoted spontaneously by it, is dishonest, artificial, a lie to ourselves and God, and will never work."

The best life, then, could not be defined by rote adherence to rules but rather by the "expression" of a true self. Once again, he separated that capacity from a necessary connection to Christianity. "The natural, spontaneous, genuine respect for personality seen in many non-Christians," he concluded, "the politeness of some common men, etc., is much better than the artificial, schooled respect for pers[onality] of many Christians." He saw this not as an "apologetic for the self-expressionist school" or the "libertine." Discipline, too, was a natural and genuine part of personality. At its heart, however, must be an appreciation for one's own genius.

Rollo kept writing, attempting to summarize somewhat formally what he called "My Theology." He began with "God is father," that "we inherit part of him," and that at "the very I, [the] very center of each person, the thing of worth, is the personality." That personality is "God in us." "I, then, am an expression of God," he continued. "It follows that my highest destiny in life, my goal, is to express God." That expression, Rollo argued, involved not only "serving" God, nor only "being," or "believing," or "loving," but all these states. "The 'summum bonum'—the best life," he concluded, "is to be gained when these things are allowed free, spontaneous expression." The problem came when even the best-intentioned Christians did not have the confidence to believe in spiritual freedom.

And what of May himself? He felt "revulsion . . . [with] the unclean feeling of ungenuineness" as he remembered the times he attempted to convert his friends at Michigan State and Oberlin. Not yet psychoanalyzed, he nonetheless traced such problems to the influence of his father: "concerned with 'should' and 'ought,' duty-driven largely. Did not know how to abandon self. Did not know how to talk. (Tho' a man of great character.)" He felt he had imitated these traits all too well. In high school, he "like[d] to do jobs well, and used others as means to these ends." At Oberlin, he "went after studies with great zeal," but his "ulterior motive" was "doing job well" rather than "int[erest] in studies."

He vowed to change. No longer would he pray in the morning simply because he "should be doing it" or because it "would look nice." "Not a prayer gets by," he commanded, "which is not genuine." Nor would he engage in ungenuine chat at the breakfast table. "'Good morning' at breakfast table often ungenuine," he concluded. "Let it not be spoken, except in answer to others." Finally, in class, he would seek to "objectify teaching more" by becoming less "hyper-sensitive to class attitude" toward him and therefore more distant from students. For God and his students, only "genuineness" would do.

May's mountaintop revelations prefigured the question of authentic selfhood that would dominate his writings decades later as he moved from Christianity to the vision of existentialism. Indeed, his youthful meditation on the mountaintop, though clearly rooted in spiritual pain, showed its liberal Protestant character to the point of not being quite sure where evil fit in the world. Rollo emphasized liberation, pure and simple, and only as an aside wondered whether "bad things are also spontaneous expression of man—don't know. But, if so, way of life is to express good and not express bad."

In a twenty-three-year-old, this obliviousness to evil might seem unremarkable except for the fact that later in life May attributed the beginnings of his palpable sense of the tragic to his years in Greece. There he had observed the results of political upheaval and genocide and had come to understand the depth of tragic wisdom gleaned over millennia of history. He attributed his "nervous breakdown" in part to the challenge that living in such an environment made to his thin shell of American optimism. Yet his ruminations included no reference to the darker themes of Europe—no refugees, no poverty, no ethnic bloodlust, no tragedy. Clearly what mattered most on Mount Hortiáti was the recovery of self. Unfamiliar surroundings were the catalyst, but the meditation remained largely self-contained.

To change his life in earnest, May had replaced the old rules and tools inherent in the routinized Christian life with the hope of a renewed faith based on authenticity. What more specific understandings of the spirit would guide this intuitive sense? What realizations of spirituality in action would define the authentic life? These were as yet unanswered questions as Rollo descended the mountain with an audacious sense of new beginnings.

4

Art and Adler

Rollo devoted most of the next two years to trying to live the authentic life in word and deed. He still envisioned a calling in Christian "religious work," but inspiration came less and less from the Bible and other "religious" sources. Instead, he cleaved to the late Victorian and early twentieth-century writers whom Johnston, Weaver, and Wager had portrayed as spiritual prophets and felt most drawn to their yearning for assurance in the face of doubt. May quoted their verse in his diary and fashioned the romantic self-image of a seeking spirit. Matthew Arnold's "Dover Beach" crystallized for him the modern menace, "The Sea of Faith/ . . . Retreating, to the breath / Of the night-wind, down the vast edges drear / And naked shingles of the world."[1]

May's idealization of the artist as arbiter of the eternal was but one example of a crucial cultural tendency that reached far more deeply and widely in the lives of individuals. The critic Joseph Wood Krutch identified it in 1929 as the "Modern Temper." He argued that science "had torn asunder any basis for faith." Krutch noted that many had turned to the artist as a substitute "God" but that this was a futile move. May was one of those many individuals passionately embracing the notion of art's capacity for spiritual revelation as an antidote for what artist Wassily Kandinsky called the "soulless life of the present."[2]

May felt it was insufficient simply to appreciate works of art in a museum. Only the process of creation allowed one to commune with that Godly part of himself. May possessed some native talent and had taken a studio class in college. Line drawings sometimes adorned his letters from Istanbul the year before. However, in the spring of 1932, he began consciously to see art as an expression of his unique personality. He could encounter the world anew through sketchbook and brush. It was a theme he would take up periodically in his life—much later, he would celebrate the "courage to create" as a path to one's unique self.

Indications of this new sense of spiritual openness and expression began to appear almost immediately after his mountaintop revelations. In April 1932, over the college's Orthodox Easter break, May traveled to Mount Athos with a group of Anatolia's teachers and students. The peninsula was a well-known if esoteric attraction. Athos had been inhabited by a few monks in the sixth century and deemed their exclusive preserve by the Byzantine emperor in 885. In 1060, the government, in a measure to ensure that no carnal temptation sully the monks' contemplative life, banned women and even female farm animals from living on or visiting the peninsula.[3]

May recounted his journey to Athos mainly through a letter to his parents. He described it as a land both shabby and austere, its pervasive silence punctuated only by the whispers of its swaying forests, the crash of waves along its craggy shore, and a pulsating cacophony of bird trills and choruses. He joked about the primitive overnight retreats, the "totally springless" beds with blankets that "smelled like a stable." Rollo and the monks made for strange bedfellows given the vast chasm between their religions. Yet, in another sense, Rollo's deeper sense of spiritual worlds allowed him to romanticize an indefinable, almost mystical kinship as he faced the rude sleeping quarters: "It is amazing how little difference these things make when one has gotten into the monastic mood and accepts nature as the monks do."[4]

May's new embrace of the world appeared as well in his boldly etched renditions—in word and image—of those he met on Mt. Athos. There was the Serbian journalist with a "wee, turned-up nose" and the "huge-bodied monk" whom one of his companions christened Friar Tuck. Drawing the monk, he managed to capture a certain sparkle and elusive smile under his thick beard. Compared to the simple illustrations of boats and battlements in prior letters, his picture of "Friar Tuck" seemed courageously intimate. May had drawn himself into a new, compelling, risky face-to-face appreciation of the Other.

A few weeks after returning to Anatolia College, as he hiked through the fields around the school, May experienced an artistically inspired awakening in some ways as intense as any of his prior religious experiences. "Ascending one hill I found myself suddenly knee-deep in a field of wild poppies covering the whole hillside," he recalled. "It was a gorgeous sight: brilliantly crimson and scarlet, the poppies were lovely forms as they bent delicately in one direction and then another. . . . I stood there, intoxicated, wholly captivated by this sight." Wordsworth's description of ten thousand golden daffodils, "tossing their heads in spritely dance," came to mind. He felt compelled "to kneel among the poppies to sketch them."[5]

This was, at least, how he wrote about the experience over forty years later. At the time, he cautiously wrote home about his newfound passion: "My painting is coming along—probably will do quite a bit this summer—will send you some. Painting and drawing will be a companion, a hobby to keep me from getting lonesome, will be lots of fun, a help toward seeing the country more accurately and maybe some half-way decent paintings and drawings will result."[6]

Almost in passing, Rollo also reported to his parents that, between June 20 and July 4, he would be traveling to Vienna to take a course in psychology with the "world-famous Dr. Adler." As he would recount it later, May noticed an announcement for the Adler seminars posted at Anatolia College and jumped at the opportunity to learn about the new science first-hand. He had heard of Adler at the Y College but had never referred to him in any prior diary entries or letters. Nor had he ever mentioned the words psychotherapy or psychoanalysis. May might well have seen such a diagnosis, delivered by a minister, not as the "science" of psychology but as an aspect of "religion"—albeit a liberal religion eager to incorporate the latest understandings of human consciousness. In his new quest for personality, what could be more natural than May being drawn to the original source of such insight?

That Adler's theories could be so easily integrated into liberal Christianity indicated how the "modern temper," so threatening to traditional culture, might provide new means of spiritual nurture even from non-Christian sources. After all, Adler's world and life were in most definable ways strikingly different from May's or the liberal Protestants who eagerly embraced his theories. What they shared was a common interest in social mission and optimism about the possibility of change. Born in 1868 to an assimilating Austrian Jewish family, Adler pursued a career in medicine and developed deep socialist convictions. He set up a practice in a working-class Jewish section of Vienna, where he familiarized himself with the problems of the working poor. His first major publication, *Health Book for the Tailor Trade* (1898), instructed tailors on health hazards common to their work and argued for increased activism on the part of the medical profession to make these dangers known.[7]

Soon Freud invited the young physician to participate in an informal discussion group that came to be known as the "Wednesday Psychological Society." The group met at Sigmund Freud's home in the largely Jewish Leopoldstadt section of Vienna. Adler found the meetings both exhilarating and frustrating. Freud's insights convinced the young doctor of how deeply ingrained the behaviors that he once had seen simply as the product of objective social conditions were. Despite Freud's resistance, Adler adapted Freudian theory to the struggle against what he saw as the emotional misery inflicted by society and the economy on common men and women. He moved the battlefield from the unconscious to the worlds of home and school. His brand of psychotherapy hoped to correct the deleterious influence of cruel, doting, or neglectful parents, as well as the crippling wounds of poverty and disease. By the time May encountered him in 1932, his theory of "individual psychology" had become a powerful force in psychological practice and popular consciousness in Europe and America.

At its center lay several interconnected ideas. Adler argued that human existence revolved around a basic urge to move from helplessness and inferiority to mastery and superiority. The drama began with the totally dependent infant at the mother's breast. Disease, heredity, social conditions, faulty parenting, or accident might distort an individual's sense of self in relation to others as he or she grew to adulthood. An "inferiority complex," a hardening and routinizing of inferiority feelings, was the major source of trouble. It prevented a person from overcoming a sense of helplessness by keeping him or her in a world of narrowed action and inauthentic compensations, often wrapped up and hidden in a secret or openly proclaimed myth of superiority. Such a "guiding fiction," only faintly understood on a conscious level, shaped an individual's response to the world.

While Freud envisioned the individual psyche in an inevitable and eternal struggle between instinct and society resulting in repression and sublimation, Adler saw a drama of neurotic, protective self-absorption as symptomatic of a cultural malaise that could be ameliorated. Freud's modest goal was a compromise between instinct and the internalized strictures of culture. Adler's loftier aim was a happier understanding between the individual and society, a congruency between the needs of others and the individual. In Adler's vision, changing the culture through reeducation could liberate the individual to embrace salutary social feeling instead of self-doubt and its consequences. Particularly in America, where he received growing acclaim in the 1920s and early 1930s, Adler's optimistic plan for social change proved more acceptable than Freud's radically pessimistic vision.

May settled into a modest pension near Adler's compound in Semmering, in the hills outside Vienna. He felt a little anxious and lost (as he put it in some personal notes, "loose . . . unintegrated . . . no plans") and all the more ready for a new view of himself and the world. Classes began early on the morning of June 21, 1932, and lasted until early July. They included general lectures about life by Adler and others, workshops in therapeutic technique, and a personal analysis by one of Adler's assistants.

May's lecture notes indicated the ease with which the Viennese psychologist's vision could be integrated into the young American's nascent conception of personal spiritual life. Adler began with a somewhat mystical definition of the soul. May's notes record Adler saying that it was "part of the sun—of the cosmos. It is not made by social relationships, but *for* them." He was also struck by Adler's comparison of his own and Freud's view of the infant and, by extension, humankind. "Freudians say child is cannibal at birth—eating mother," Rollo dutifully wrote. "No—child waits to be given breast; factor present is *co-operation*." Against Freud's darker assessment, Adler set forth individual psychology's vision of "an ideal world, a goal in which everyone seeks to relieve and embellish lives of others." He asserted that the "faculty to dev[elop] soc[ial] interest is inherited, *belongs to all human beings*." It was a doctrine that lay at the base of liberal Christianity and the efforts of the YMCA. In fact, Rollo jotted in the margins next to this particular note, "cf. Kingdom of Heaven." In a later lecture, one of Adler's coworkers declared that the chief cause of disturbance in the world was inequality and that the goal of individual psychology was a "United States of the Planet" in which (according to Rollo's lecture notes) "Equality = esteem human dignity in every person."[8]

Most compelling to Rollo, however, was Adler's analysis of personal symptoms. In the psychoanalyst's description of the relation between impaired social feeling and "organ inferiority," May could not help but think about his childhood diagnosis of a heart problem (tachycardia) that he never had thought about in relation to his personality. "My heart trouble an excuse to escape physical responsibilities?" he asked himself. Nor, seemingly, had he ever admitted to competition with his brothers and sisters. A lecture on sibling rivalry, however, jogged his memory and made him wonder: "Satisfaction at failing of Ruth?"

May's consulting analyst at the seminar, Leonhard Seif, dug even deeper into his physical symptoms. Seif was the leading voice of individual psychology in Germany. Unlike Adler, who often told jokes in his lectures and chatted with patients, Seif specialized in somber truths. He told the young American that his shyness, childhood bedwetting, and masturbation originated in his being a "spoiled child," typical of a first son coming after an older sister. This was no taunt but rather an explanation for a puzzling combination of feelings—self-consciousness, exaggerated sensitivity to what others thought, helplessness, distance from others, and simultaneous feelings of inferiority and superiority.[9]

Of course, Seif blamed a faulty upbringing. May's bedwetting, which caused no end of misery and shame for the young man, originated as an "organ dialect," a way of "saying no" to his parents' stressful demands. Seif was also struck by May's vanity, his narcissistic attention to detail of dress, and his worry about particular aspects of his anatomy—for instance, Rollo thought his nose was too small. As May wrote in his diary, Seif surmised, "Something must have been said to you as a child that led you to overemphasize aesthetic detail." His advice?

> Because you are a spoiled child, you demand too much of life, and have an exaggerated opinion of your own inferiority. The more you learn to affirm the planet, the world, and yourself, the better off you'll be. Your inferiority feelings lead to seeing and dwelling upon weaknesses of others.

Dr. Erwin Krausz, another of Adler's coworkers, further complicated Rollo's personal analysis. After reading May's self-analysis, he congratulated him on its brilliance but also noted that it was itself a symptom to be analyzed. "If one is introspective," he said, "it is for some reason; find out the reason, do not fight the introspection." Krausz suggested that he ask, "What happens when one is introspective?" What direct action or realization was May avoiding by turning inward? Krausz's questions stuck with May and prefigured some basic tenets of his version of existential therapy: What are you feeling right now? Why?

Adlerian theory also had a special approach to dreams.[10] Freud emphasized remembered dream fragments as a door to an ever-present unconscious world of fear and desire, one whose images and feelings could be mined endlessly for insight into the psyche. Adler accepted Freud's stress on the usefulness of dreams and dream analysis but thought his interpretive framework too narrow. Instead he argued that dreams were confused or disguised extensions of common consciousness. They might be useful but were hardly crucial to individual psychology. He was sure that as neurotics got better, they produced fewer and fewer dreams. Indeed, when an American colleague once began a breakfast conversation with the simple remark "I trust you had pleasant dreams last night," Adler said simply: "I *never* dream!"[11]

Nonetheless, Adler encouraged participants at his seminars to preserve and interpret their dreams. It was a totally new experience for May. Painful self-scrutiny, moralism, spiritual exercises, plans for reform—all informed a consciousness cramped in time and place and impoverished in imagery and narrative. No matter what he felt without words or symbols, no matter what gripped him in nameless melancholy or compulsive activity, Rollo had defined his life in literal reality and forced upon it a simple moral perspective. What a miraculous liberation, then, the simple act of recording a dream must have been. Flat became deep; linear time became ambiguous suspension; places and names and figures, known and unknown, created surreal personal tableaux. Sensual, frightening, weirdly meaningful dreams lent Rollo's self-scrutiny uncanny dimensions and unsuspected significance.

One dream he recorded at Semmering vividly illustrated what Rollo would eventually see as the unruly creativity of the unconscious. It heralded a return to Marine City to remake his high school years in the image of newly found freedom, confidence, and desire. The dream concluded with imagery suggesting his readiness for the tasks of life and perhaps reconciliation with Ruth:

> Arrived home—Marine City, in house near B__. Undecided as to whom I should date that night. Suit not pressed and ready, finally brown suit brought pressed. Wanted to date a pretty girl whom I could kiss. . . . Drove in our Ford to another city; I drove. . . . Had buffet supper outdoors—at that time I picked out Peg to have date with; she was sitting next to the end in a line of girls. Several of us trying to get a job on a ship; I walked past the windows of the cabin of the ship, where the capt. and chief men were holding a conference, saying "you need a good treasurer." I was carrying a cat. Afterwards I was sitting with someone, both having cats—the someone was Ruth, I think.[12]

However one might analyze this dream, it owed its externalized existence to the theory and encouragement of Adler and his assistants. Adlerian analysis, with its emphasis on the broader social context of individual lives and its grand theme of overcoming feelings of inferiority that warped personal and social behavior, was an all-important if ultimately inadequate tool for teasing out all the complex meanings of dreams. Within a decade May had come to see Adler's construction of reality as too simplistic. However, his experience at Semmering marked a giant first step in his exploration of the human psyche.

May also received some direct advice from Seif. He told the self-conscious man, "Never mind others—let them act as they wish. Our selves are our business. Moralizers show own inferiority feeling, and want to dominate. You lack courage. Must have courage—to be your simple, natural self." Engage the world openly, they recommended, break through barriers of fear and shyness toward a true embrace of others.[13]

May took them at their word and worked in particular to unleash his previously shackled sexual desire. The liberating mood of the seminar, his distance from the missionary strictures of Anatolia College and Michigan, and an accident of circumstance all aided in this endeavor. The first step was to lose his virginity. The poet Susan Griffin, whose friendship May made late in life, remembered him telling the story of his loss of sexual innocence, one that clearly had been honed into a kind of fairy tale. A countess who was staying at his pension, he recalled, beckoned him to her room for some candies. There she patiently brought him to bed. He described himself to Griffin as "a gravely serious young man, shy and completely inexperienced in such matters" and "stiff and uncertain" as he entered the countess's room. "At the door she moved to embrace him," as Griffin retold it, "holding him close to her and then moving away, close and apart, close and part until an irresistible force field existed between them." This rhythmic dance, he told the poet, was among the most erotic moments he had ever experienced.[14]

5

"Courageous Evolution"

One day during the last week of the Adler seminar, as May told the tale, he was drawing the trees outside his pension window when he heard a woman call up to him from the street. The stranger, an American, asked if he wanted to join a painting expedition to eastern Europe. She introduced herself as Elma Pratt, head of the International School of Art, and invited him down to talk it over. May protested that he had no money (the $350 tuition and expenses was a mighty sum in 1932 and way beyond his means). Pratt made a deal—he could come along "as a kind of refined gigolo," he later put it, escorting the mainly female artists as they explored European nightlife, helping with their luggage, and making rail and hotel reservations. In return, he would gain the privileges of full membership in the group. He quickly accepted the offer. May became the poor but handsome artist among women largely from families whose fortunes had survived the calamity of an ever-deepening worldwide depression.[1]

Pratt and May's meeting was accidental but rich with coincidences that no doubt facilitated the bargain. Though twenty years apart in age, they were kindred children of the heartland in search of a modern Christian life. Even as Rollo searched for meaning and a calling, it was clear that Pratt had found hers and could understand his quest. May left no record of their conversation, but one thing they surely talked about was Oberlin. Born in 1888, Elma Pratt grew up in the town of Oberlin and graduated from the college in 1912. She came from a family of means and after graduation traveled numerous times to Europe. After American entry into World War I, she worked for the YMCA among Allied troops in France. Asked in 1922 how Oberlin had shaped her life, she replied that it had "engendered a deep desire to know God and to use that knowledge to destroy all that is unlike Him—and so serve my fellow man." In Pratt's case, that meant the passionate pursuit of world peace and understanding.

By the mid-1920s Pratt's missionary zeal focused on art. She took studio classes in Vienna and was introduced by a Polish Jewish colleague, Marya Werten, to the folk art of Poland—dance, music, crafts, and painting. Along with many other artists and musicians of the time, Werten hoped to preserve traditions endangered by modernity and to bolster national pride through folk tradition. Pratt was so taken with the experience that, with Werten's aid, she launched the International School of Art in 1928. They conducted study tours for American artists, exploring contemporary developments in European art as well as the folk art of rural villages. Pratt hoped to inspire in others the cultural understanding gleaned from her own engagement with the arts and village life.[2]

The tour began with a two-week residency at the studio of Joseph Binder, a distinguished Viennese graphic artist famous in the 1920s and early 1930s for his contributions to advertising and poster design. Binder infused advertisements, posters, watercolors, and sketches with modernism's bold simplicity of rich color and decisive line. In person, he exuded that peculiarly Viennese mix of joviality, blunt honesty, and sardonic wit. As one whose works had helped to define the visual world in which he lived, Binder partially fulfilled May's own vision of the artist as prophet. Binder had visited America and, like Adler, had come to admire the country's freshness and unfettered dynamism. He enjoyed May's eager embrace of every word he uttered and every technique he demonstrated. This first meeting between May and Binder led to a lifelong friendship.[3]

Binder's studio provided the setting for another important encounter. Among those in the ISA group was Isabella Hunner, or "Bets," as she preferred to be called. At twenty-eight, five years older than Rollo, she already commanded fees for fashionable portraits in her native Baltimore but yearned to embrace the life of the "real" artist. Petite, intelligent, and articulate, she was experienced in love and possessed a streak of rebelliousness that spiced her Junior League bearing. Rollo and Bets felt drawn to each other. They talked and talked and toured Vienna together—its museums, cafés, and palaces. They attended the opera and symphony, and sunbathed at the public pools in skimpy European swimsuits. Rollo truly experienced romance for the first time, as well as its attendant insecurities and jealousies. On their last Saturday evening in Vienna, the two explored the Belvedere Gardens, and, as they sat along the rim of one of the grand fountains, Bets declared her love for Rollo. He echoed back, "I love you." For the rest of the summer, they were virtually inseparable.

From Vienna the artists traveled to Veselí, a small town in the Moravian region of Czechoslovakia. Their bus rattled down primitive roads, its passengers inhaling the black exhaust as they peered out the vehicle's windows to view the majestic Czech countryside. Pratt and Werten had arranged for Veselí's inhabitants to walk its wide streets in traditional costume, and a group of schoolgirls in bright colors and fine lace gave the arriving painters a grand welcome as they stepped off the bus. The next day they toured a home, and, in broken German, Rollo chatted with its owner about the sons of villagers who now lived in America. The inhabitants staged a traditional Moravian wedding for the Americans, supplying the visitors with costumes so that they could "go native."[4]

Adler, Seif, and Krausz would have been proud of May's abandon. As the group made its way through Czechoslovakia and Poland, he danced and drank and celebrated to a state of delirium. Rollo and Bets hiked and made love in the fields. The scent of their bodies and newly mowed hay merged into an overwhelming intoxication. Almost fifty years later, May retained a feeling "as precious and delicious" as any in his life, that he had been "carried away into a new world."[5]

At the end of the ISA tour, Bets remained in Europe and traveled with Rollo for the three weeks before classes recommenced at Anatolia College. Roughing it through the Balkans down to Salonica on the wooden seats of a third-class car, feasting on boiled eggs amid a jumble of ragged suitcases and the pungent odor of unbathed bodies, they kissed and slept in each other's arms. Rollo showed her the city and the school, introduced her to the teachers and administrators, and pointed to the distant Mount Hortiati.[6]

Abandoning the necessary decorum of their visit to the college, the couple traveled by train to Athens and commissioned a cab driver to take them across the isthmus to the Peloponnese and south to a spot along the wild coast of the Saronic Gulf near Corinth. Close to Corinth, to whose inhabitants Paul had declared, "It is good for a man not to touch a woman," Rollo and Bets set up camp on an isolated beach. Crystalline blue waters gently lapped the sand beneath a clear blue September sky. They spent most of the day nude, reciting poetry, sketching each other and the wild coastal terrain, and periodically plunging into the cool water. They talked about Adler, art, creativity, and love. Rollo the loner proclaimed the rightness of Adler's "social interest." Bets the rebellious socialite held out for the alienation of the artist. He sought ideals for living; she argued for embracing life experientially. They made love by the light of moon and stars. One evening they visited the town of Nafplio and walked out on its long pier as fishing boats returned with the catches of the day. Holding hands as they gazed upon the Bourtzi, an island fortress surrounded by water tinted deep red by the sunset, Rollo remembered Bets breaking the silence with a single exclamation, "I've seen so much beauty today!"[7]

But it was already September and time to part. They returned to Athens and Rollo kissed Bets goodbye as he boarded the night train to Salonica. Upon returning to Anatolia College, he remembered, "I couldn't drink a glass of water . . . because in every primitive reflex the one response I would have, would be Betty. I would see her in front of my eyes, would feel her close to me . . . "[8] "The weakest moment was just after dawn," Bets wrote the day after he left, "when there were no pine boughs and stars overhead, and no rosy light in the East and no you and the white moon in the West, no rolling of the waves and whispering of the wind."[9] All that autumn, May mourned for that blissful world out of time and place. Never again would he experience love in such all-consuming intensity.

It was difficult to begin teaching again, and not only because he missed Bets. Love and psychology, as well as a leap into the practice of art, had exploded May's notions of possibility, and it proved painful to return to the strictures imposed upon him at Anatolia College. Rollo's jangled nerves returned. He confided to his diary in October 1932 that such nervousness was "a protest against my staying and living in Thessaloniki." He argued with himself, reciting the benefits of teaching at Anatolia and his obligation to the school but also his yearning for the wider world. In the end, he sought resolution by giving his emotions a direct order: "Therefore, let me *like* the life here."[10] Now, however, he possessed the sharpened perspective of Adler's ideas, his own unleashed creativity, and the experience of love and sexual abandon. He understood that shaping a new life would take more than a mountaintop revelation, orders from the superego, or simple self-abnegation. Rather, he must work toward a new way of living. As he wrote in his diary a month after leaving Bets: "Evolution, not sudden conversion, is the way of change. *Courageous evolution.*"[11]

One sign of new courage displayed itself in his letters home. He wrote openly in his letters to "Mother, Dad, and all" of his relationship with Bets, despite its obvious sexual dimension and the fact that neither saw it as ongoing. "She and I became very intimate friends during the summer," he revealed, "the most intimate girlfriend I've ever had. . . . We really loved each other, tho' 'twas not the kind of love that looks toward marriage since she (5 years my senior) has her work back in Baltimore and I have mine here."[12]

Another sign of change came in his diary meditations, where religious tests became psychological analyses, characterizing his nervousness as that

'ed child" who sought to "escape responsibility" and "to run home
..' He rejected "religion" as too simple a guide, at least as it was commonly understood: *simplistic*

> Is religion an attempt to make life easier? Very often yes: one has all the great
> questions answered. One has a clear standard by which to judge everything,
> which makes life much simpler. Life really isn't that simple, tho'. The reli-
> gionist usually puts his religion before truth; he violates life by making it fit
> his standard. Everything is done with an ulterior motive—nothing for its
> own sake.

"I must be willing to *abandon* myself," he declared, as Dr. Seif's advice reverberated in his mind, "willing to give *myself up to life* and take its knocks;
willing not to be thinking always and 'taking stock' consciously, but allow
my consciousness, tho[ugh]t, to play." It was an order, in short, to stop taking
orders.[13]

There lay a curious irony in Rollo's trading the language of Christianity for
that of psychology. As Krausz had noted during the Adler seminars, introspection might be for May as much a neurotic trait to be observed and analyzed as it was a useful analytic tool. The very process of analysis encouraged
Rollo to "take stock" all the time, aiding and abetting in a new form what had
once been recognized as a sign of Christian piety. In fact, he remained all
his life a man wedded to obsessive self-scrutiny. The theories and terminolo-
gies of Adlerian analysis helped him to tame his tendency toward verbal self-
flagellation, but a new vocabulary could not quite extinguish the moralistic
purpose of an old habit.

Psychological analysis did allow May to think more clearly about voca-
tion. A person of his spiritual passion did not simply need a job. He needed a
calling. Until the summer of 1932, May had routinely described that calling
as "religious work," by which he meant the ministry or a lay career in an organization like the Y. His recent psychological awakening and increasingly
critical view of most religion opened up a confusing if rich array of new
options. One obvious choice was to be a psychoanalyst. Life as an Adlerian
therapist fit both his spiritual commitments and intellectual curiosity. In
November 1932, he tried out the idea on Bets and enclosed a similar letter
for her to send on to Adler. Bets professed excitement about his choice but
declared, "That's certainly your field—in all ways but one." She remembered
their long discussions on life and "the various signs of the differences in our

ages and experience." He needed to "*live* a great deal" before he could "*really*
understand others' troubles."[14] Adler had more practical doubts. Without
questioning May's fitness for psychotherapeutic practice, he noted that in
America he would need to become a doctor first, and "of course to study
medicine would be hard work. It needs at least 5 years."[15]

Bets and Adler's lack of encouragement forced May to consider the question more systematically. In early 1933, he drew a diagram to find "that
point where the needs of society intersect with my personal capabilities."
His talents included "working with people" and helping them "by means of
ideas." He needed challenging endeavors in which he couldn't "baby" himself.
He needed "stimulating, likable associates" and the "cultural stimulation" of
reading and learning. The "jobs open to such a person" included teaching,
preaching, Y work, and social service. Rollo doubted that as a teacher he
could work with the "*real vital* aspects of a person," and the church did not
seem capable of making a "real, vital contribution" to society. Possibilities
remained for the Y and social work. He felt moderately useful at Anatolia
College but longed to return home to see family and friends and "to get stimulation of life among my own people, where people *do* things." He would
continue his formal education. "I must study," he noted, "to get up in world"
and to find out what he wanted. Besides, he was "mentally hungry."[16]

May's ongoing, self-obsessed debates over calling revealed not a smidgen
of reference to the fact that in early 1933 the world's economy was bottoming
out around him and that unemployment, political unrest, and human misery
had been for some years the order of the day in Europe and America. It
was not for lack of information. Just before New Year's 1933, May solicited
wisdom from Bets and Charles Wager concerning a return to America. From
Baltimore, Bets advised against it, especially since a commission appointed
by President Hoover had just admitted that the country was "headed for
chaos, revolution." She thought that Franklin D. Roosevelt's inauguration
in March 1933 wouldn't change conditions very much.[17] When, a few days
later, Rollo wrote that he was considering a return more strongly because of
trouble in his family and his mother's urgent plea to come home, Bets reiterated her view that he should stay in Greece. "You can't have a true picture of
what this country is like," she emphasized. "No matter how much your family
needs a peacemaker—reconsider. Don't forget, your future must be considered for their sakes as well as your own, and there is no future here now."[18]

Wager, with whom he had not corresponded in over a year, responded
with a series of intensely personal letters beginning in dark whimsy and

ending in despair. Wager yearned to see Rollo but like Bets thought he should stay put. Jobs were scarce, and the college had already fired many instructors in English and music. "We've had an election, as you may have heard," he quipped concerning Roosevelt, "and now we shall be drinking all the three per cent beer we like, or can stand." In March, pleased that Rollo had decided to stay at Anatolia College, he wrote of his personal confrontation, as chair of the English department, with the calamity of the Great Depression: "I have applications from destitute and desperate *married* doctors of philosophy every week of my life."[19] By late April, despite Roosevelt's brave inaugural and initial emergency measures, Wager was more pessimistic than ever. "For my part," he wrote, "I can't see any hope. I don't know how much you have heard of what is going on over here, but believe me, young 'un, the outlook is not rosy.... We are skating—everybody is—on very rotten ice, and the water underneath it is cold."[20]

Such dismal appraisals of the situation at home not only heightened May's worries about the future but also wore down his self-confidence. He felt rushed, bored, confused, and trapped and, with a penitent's penchant for "taking stock," began once again to catalog his sins. Most of all, he felt deep loneliness and self-alienation. As he bore into his soul, searching for a path to truth and meaning, this time he employed Adler's psychological theories to "objectify" his situation. No longer would he mistake platitudes for his real self, he decided with unintended irony, but instead confront self-delusion as if his life depended on it. Struck by a chronic inability to feel comfortable with others, he looked back even on his "radical" and "unconventional" moments at Michigan State and Oberlin as a "conventional unconventionalness," more formulaic than authentic. "I was attacking the crowd (because I felt outside of it)." This habit he judged "1 degree worse" than simply "following the crowd."[21]

Nor was May happy with his "*Ethics Concerning Sex*" and analyzed the most recent "experimental data." By contrast to the loving passion he felt for Bets, one based on "natural desire, in turn based on mutual love," two recent unfortunate adventures in Salonica proved less edifying. Neither woman "want[ed] it," and one felt "great remorse (for weeks afterward)." He had been driven by desire, he realized, to treat these women as objects.[22] What "it" was we will never know, since in his diaries "it" covered everything from a passionate kiss to petting to intercourse. Clearly Rollo felt he had forced these situations and felt guilty about breaking his cardinal rule to treat individuals as unique personalities rather than objects. Yet the quality of his guilt, at least as he allowed himself to confront it in the privacy of his diary, ultimately had little to do with the women involved. The unpretty limits of ethical revelation in this regard were only underlined when he moved quickly to what he thought was an apt comparison: "A person feels self-conscious the next morning after having masturbated at night because he has used himself as an *object*, not *subject*. . . . This has lowered his opinion of himself—hence lack of courage, which leads to self-consciousness."[23]

Rollo's loneliness and, indeed, self-alienation led to an obsessive search for new means of analyzing his condition. He evinced a hunger for knowledge and insight that moved well beyond the identification and correction of sins. He watched his moods closely for rhythms of clarity or confusion as well as happiness or depression. He turned to Mary Baker Eddy's *Science and Health* for wisdom. He admired the enthusiasm and direction that thinking only "good thoughts" brought to the Christian Scientist's life, but also felt that closing one's eyes to evil would end in disaster. Indeed, he saw the "scheme of thinking only right thoughts" as a problem for some of the college's missionary leadership as well.[24]

He even welcomed knowledge of religions outside Christianity. In a visit to the home of Paulette Varsons, a local Jewish woman with whom he had become platonically attached, he listened with rapt attention as her mother explained Judaism's history and beliefs. "The Jewish religion and Protestantism are very similar," he noted, but added that "Christianity makes its followers lazy—'Remember the lilies of the field, they toil not, etc.'"[25] While Rollo remained surprisingly unreflective on the impact the economic depression might have on his own life, he began thinking in earnest about broader questions of peace and the just society. He embraced Bertrand Russell's "principles of social reconstruction," which sought to end to war by creating societies that encouraged the positive passions of human beings rather than restricting them and turning them toward destruction.[26] From Albert Schweitzer, he imbibed a vision of civilization in decline since the Great War, but one in which individual action might still rescue humankind.[27]

He now pondered not only personal genuineness but also how to be that "man by the side of the road" in the complex and dangerous world of the twentieth century. May sought heroes for this widened sense of his life. He had already shed his father as a model and now rejected even Jesus as models of action: "Why not better say, 'Would Compton [Anatolia College's heroic president] do this?' or 'Would Schweitzer do this?'"[28]

The question remained, however, *what* to do. As Rollo's twenty-fourth birthday approached, a new book caused a stir in Christendom and channeled May's career planning back toward the ministry. *Re-Thinking Missions*, the report of a commission appointed by the Layman's Foreign Missions Inquiry, criticized the narrowness and intolerance of past endeavors, especially in relation to native cultures. Broad-minded and cooperative, it reinterpreted the general aim of missionary work: "To seek with people of other lands a true knowledge and love of God, expressing in life and word what we have learned through Jesus Christ, and endeavoring to give effect to his spirit in the life of the world." The report reiterated that such an enterprise called "for not only a self-sacrificing spirit and an utter devotion, but for moral courage, a high order of intelligence, and a love of adventure."[29]

These recommendations hardly sound revolutionary today, nor were they new sentiments in 1932. However, they struck at a problem endemic to the twentieth century in general—the validity of a single religious Truth and, for that matter, notions of cultural superiority in a world of many peoples and faiths. *Re-Thinking Missions* touched off debates in local churches as well as in missionary societies and garnered much public notice. A discussion that took place at Anatolia College in late March and early April 1933 helped May to refine his discomfort as a "missionary" and, paradoxically, to rejuvenate his interest in "religious work." "In this missions business," he declared in his diary, "there are two decidedly different camps—those who know, and those who aren't quite as sure they know all." He could find both kinds at the college and sided with those who were there "only to help in the search, a humbler position." Those in the know seemed "to have less of a good grip on life." More generally, he declared simply, "The greatest shortcoming of the missions movement is *arrogance*."[30]

One injunction from *Re-Thinking Missions* held special meaning for May: "the capacity truly to understand and genuinely to love and sympathize with the people among whom he works."[31] Yet May's own limits in truly living by such a creed revealed themselves as he and a companion roamed central Greece in mid-April 1933. Near the city of Larissa, they encountered a Roma encampment of about forty tents. May thought that it must have been a traveling circus, since amid the tents were chained four bears, two monkeys, and "countless fierce dogs." He was drawn most of all to the women. He watched as one young teenage girl shouted at a peddler on the road, bolted from her tent in a whirl, and began to bargain with him. Another girl of about seventeen, carrying a large brass can full of water, approached Rollo for a cigarette.

Entranced by her large, deep brown eyes and "soft and rich" skin, he quickly sketched her. He also drew a "beautiful" woman nursing her infant. She laughed as he painstakingly penciled in the details of her ragged dress.

Completely ignorant not only of their culture but also of their history of enslavement and isolation, May projected his own concerns onto the impoverished band. He contrasted them to eastern European peasants, whose nobility and reserve, as he saw it, marked the "bulwark of civilization." By contrast, the "free Hellenic life of the Gypsies" provided the "frosting." Rollo mused on the "interesting psychological characteristics of the gypsies":

> They look at you full in the face, never a care for who you are. The nomad life from which comes art . . . a life of forgetting everything that has gone before, living for the moment. Following the impulse of the moment. A life free from inhibitions. A lazy life (children certainly are dirty in some tents) from standpoint of things accomplished—yet what a contribution to life in art, in stimulation toward the free in romance suggested to the rest of conventional living people.[32]

Such observations revealed how difficult it might be to achieve the goals of *Re-Thinking Missions*, no matter how heartfelt the commitment.

The end of spring term brought memories of the prior summer's adventures and a keen desire to live their spirit, so Rollo headed to Vienna to see Adler and to begin another tour with the International School of Art. "Same Viennese," he wrote, "'everything is hopeless, but not quite'—and so they dance their little while and laugh and cover existence with as much gayety and beauty as possible."[33] Rollo strolled through museums, attended performances of the Vienna Philharmonic and the Vienna State Opera, listened to a series of lectures by Adler, rekindled his friendship with Joseph Binder, and admired the beauty of young women as he sipped coffee in the outdoor cafés.

Yet amidst the pleasures of Viennese street life, the economic depression and the heightened clash of left- and right-wing movements in Austria contributed to a sense of impending chaos. Attuned to anti-Semitism by Madame Varsons and appalled by the anti-Jewish violence that accompanied the Nazi takeover in neighboring Germany, May could hardly contain himself at a café as a "sandy-haired, red-faced Austrian" told him (in defending the Nazis) that the "Jews control newspapers (as cinemas), and so are always 'tooting their own horn,' inciting animosity of gentiles."[34] Rollo chatted with an American student at the University of Vienna, who told him of an anti-Semitic incident he had actually witnessed. "He remarked," Rollo noted in his diary, "how sickening to see fifty big Nazis attack a little Jewish student." Such shocking moments mixed almost seamlessly in his diary with the sensory delights of Vienna. A painting or building, anonymous men and women on the street or passing acquaintances, the glitter of the opera—Rollo sketched each with words that fairly glowed with life.[35]

By July, May was off to Kitzbühel with "Jolly Binder" to begin the art tour. As Elma Pratt's students arrived in the postcard-perfect town, his enthusiasm reached its peak. He sought out the women on the tour and (by his own account at least) seemed irresistible to them. First there was Isabell, with whom he went swimming the very day of her arrival and with whom, the next day, a deep philosophical conversation turned physical—"Bang! We were off necking." With others he made auspicious beginnings. Indeed, the electricity of this process of "'becoming part' of one another," as he put it, elicited a giddy but anxious dream in which Rollo was precariously stranded on a very high spot.[36]

Perhaps, unconsciously, May knew he was headed for a fall. A week later he tried his luck with a woman named Ada, romancing her with his view of life, as they walked along an "entrancing stream." She was anything but entranced, accused him of preaching, and asked him not "to drag his philosophy into every conversation." That evening, another woman turned down his advances after a dance at the Grand Hotel. What had been an expectation of sensual delight collapsed. He tossed and turned but couldn't sleep. Europe now seemed a waste. The School of Art "didn't interest" him. He wanted to go home. "Visions of meeting Mother, Dad, Don, and all the family coursed thru my imagination," he wrote in his diary. "The world was suddenly alive and colorful and full of promise." Only a conversation the next morning with Elma Pratt kept him from leaving immediately. He consulted with Binder, who responded with Viennese terseness: "I think you waste your time in Greece." By the next day, he had decided that, at the very least, he would not return to Anatolia College.[37]

However, rejection and homesickness were not the only factors that led to his wish to return home. He also felt that he had been "out of the mill and rough and tumble of life long enuf." "My call was back to America," he declared to his diary, "I wanted most of all to study; I resolved to canvass all people I knew in America to borrow enuf money to go on to Union [Theological Seminary]. . . . Courage said go back into life." Pratt helped by offering him a job at the School of Art office in New York. Confirmed in his decision, Rollo resigned from Anatolia College and asked that his clothing and other belongings be packaged and sent to New York. The college wrote back to say that they would be happy to pack up his things and send them, but at the bottom of the typed letter the dean appended a longhand note excoriating Rollo for taking his commitment to the college so lightly.[38]

Within a week, Rollo was back in Vienna with the School of Art, preparing for one final art outing to Budapest and then a return to America. He also found time to look up Alfred Adler:

> I can almost say I love that man! Such a warmth as filled me on shaking his hand—such comfort feeling of being perfectly at ease, as I enjoyed talking to him then!
>
> He gives you courage when you meet him. He believes in you; you are fortified, and can speak out. You cannot get embarrassed in his presence. Such is a personality after a life devoted to understanding people and helping them. Meeting a person like Adler . . . gives one a flow of love for others, a contagion from the love in their souls.[39]

Rollo booked passage to New York on the steamship *Europa* with Joseph Binder as a travel companion. Fearful of events in Germany and Austria, Binder had secured two years of teaching at various art schools and universities in America. As they traveled by train across Hitler's Germany to the port of Bremen, May casually noted, as he looked out at the fields, that he had expected to see "daggers" instead of grass. Binder immediately dragged him to the men's toilet and whispered that he could not make such remarks safely in Germany.[40]

It was with some relief that they boarded the ship, leaving the increasingly violent climate of Germany and Austria for a more benign if troubled America. For Rollo, there was even time for one last, mostly innocent shipboard romance, this time with a young dancer of Binder's acquaintance. In late August 1933, the *Europa* docked in New York.

6

Toward the Unconditional Realm

May came back to America in the summer of 1933 anxious to plunge into life, to fashion a calling from "religious work" and psychology. Steered away from training in psychotherapy, he chose to continue his education in the progressive religious setting of New York's Union Theological Seminary. He had already dismissed the idea of becoming a minister and months before had set forth his ideal of modern religious preparation, forged at last in a deepening recognition of the Great Depression: "Let there be a minimum of theology, and a maximum of teaching of how to cope with social and economic wrongs of the situation. Train *social workers*." Although Union was a bit more traditional than the seminary of his dreams, it represented the cutting edge of liberal Protestantism and Christian social action. Nor could one have selected a more vibrant city in which to seek a place in the world of advanced thought.[1]

Still, from almost the moment of May's arrival in New York, a series of challenges and complications arose. Upon receiving word that his family was in upheaval, he was forced to make a quick trip to Lansing before starting classes. What he found was appalling. Don and E. T. had come to blows, and his parents were locked in combat as ever. Worst of all, Ruth had recently run off to Memphis, picked up a stranger, and promptly slept with him. Just as quickly, he had robbed and abandoned her and, it turned out, left her pregnant. E. T. and Matie drove Ruth to Detroit to have an abortion, and Don accompanied them literally to protect his sister from their mother's abuse. The household reverberated with guilt and recrimination but, for the moment, remained intact.

May did not find New York an easy place to love, at least at first. It was at once one of the most exciting cities in the world and an often exasperating challenge for a young man from small-town Michigan. One of the great centers of cultural and political ferment, it dwarfed every other place May had known in every way—population, noise, and contrasts of wealth and poverty, as well as racial and religious diversity and tension. In 1930, one-third of all New Yorkers were foreign-born; five million, about two-thirds, had at least one foreign-born parent. Russians, Hungarians, Irish, Italians, Poles, Germans, French, Chinese, Greeks, eastern European Jews, and myriad others had turned Protestant America's greatest metropolis into an immigrant city. Catholics and Jews collectively comprised over half its population. As important, African Americans from the South, as well as immigrants from the Caribbean and Africa, had transformed Harlem—which abutted Union Theological Seminary—into what its inhabitants and many others considered the capital of the black world.

Arriving at the depth of the Great Depression, May faced a city that bled misery. One-quarter of its working population was unemployed, and hundreds of thousands of families survived only because of government relief. New York's vaunted financial community had crumbled. Dreary soup lines and "Hooverville" encampments amid elegantly landscaped parks offered a stern rebuke to Manhattan's façade of wealth and splendor. A few blocks from Rollo's dormitory at Union, Harlem had suffered 50 percent unemployment rates as early as 1930, and matters got progressively worse as the Depression deepened. Every day, city authorities evicted ten to twenty black families from their apartments, leaving them to sleep on the sidewalks surrounded by their meager belongings. Many were able to eat only because local businesses and charities organized food handouts and soup kitchens.

The gloom of 1933 evoked May's sympathy but also triggered provincial fears. A scholarship and room and board in a small oasis of Protestant gentility afforded him little protection against the rude shock of human privation. He chafed at the tough veneer of New Yorkers and concluded, "The surroundings of the people of New York are so ugly how can one expect politeness?"[2]

Nor did the school year begin well. Almost immediately Rollo experienced a relapse of malaria doctors said he must have first contracted in Greece (though no sign of the disease surfaced in his diaries or letters home). It landed him in the hospital for most of October. High fever, chills, and frightening hallucinations barraged his body and psyche. A dream he had in the hospital summed up his state: "Me in a room which was being assaulted by enemies. I locked all the doors, barred the windows,—but made no attempt to fight."[3] A week later, he had a dream that indicated his strength was returning but that his life was no less embattled. "An armed person entered a room," recorded, "where mother, Dad and I were; I grabbed a gun and exchanged shots with him, without fear." As he put it in his diary: "This past month and a half—a nightmare."[4] He found the rest of the semester predictably challenging. May returned to classes exhausted, took incompletes in three subjects, and excelled only in a course on the history of religion.[5]

Despite a rocky start, May felt a growing sense of exhilaration from being at Union. He had thrust himself into the eye of a storm that continued to buffet the religious life of the nation and impinged increasingly on civic life as well. Since the Civil War, pluralism, science, theological modernism, and the economic inequalities wrought by industrial capitalism had eroded any semblance of religious or social unity in Protestant America. Fundamentalists and evangelicals battled liberal Christian attempts to historicize the Bible and turn toward more personalist conceptions of God's existence and power. Schisms within and wars across denominational lines developed over the nature of religious experience, biblical literalism, and how (as well as if) the church should respond to the fearful social and economic situation of the 1930s.

Rollo had already been exposed to personalist and social activist aspects of liberalism within the Y and at Oberlin. However, coming to Union at this particular moment put him at the very center of the movement. Founded in the nineteenth century by New School Presbyterians, in the modern era Union had moved decisively toward the fusion of faith and the broad historical and philosophical study of religion. Henry Sloane Coffin, Union's president since 1926, presided over a faculty that included some of the most influential Protestant theologians of the era: Reinhold Niebuhr, his brother, H. Richard Niebuhr, who taught at Yale, Harry Emerson Fosdick, and, beginning in late 1933, the great German radical theologian Paul Tillich. Despite some disagreement over means and theological underpinnings, they were united in their affirmative response to the question posed by the title of Reinhold Niebuhr's book of 1927, *Does Civilization Need Religion?*[6] Even as they trained a new generation of ministers and lay leaders, each preached to the nation in newspaper columns, magazine articles, radio broadcasts, and popular books. Each helped to revolutionize Christianity in America and its place in public discourse.

In doing so, they spoke directly to Rollo's developing sense of mission in the world. His diaries document a daily infusion of new ideas and visions, ones that shaped and sometimes piqued his usual stream of mordant introspection. Rollo was especially impressed by Harry Emerson Fosdick's legendary sermons at Morningside Heights' Riverside Church. Fosdick, an independent and modernizing Baptist, had become a hero to liberal Protestants as he forthrightly defended liberalism against the early twentieth-century fundamentalist insurgency.[7] Most Americans knew him, however, as the author of a series of successful books that guided souls through the crises of everyday life. He became a spokesperson for an optimistic, personality-centered vision of Christianity and, not incidentally, one of the most popular American preachers.[8]

May was already familiar with the basics of liberal theology; however, he had never heard it stated more succinctly than in Fosdick's direct definition: the aim of liberal Christianity was "to put first things first in religion, to subordinate the details of ritual, creed, and church to the major objects of Christianity—the creation of personal character and social righteousness."[9] No wonder then that May "felt [himself] being called anew to religion by Fosdick's preaching." One of the first Fosdick sermons Rollo heard caused him to set forth his own standards for "any good and acceptable religion for me [and] for us moderns." That faith must "demand and use man's courage," encourage "a solidarity among mankind," and "must not go counter to— rather work in partnership with—man's intellect." May was drawn especially to Fosdick's notion that "ultimate worth" could be found in "personality."[10]

May also noted insights from Fosdick that seemed to describe his own struggles. He had always felt he was what would later be called an "under-achiever," a sense his wobbly first semester seemed to confirm. Yet, as Rollo noted in his diary, Fosdick reminded his congregants that "Edison, Watts, Newton, Darwin, Hume . . . were all said to be unpromising and dull when young. 'Something great laid hold upon them.'" Fosdick also addressed the question of meaning in a world turned upside down by war, depression, and the rise of bloody dictatorships. As May listened to "The Sane Individual in a Crazy World," he felt gripped by Fosdick's insistence that much of the "crisis" in society was "really *internal*, not external," and that one could still imbue personal relationships with meaning.[11]

That such an idea could seem revelatory and not a simple cliché spoke to the freshness of psychologized religious culture in 1934. It also implicitly reflected Fosdick's turn inward as a result of World War I. He had been a zealous supporter of the war effort, only to face its calamitous results in death and destruction and the mean-spirited Treaty of Versailles. Indeed, the war experience turned him into a pacifist.

More politically attuned and less openly warm than Fosdick, Reinhold Niebuhr was by all accounts a man on fire. The very first thing Rollo noticed about him was his "complete absence of repression . . . [and] his being completely absorbed in the thing he is talking about."[12] Niebuhr's career began in 1912 as minister of Bethel Church, a small "frontier" German American congregation on the outskirts of Detroit. Like Fosdick, the young Niebuhr enthusiastically supported America's participation in World War I (and roundly criticized German Americans who didn't) but became disenchanted with the harsh peace and with war in general. He was a confirmed pacifist through the early 1920s. However, he took a less sanguine view of human capacities for good than Fosdick and, as early as the mid-1920s, was developing a critique from within of what he saw as an all too sunny liberal Christianity.

This vision of the world came in part from Niebuhr's perch at the Bethel Church, where he witnessed Henry Ford and others transform Detroit from a pleasant city to a crowded, dirty, and poverty-infected factory town. Niebuhr began to preach that a Christian had the duty to act, however imperfectly, against social injustice. Soon he rejected what he saw as a utopian strain in the social gospel in favor of Marx's vision of class warfare. By late 1929, Niebuhr joined the Socialist Party and even stood as its candidate for Congress in 1932, when the Party assumed that it would gain a significant following because of the worsening depression.[13] That they were trounced, from presidential candidate Norman Thomas down to Niebuhr for Congress, came as a disheartening surprise.

Niebuhr's radicalization moved him decisively away from pacifism. By the early 1930s, he advocated coercion instead of Christian love in the battle for the rights of labor, social justice, and international peace. In one of his most influential and greatest works, *Moral Man and Immoral Society*, published the year before May's arrival at Union, he took the giant step of entertaining the idea that even outright violence might be justified in achieving social ends or in resisting aggressive evil.[14]

Niebuhr's abandonment of pacifism shocked his friends and colleagues. Some assumed he was moving away from Christianity and toward secular politics, so strongly did his views challenge the reigning assumptions of liberal Christianity. However, Niebuhr's newly darkened view of human nature sparked instead the conviction that humankind desperately needed the guidance of faith. He argued that only through the grace of God could human beings act morally. In short, he envisioned a "neo-Orthodox" theology that at one and the same time embraced the sovereignty of God and inspired imperfect men and women to struggle against ignorance, poverty, and tyranny. More than any member of the faculty except Harry Ward (Union's senior ethicist, radical pacifist, and cofounder of the ACLU), Niebuhr kept the social and economic crisis of the 1930s on the agenda for both colleagues and students.[15]

Although May and Niebuhr were never close, the theologian's class on Christian ethics led Rollo and many other students toward social activism at the seminary and in the broader community. "It may be necessary to bring the revolution about," Rollo wrote at the time, "one could not sit under Niebuhr three hours a week and not think long thoughts on the subject."[16] In early December 1933, he and several other seminarians joined members of the radical Intercollegiate League for Industrial Democracy in picketing Sunday services at the fashionable Church of the Heavenly Rest. Its minister, the Reverend Henry Darlington, had publicly supported the governor of California's endorsement of a lynching in San Jose. Rollo took turns carrying a sign that read: "HOW MANY TIMES MUST HE BE CRUCIFIED?"[17] Less controversially, he played trombone for the poor and homeless at Jerry McAuley's Rescue Mission. In early 1934, he also worked for Pioneer Youth, a labor-socialist organization that provided recreation to the children of factory workers and the unemployed.[18]

Rollo mostly viewed his participation in these activities as a sign of Adlerian health and Christian virtue, submerging one's self in activities for social good. He feared, though, that he might also lose his authentic self in the crowd. He was in a quandary, and wisdom gleaned around the seminary didn't help much. Listening to one guest speaker, he agreed with the motto "Try helping other people" as a cure for unhappiness. A week before, however, another lecturer had taken a different tack—"follow your inner light at all times." Both made Christian and psychological sense, each in tension with the other. In one case, feeling his own beliefs deeply compromised, Rollo left the highly politicized Pioneer Youth after three months of service and shifted his energies to an assistantship with the Reverend Herman Reissig, a minister in Brooklyn interested in social welfare.[19]

Politics became even more troublesome for Rollo when the issues concerned Union Theological Seminary. In the winter of 1934, a group of radical students who had already picketed in support of workers at the Waldorf Astoria hotel turned its attention to the seminary. They accused its leaders of mistreating its own employees and campaigned to raise the pay for refectory staff. A majority of students signed a petition that urged creation of a faculty committee to look into working conditions. When the committee returned what some deemed to be an insufficiently critical report, the radicals loudly ridiculed it and responded with a daring prank. On May Day, a radical activist climbed atop the seminary's main building and replaced the Stars and Stripes with a red flag. Unamused, President Coffin and the trustees publicly denounced the activists.[20]

These events brought May to a defining moment. Whatever his socialist sympathies, he had become deeply attached to Union and its mission and came to resent the Communist left's disregard for the institution. When an article in the *Christian Century* ridiculed the administration's criticism of the activists, he responded with an unpublished letter to the magazine. He rejected the implication that Coffin had sought to limit free speech and political action. Taking the offensive, May charged that the radical students did not care about Union's basic mission. He reported that one radical had remarked to him, "I never should have come to a seminary anyway. I don't want to be a minister; I ought to have become a doctor." May's views represented those of many liberals at Union who felt themselves caught between the rival ideals of social justice and respect for Union as an institution. Even Niebuhr thought the radicals had gone too far.[21]

In all, the first year at Union, despite or perhaps owing to its heightened politics, confirmed May's commitment to religion. He took stock in April, a few days after his twenty-fifth birthday: "Last fall I considered myself a humanist. Now God is my personal friend. Last fall I hesitated to believe anything of which I was not certain in the everyday, material life. Now I live, if not all the time at least the times when I am most alive, in the transcendent, 'unconditional' realm as Tillich would say." May's affirmations of faith would come and go, but this new commitment to religion could not have come at a better time. Furthermore, that he reached for Tillich's compelling abstraction—the unconditional—to describe that aliveness pointed toward what would become the unswerving direction of his spiritual life.[22]

7

"I *will not* become a
professional Christian"

Late in the spring of 1934, as he was finishing his second term at Union, May received news from his mother: E. T. had left for good. It could not have been entirely surprising news, but it left Matie frantic. She pleaded with Rollo to come home, even for just a little while. He couldn't refuse. He arrived in East Lansing in September 1934, hoping to stay a few weeks and then resume his studies. Instead, he remained for most of the next two years. What began as a simple mission of family rescue became a crucial turning point, one in which he found and began to practice what would be his life's calling.

Rollo returned home reluctantly. He knew when he arrived that it was up to him to keep the family afloat. The biggest problem was Matie. "Mother seeks to hold all to a 15-year ago level," Rollo noted in his diary, "where cowardly life fears any move upward and outward." Although every day revealed new signs of his mother's psychological devastation, his memory fixed on one incident for the next sixty years. He and Yona were in a heated argument with their mother when Matie, with what he later called a "schizzy" zeal, threatened to show them the "baby in the attic." Rollo turned to nineteen-year-old Yona in puzzlement. His sister explained that Matie had preserved Ruth's aborted fetus in a jar and, when enraged, would retrieve it and wave it threateningly at E. T. or the kids. Rollo bounded upstairs to the attic, grabbed the jar, and promptly buried it in the backyard.[1]

Rollo vowed to be as present in the family as E. T. had been absent and to shield his sisters and brothers from Matie's rage. He became Yona's loving protector, feeling deeply drawn to her helplessness before her mother's barrages and in love with her gentle face and demeanor. When Matie refused to replace Yona's threadbare clothes, he took her downtown to buy a new coat. Later, he helped finance her attendance at Michigan State, even though he himself was building up his own personal debt. He helped pay Don's tuition to art school as well. And he became twelve-year-old Pat's surrogate dad, escorting him to father-son events at school and encouraging him to see beyond the emotional prison of home. Ruth was the toughest challenge, as the intense web of love and anger that bound them was further complicated by Rollo's responsibilities as the family's guardian. Ruth had become progressively more unbalanced after her abortion, and on several occasions Rollo rescued her from near calamities. Once, she left for Florida after being abandoned by her latest lover and attempted suicide. The police in Florida intervened and called Rollo after finding his phone number on a note in her pocket. When she returned, he tried to soothe her with words of faith and hope. Ruth had a simple reply: "Don't Shit Me, Big Boy."[2]

The family needed him to stay as long as he could, and an exceptional professional opportunity allowed Rollo to remain in East Lansing until 1936. Buck Weaver, now teaching at the University of Michigan but still connected to Lansing's YMCA, helped arrange for him a package of three part-time jobs: college counselor at Michigan State, student director at the Peoples Church, and student secretary at the YMCA. Any employment would have been a blessing in 1934, but these positions were an extraordinary, unexpected opportunity for May, allowing him to combine "religious work" and counseling with little constraint or supervision.

The religious mission was foremost. As he wrote to the Peoples Church board in October 1934, he aimed "to make religion indigenous to the campus." He saw as his first task attracting great numbers and varieties of students to events at the Y and the church. He instituted a series of Sunday-morning religious classes in order to give students "inspiration and religious experience." He created a "Frosh Council" to teach college traditions at meetings that he proudly noted had "hit the headlines of the college paper several times." Early-morning devotional meetings, Friday Night Fun Nights (with dancing), and a Sunday noon "Spartan Y Forum" featuring faculty or Rollo himself discussing "religious or character-building subjects" filled out the week.[3]

Rollo programmed educational events that emphasized the development of individual personality and the commonality of religious quests. For instance, a lecture series called "What Can We Learn from Other Religions?" ranged across the spiritual map: Theosophy, Catholicism, and Confucianism, as well as talks titled "The Religion of Gandhi," "Hebrew Religion," and "Mohammedanism." The lecturers comprised professors and graduate students as well as a rabbi and a priest. He also promoted the social mission of Christianity and a Niebuhrian political agenda. The Spartan Forum presented talks by the 1934 Socialist candidate for governor of Michigan and an African American civil rights activist. With a mixture of trepidation and self-satisfaction about the radical political tone of the series, May scrawled on a Michigan State News story about the lectures, "This series is getting us in hot water."[4]

He also devised an ingenious interview project to advance the institutional goals of the Y and the church, inviting every fifth male in the college directory to be interviewed about his religious life. Rollo asked each a few leading questions but mostly listened as each student "just turn[ed] on the gas and talk[ed]." He conducted more than 150 half-hour meetings with a wide variety of students:

> President of the "wettest" frat of the campus, football heroes, intelligent students who have thought religion through and believe it the more firmly, nice boys who come to all church activities but never know why, atheists who go around always "blue" on the campus, hide-bound Lutherans whose pastors forbid their having anything to do with the college Y, church-soured Dutch Reformed, watered-out Unitarians, "A" students and flunkers . . .[5]

May's report emphasized the basic friendliness of the student body to liberal religion and the need on campus for appropriate activities. The upbeat tone of the survey marked the degree to which May had adopted not only a cheery sense of organizing but also, despite his embrace of *Re-Thinking Missions* in Greece, a missionary's contempt for those who failed to see the light. In an unpublished manuscript, he caricatured the various "thems" who resisted the "us" of the Y and the Peoples Church. "The Purposeless Student," a cliché of 1920s college life, mostly indulged in "drinking, carousing and cutting classes" and attended college because he had "nothing else to do." Rollo noted that though the economic depression had diminished their numbers, they still could be recognized: reasonably bright, rich, and happily unmotivated. He argued that they were actually secretly "melancholy" because "life h[eld] no meaning." A typical "purposeless student" rarely went to church, "never attended Sunday School or Young Peoples Society," and thought students who did so were "intellectually his inferiors." May noted that Jewish students were "often in this group."[6]

Quite as problematic were "fundamentalist" students. Typically, they came from small-town northern Michigan or the Upper Peninsula, were raised in a larger-than-average German American or Scandinavian American family, professed Lutheranism, and attended Michigan State specifically for job training rather than cultural enrichment. Such a student felt "apart from the campus, tend[ed] to be an individualist," rejected "interdenominationalism," and could not imagine Abraham Lincoln to be "a fit subject for a sermon." He believed that "religion is primarily creedal," was not "interested in discussing religion with other students," and felt "he already ha[d] the 'one true religion.'" May even attributed problematic physical and behavioral characteristics to the devout Lutheran student, noting that he shook hands "hesitatingly and jerkily" and was "ill at ease" when he talked. Such reflections illustrated not only the combative side of Rollo's liberal Christianity but also a merger of that vision with Adlerian psychology. The clannish "fundamentalist" no less than the "individualist" was an enemy of a commonly understood social good, and the miseducation that had led him to that position literally revealed itself in his physical way of being in the world.[7]

Illuminating his perceptions of the enemies of liberal religion, the report and its methods nonetheless seemed to be at odds with May's once-expressed concerns about "using" individuals for ulterior personal and organizational motives. He exploited intimate counseling meetings with hundreds of students for a specific advocacy hardly congenial to all the interviewees. Not incidentally, May also published an article based on the study, "Portrait of Men Students," in the national journal *Christian Education*. It was his first professional publication.[8]

May knew from the beginning that such a job might involve straying from such purist principles as never objectifying the individual. A frank conversation with Buck Weaver helped him to see the usefulness of such activities. Still, he worried that dishonest motives might make someone "rotten at the core." "I *will not* become a professional Christian," he declared in his diary, "If I can't be genuine—be a real man—in the ministry, then I'll get out." He believed that a minister, director, or counselor could stay "absolutely honest" despite temptation and that being an honest Christian also meant that he would "tolerate no barriers between people."[9]

If the practical matters of working within an institution meant that he could pursue such genuineness in the world with only mixed success, in private moments he could employ "absolute honesty" and reap its rewards. Thus a September 1934 diary entry:

> My covenant with God—the covenant which we made last June when I got the job—was renewed: I shall do it all for *him*. Every task I undertake in this job, I shall go into with the understanding that I am doing it for him.[10]

And another from October:

> Yesterday I lived every moment like one in love. Overflowing with a strange happiness, I could scarcely restrain myself from running—joyous energy abounded in me. I kept saying to God over and over again! I love thee![11]

Rollo gained confidence in such avowals of faith through a series of religious experiences "in the woods."[12] In one such episode in October 1934, he "jotted down" the transcendent scene he viewed and the prayer he made, which ended: "May I understand, and know the answers to life; may I be respected by people, that being necessary to influence; and may I abandon myself in joyful service to these young men."[13] He attempted to structure such aspirations into everyday life: a regular routine of exercise, meals, rest, reading, and meetings with students.[14] Ostensibly secular concerns, in the life of a religious virtuoso like Rollo they became the tools of holiness.

That meant he must continue to sort out what his essential work should be. He had come to see himself as more than an "organizer of programs" or "a spreader of good cheer." He chose instead a mightier mission, a "great place," one particularly challenging for a young man of twenty-five. He would be "a teacher, counselor of religion," a role in which one "must *know the answers* to life, and pass them on." He needed to meditate on his own life and to study religion, psychology, and philosophy with utmost seriousness. Then he would be prepared to know and help his student clients.[15] It was neither a small nor a simple task. For one thing, May felt the need to be an exemplar to his students. In January 1935, as he commenced his second semester as a counselor, Rollo vowed that he would lead "as simple a life as possible," with "renunciation" as a key theme in order to support his broader mission. This included his romantic and sex life. Previous obsessions over one or another woman disappeared from his diary entries, and only occasionally yielded a reference to a not entirely successful war on masturbation.[16]

His public admonitions to students highlighted "healthy" outlets for "tension" and avoidance of the compulsive search for sexual satisfaction. Some indication of the advice he gave to students appeared in "Make Your Recreation Creative!," a short article in the February 1936 issue of *Recreation* magazine. E. T. himself could have written this plea to provide adolescents and young adults with innocent entertainment lest they be drawn to a seamier side of life:

We cannot remain placid while our young people run off to beer gardens, frequent the public dance halls, and plunk down their quarters at a mediocre movie out of sheer lack of any better way to spend a Friday evening. . . . If all your son or daughter can find for amusement is dancing in beer gardens or absorbing a steady diet of sex-stimulating movies, then all the preaching or moral counsel in the world won't do much good. We can be sure of this, I am confident; that promiscuous petting is a result often of the fact that our young people have nothing more interesting to do. The necking party is much more likely to follow a flat, empty evening than a happy, really recreative one.[17]

If "Make Your Recreation Creative!" demonstrated the enduring power of the YMCA on Rollo's vision for the public, it was somewhat at odds with the more frank and ambiguous setting of counseling. Confidentiality and the passage of time have closed off the possibility of knowing much about May's counselees, his techniques, or specific successes and failures as a counselor. Little could have been based on the contemporary training of counselors for two simple reasons—training programs were in their infancy, and no widely used text existed. Besides, Rollo had no formal training for the job. He did count himself lucky to have encountered such inspirational models as Buck Weaver and various counselors at Oberlin and the YMCA College. His exposure to Adlerian theory and practice at Semmering permanently widened and complicated his sense of the psyche. The overriding goal of his counseling was to allow the fullest discovery and expression, in the liberal Christian sense, of the student's "personality." And more than a few students took up the challenge, discussing with him major dilemmas and fears, choices in love and work, in single meetings or over three or four sessions.[18]

Clearly, as May declared in a report to the Peoples Church, he found counseling "the most gratifying" aspect of his work. He perfected his approach through endless, compulsive meditations on his own ambitions, defenses, faults, faith, and much more, and how they might affect his counseling efforts. And he cared deeply for those he counseled. He took time in his diary entries to ponder their fates and futures. Lee needed "coaching—which I must give him," while Harry needed "much change, either gradually or by 'cracking.'" Sometimes he even congratulated himself: "You were right in diagnosing Gertrud _____. (You read people largely by their actions and behavior)."[19]

May's approaches to "religious work" in Lansing thus reflected at least one deeply embedded tension in twentieth-century liberal Protestantism and, for that matter, American culture: reconciling the needs of the individual with those of the community. As a liberal Christian in a counseling setting, he could allow himself great latitude of experience, thought, and personal advice in the encouragement of personal growth. He sought to engender genuine "personality" in himself and others. As a spokesperson for an institution and to a public, he could find no better language than one of moralistic generalization. May could not yet define, as he later would, a suitable solution.

Even as he articulated a mission for the Peoples Church, Rollo worked on what he considered his most urgent personal issues. He felt crippled by "certain character weaknesses" (the personality faults he had been working on since his sessions with Adler), most "having to do with 'spoiled child' trend." If he could overcome them, he surmised, he might have a life of "great success." If not, he could only count on one of "moderate success, but always baffled, such as Dad's." He knew that to be a "great success" he would have to not only resolve the contradictions in his character but also study great ideas with great men. He had met those men at Union, and it was back to Union that he went for a summer session in 1935.[20]

"Rasputin, Shelley, Van Gogh
and Fosdick in One"

We cannot know May's thoughts as he boarded the train in Lansing for New York in July 1935, but his success at helping his family and becoming a small celebrity on campus fed a sense that he was destined for greatness. He planned a return to Lansing in the fall, but he hoped that taking summer courses at Union would further ready him to make an impact on the world. At twenty-six, he was ready to engineer a "psychic advance" for humankind. His diary revealed a young man on a roller coaster of creativity, desire, tortured self-consciousness, and intellectual boldness. It also betrayed a lonely, competitive meditation on self in the guise of artist-genius. He prefaced his own entries with telling epigraphs from great minds, including a paraphrase from Goethe: "No great creative thing was ever done except in solitude." And Jung: "Every psychic advance of man arises from a state of mental suffering." Quotations from Santayana and Wagner offered similar wisdom. "I am growing!" he exclaimed, and, as if in an intellectual foot race, named teachers and contemporaries whom he had already "grown past."[1]

May's dreams of greatness were hardly unusual for a talented, creative man in his mid-twenties whose sense of specialness and mission had been fostered from birth. Yet his obsession with personal destiny also revealed Adlerian symptoms that had not been part of his personal analysis at Semmering. Adler and his assistants had shocked May into an awareness of crippling aspects of his personality, especially childhood senses of inferiority that encouraged him to avoid close relationships. The Adlerians imparted a new narrative of his life but, as his experience with women showed, hardly completely cured him of his fear of their domination. Always holding the cards—the teacher, the counselor, or the savior of his family—he felt safest practicing an altruism built on power and distance. Adler would have talked about it as a distorted *Lebensstil* (literally "lifestyle," but with more profound meaning than in today's English usage), a set of behaviors that humans develop from childhood and build upon as they find a way of relating to others and to society at large.

May hoped that a summer at Union would help him work on those "certain character weaknesses," as well as expose him more deeply to the intellectual currents of the day. He pursued his courses with vigor, gleaning a bounty of rewards in classes like Eugene Lyman's Current Trends in Religious Thought. Lyman's readings included selections from Karl Barth and Emil Brunner in theology; John Dewey, Walter Lippmann, Alfred North Whitehead, and Henri-Louis Bergson in philosophy; and a half dozen books by less well-remembered philosophers, scientists, and theologians. May also took a religious education class, for which he wrote a paper reviewing Jung's recently published *Modern Man in Search of a Soul*. His reading of Jung revealed a growing understanding of modern psychological theory as well as a penchant for the vernacular when it came to illustrating complex ideas or consequences.[2] For example, contrasting Freud's conception of dreams as wish fulfillment to Jung's more multivalent notions, May noted that for Jung "the dream [played] the teleological role of 'giving gas' to the style of life of the person."[3]

He also felt drawn to Jung's therapeutic approach. As opposed to the Freudian probe into sexual impulse and the Adlerian concern with the "unconscious workings of the drive to power," Jung outlined a more spiritual structure of stages: confession, explanation, education, and transformation. In reality, the process was not so different than in other therapies, but Jung spoke in a language of spirituality congenial to May. "The meeting of two personalities is like the contact of two chemical substances," wrote May of Jung's psycho-alchemy; "if there is any reaction, both are transformed." As May noted, the "human quality of the doctor becomes the important consideration in the treatment."[4]

May thus underlined a core issue in the marriage of religion and psychology, that of moral judgment. He saw confession as one of the most important stages in therapy and credited the Catholic Church with recognizing its power. However, he wondered whether a Protestant minister could "divorce his own personal moral bias from the confession." To judge the confessor would be "fatal to any treatment, for the patient will not confess frankly against a moral judgment already pre-supposed in the minister." In addition, a minister untrained in psychological techniques might well be sympathetic "subjectively" but not know "when to withhold sympathy in spite of the demands of the patient." Nor did May think it would be easy for the minister to open himself to self-change in the "transformation stage." "This demands much greater moral flexibility," he wrote, "much less stereotype on the part of the minister if he is to be an effective counselor."[5]

That May called the object of a minister's attention the "patient" indicates how compelling he found the psychotherapeutic worldview, but he wrote the paper in a course on religious education and also drew some lessons for that field. Recognizing the power of the unconscious, he doubted the efficacy of religious training that emphasized "external rules" and favored giving the greatest opportunity for creativity. "Jung has a valuable contribution to make to us in pointing out the essential hypothetical character of our basic assumptions," he added, "and hence leading us to be less dogmatic about our so-called universal laws." Indeed, May argued for the validity of "hints, hunches, warnings."[6]

Jung's chapter "Psychology and Literature" elicited Rollo's lengthiest and most sensitive summary as well as his deepest identification with any part of the book. "I find myself in agreement with the essential points in Jung's theory of art," he wrote; "the ideas that he has so well expressed have been running through my mind for several years, though I have always been aware of the impossibility of logically substantiating any theories of art that endeavor to pierce as deeply into the inner sources of art as do these." Jung placed the artist—whether painter, poet, writer, musician, or composer—at the very crossroads of individual and cosmic consciousness. A quirk of circumstance and heredity gave the artist the power to tap the "collective unconscious." Jung's artist expressed the mind of "collective man" through individual creativity. May thus sided with Jung in correcting the public's jaundiced view of the artist. "The man in the street" saw them as "maladjusted to life" and marked by "egocentricity." Yet, despite surface appearances, May argued, they expressed "the deep fears, inner hopes, joys and sorrows, and all psychic experience of mankind. He therefore is the *most* social of men."[7]

May carried on a parallel discussion in his diary. He asked, "Am I essentially an artist?" and adduced as evidence his love of art and literature as well as testimony from expert witnesses. He recalled that Wager had called him a "poet in action," and Harry Emerson Fosdick said his practice sermon "went on like music." May even termed his student survey project and speaker series at the Y "essentially works of art: conceived in inspiration, executed in great travail . . . as one does a great statue." He argued as well for the crucial role that psychoanalysis might play in modern spirituality. "With its acid-like analysis of human motives," he noted, "psychotherapy presents to us in bold relief the essentially selfish foundation of much of our modern religion. . . . We are then in a position to wash away the dross and retain the gold." In a grand turnabout of Freud, psychotherapy became the royal road to true religion. Jungian therapy supported belief in "God, human freedom, and immortality." May found a role for Adler as well, concluding that "religious leaders . . . partake themselves of the beatific treatments of psychotherapy and become cured once and for all of their inferiority complex as regards their profession."[8]

May's own "inferiority complex" affected his sexual and romantic life more than his professional one. He remained self-conscious, vulnerable, and deeply craving of success with women. These obsessions, which had taken a back seat to family and work during his initial return to Lansing, came back in force when he came back for the summer session at Union. He felt he had made some progress; he noted, "So far as girls go and my ability to attract them, I am growing."[9] He wouldn't be happy until his creative, spiritual, and amorous natures merged. May vowed that he would both "love a girl more passionately than I have ever heard of man loving" and "write the world's best poetry to her." In short, he would revolutionize not only religion but also courtly love.[10]

Yet as fantasies of sex, love, and marriage consumed Rollo's conscious and unconscious life, reality interceded in sobering ways. He was smitten with a fellow student—dark, sexy, and seriously intellectual—who in their time together was fully a match for May. He fantasized about marrying M., but she reminded him too much of his brilliant if unbalanced sister Ruth. She was too masculine, too neurotic, too competitive, and too willing to provoke jealousy (when May talked to her about psychology, she countered with the authority of another man, her "friend the psychiatrist"). Still, the thought of committing to a relationship led to ritual self-evaluation worthy of a combination narcissist, striver, and saint. He inspected himself before a full mirror and vowed to stand, sit, and walk with more assured straightness. He puzzled over his smile after M. made fun of his "grinning." He practiced looking others in the eye and speaking straight. Sizing himself up against fellow student religious workers at a conference, he felt "distinctly superior . . . in intellectual ability, imagination, charm of personality, energy and initiative." However, he added with a saintly pause, that was no reason "for self-satisfaction or pride."[11]

Not surprisingly, issues of love and lust invaded his dreams. In one, Rollo fixed an old Ford and drove it wildly and dangerously down the street. He remembered feeling that next time he had better "get inside and man the controls in the regular way." In another, he and M. searched for a place to settle down and found "one—old—baroque" place, where, in another urge toward self-control, he immediately covered up the ornate curlicues with tapestries. In another nocturnal drama, he sat next to her in a class taught by a famous person's "sissy" son. The teacher asked him to leave the room because May was talking to his woman friend. " 'God damn son of a _____ '", he shouted to the teacher, "then said nothing but took my things slowly and walked out. . . . I had a secret pride that I had blurted out in this manly, rough fashion." May wanted to prove that, despite being the son of a well-known Y man, he was no "sissy" but a "manly" man. Still, rather than celebrate his triumph, he noted the "danger of being exhibitionist in unconventionality."[12]

The day after this dream, he recorded a set of striking images in his diary. He recounted how M. waited for him after class, "the girl of full arms and breasts and curly brown hair that flows back in riotous abundance." However, his focus shifted to another woman, "her waves of golden hair reflecting flecks of light, her scarlet lips, matching bright hues in that multi-colored dress and contrasted to pure white teeth, wide in a smile made lovely by clear blue eyes." M. found her rival in the marble-like, classically feminine poise of a new love interest: Florence DeFrees.[13]

Rollo's summer in New York lasted less than two months, but he returned to Lansing more focused, confident, and self-possessed. He admitted that before the summer session he had been " 'don't careish'—slightly cynical." In September 1935, he was ready to make a great and authentic contribution to the world. He contrasted this sense of personal destiny to his father's "ingratiating approach, groveling attitude" and the "general Y-man ungenuineness," both of which Rollo still detected in himself and sought to "eradicate completely." Paradoxically, that meant he must devote himself to remaking the Y and the Peoples Church in the spirit of authenticity: "Do I seek to serve God? Let me do it by serving students, doing my job well."[14]

That was what serving God meant in September. After some months, however, May became increasingly impatient with the small world of Lansing and anxious to challenge its narrow confines. He became bolder, giving student groups talks about dating and intimacy—"sex dope"—based on his own European experiences rather than even the most progressive Y texts. He continued his self-education, exploring the recent work of Otto Rank, the renegade Freudian whom he found more compelling than either Freud or Adler because of Rank's emphasis on the uniqueness of individual human beings and on a therapy that sought to liberate personal spiritual and creative potentialities. Inspired by Rank, May created a new watchword in his diary: "Living in present, courageously, adequately, is to free one's self from the past."[15]

May sometimes framed his sense of destiny through the lens of literature. He read Joyce's *Portrait of the Artist as a Young Man* and memorized its famous penultimate passage as if it reflected his very soul: "Welcome, O life! I go to encounter for the millionth time the reality of experience and to forge in the smithy of my soul the uncreated conscience of my race." Joyce's words inspired in Rollo a rebellious cry: "This wild arrogance, which would do everything, experience everything, love everything—to which humility seems putting on the brakes. Keep this *insurgent arrogance*."[16] He evinced a manic appetite for "everything." The magnetic future, "infused with a brilliance that inspires me toward it," inspired a "Faustian thirst." "I plan to read all and know all," Rollo declared, "then, to serve magnificently." He vowed to finish his degree at Union quickly so that he could unleash the "great powers surging up within."[17]

"For possibly the first time in history," he declared, presumably referring to his personal history, "I feel I have found myself." He experienced this discovery as a transcendent state, breaking "down the barriers of one's subconscious, and repressed ideas leap forth." Perhaps he had remembered Jung's startling statement in *Modern Man's Search for a Soul*: "Are we to understand the 'imitation of Christ' in the sense that we should copy his life and, if I may use the expression, ape his stigmata; or in the deeper sense that we are to live our own proper lives as truly as he lived his in all its implications?" Yet a persistent loneliness laced his enthusiasm and increased his need to see himself as a solitary soul possessed of special powers. In mystical moments, he was sure that he possessed psychical insight: "I can feel out my appearance by psychic transference from the mind of people I meet."[18]

He sought to share the experience of his "true" embrace of "everything" by offering an audacious and inspired course, Religion in Modern Life, twice a week at the YMCA. May traversed the realms of psychology, art, and politics as he focused on the most profound and controversial issues in contemporary culture. He began by introducing individual philosophers, moving from the Greeks through Spinoza, Kant, William James, Dewey, Whitehead, and the "religious realism" of William Ernst Hocking and Eugene William Lyman. Then came topical units: "Science and Religion," "Religion and Modern Culture," and "Religion and Modern Social Issues."[19]

He structured each topic as a troubled crossroads whose debates none-theless promised progress and renewal. His lively discourse on modern art underlined the aim of the painter "to pierce underneath the surface and paint Beauty itself," not the surface of the thing itself but its "balance, harmony, rhythm, variety, and unity." As for "religious art," he followed Kandinsky in arguing that it dealt not with the depiction of "religious subjects" but rather with the "meaning of life." "That which is good art is religious," he declared; "that which is bad, ugly art is irreligious, no matter what the subject of the picture." Faith itself took on a distinctly modern flavor: "To believe in the principles of beauty as fundamental in the universe is to have a religious atti-tude toward life."

"Life" included politics and society, and the expression of a religious ap-proach to seemingly "secular" issues allowed May to emphasize the prophetic tradition in Judaism and Christianity and its relevance to contemporary so-ciety. War, for instance, was a central challenge to the Christian conscience in 1936. Despite "Organized Christianity's" endorsements of wars throughout history, he stood with thousands of Protestant ministers and many layper-sons who "refuse[d] support of war." On other issues, Rollo noted that "out-standing" Protestants favored birth control but admitted that the question was "hotly disputed" and theology provided no clear guidance. As for the central question of labor's relationship to management and the future of capitalism, Christians were "torn between the desire to retain the financial backing of the class who owns the factories and the duty of supporting the workmen in strikes, etc. for fairer wages." He also noted the ambivalence of the Christian left, most notably Reinhold Niebuhr and the Social Gospel tra-dition, toward Communism and other movements that eschewed religion. May himself thought it was less an issue of faith than one of action: "It is de-batable whether communism is atheistic. . . . In many ways the communists manifest more 'religion in action' than the bulk of Christians. The more alert ministers are adopting an open-minded attitude toward Communism and other political economic systems."[20]

On the question of science and religion, he rejected the "mechanistic view" that assumed a naturalistic cause and effect for every human action. Instead, he noted that the best of the new science argued that determinism held true for only a "limited field of human experience" and could not account for the most important aspects of human consciousness. As for Christian beliefs concerning immortality, May agreed that corporeal survival seemed doubtful but asserted that "nothing essentially good, true, or beautiful is ever lost." He admitted this was mostly a matter of faith and conjecture but that "psychic research (telepathy, etc.)" offered some hint of immortality.

The Religion in Modern Life lectures were a tour de force of synthesis, interpretation, and speculation. Though he saw room for improvement, Rollo seemed happy. Those who attended—both college students and adults from the community—had gained "many ideas," "a conception of the important role of rel[igion]," "a new idea of what rel[igion] is." It inspired a rare moment of unalloyed satisfaction. "Very enjoyable—*to me*," he added, "and I think *to them*."[21]

The success of the course bolstered what May had come to recognize as an ambition informed not only by genius but also by a certain madness. In the spring, as he counted down the last weeks of his stay in Lansing, Rollo indulged in a celebratory and romantically narcissistic bout of self-reflection. He saw himself now as "a curious person—half demonic and half angelic; half soft and sentimental and desirous of dodging the most trivial pain, and half strong and stubborn and 'sinning continuously.'" "Ah," he exclaimed, "Rasputin, Shelley, Van Gogh and Fosdick in one." Despite these contradictions and excesses, however, he needed to remind himself that he had pleased the authorities, a YMCA trustee calling him "one of the finest student leaders on any campus." Most of all, he had led the family to stability: "Don is made! Yona anchored. Mother calmed."[22]

He continued in the third person, indulging in a burst of self-fascinated personal history to justify his emotional indulgences:

> Look at the past—that contortional, volcanic past! An unhappy family— a lad with an inferiority complex—three rainbow years in Europe with brilliant strokes of life, and psychology and art—then that year of dogged fight against ill-health and a dozen other things in New York—then returning . . . to take over the fragments of a broken family. And not only a broken family, but also broken persons in the form of a neurotic mother and brothers. Ha! What calm normality would naturally and placidly arise from that background![23]

He termed his two years in Lansing "a sort of penance" and "a period of enslavement," an expiation of sins for the entire family. As for his time at the Y and the Peoples Church: "I have strewn my life blood upon this ground, and it has made it fertile." However, martyrdom had its value. "I am bigger, stronger, more seasoned, more understanding," he noted, "because I labored here."[24]

Continuing these reflections a few days later, May identified his radically shifting moods as intrinsic to his creativity. "I am neurotic!" he declared, but not as a "crushing" and "final" diagnosis. Instead, it was "an objective comment on a certain curious kind of life, this strange person that is I," which was the key to true creativity. Great art and the artistic touch in any realm were forged in the struggle to overcome neurosis. No neuroses, no art.[25]

Narcissistic flights of fancy about love were another manifestation of Rollo's neuroses, though they hardly rose to the level of art. His summer involvements with M. and Florence made him more confident with women, but when he returned to East Lansing, he had found few opportunities to hone his amorous skills. Perhaps it was the very lack of recent experience that encouraged him, in May and June 1936, to cast the history of his "affaires d'amour" as the "chaotic" and "capricious" life of a "modern Byron." No matter that in his Religion and Modern Culture course, he had criticized the "abnormal and pathological interest in sex in the post-war decade." He now proudly portrayed himself (to his diary) as a Don Juan in search of true love.[26]

Yet he saw himself as a Don Juan with a difference, a Christian knight ready to perform "a deed of unselfish service that would be more laudable than any yet thought of." He had in mind a singular endeavor, though he fully expected "vehement social disapproval and complete misunderstanding of this act." The height of altruism would be to give one's male body in sexual love to a woman who had never experienced the interest of men nor any form of sexual joy. It would be no different from giving oneself in other ways except that it would be "a much more rarefied form of unselfishness—hard for mortals to grasp."[27] The problem was finding a woman worthy of such a gift, and in East Lansing he had found only one who suited his higher artistic tastes. Frances had a "Grecian molded head and . . . lavishly curved breasts and hips," but most of all she had a "color, a charm" and intelligence: "the first girl I have met in E. Lansing to whom I do not need to 'translate.'"[28]

This unbridled world of lonely introspection and fantasy, so overbearingly self-interested, allowed May to mark out an extraordinary destiny for himself. In a diary entry from July 28, 1936, labeled "Thoughts for My Seminary Career," he remade himself into a prophet. "I hear you calling, Frances, I hear you calling—'What can I believe?'" he proclaimed to his latest love in the privacy of his journal; "and I, Frances, shall lay myself on the altar of finding these answers for you." This vision of destiny reached a crescendo in early September as he rested in Colorado and declared his life's goal:

I definitely feel a call to a high work in the field of religion and modern culture. Whenever I tire or faint I shall look forward to that work. I <u>must prepare myself well</u>. Modern culture calls me, we are at the threshold of a rebirth—in art and psych and lit and phil and pol etc and in religion. But religion especially is in crying need of its leader. I am fitted to be that leader. I feel called to it. I shall prepare myself thoroughly, then we shall see. More than anything else do we need religious enlightenment and leadership. The world calls—I must give.

I shall be in a great succession—Whitman, Ibsen, Van Gogh, Adler and Kunkel and Rank and Jung, etc., etc.

I hear all these persons [friends and counselees] crying: Lead me to the beautiful and the intelligent and the good way of life: let me see and love a good God.

And thru them all people the world over are calling. I love them—I love all people—I shall furnish an answer. No longer do I need much for myself—it is for the work of God.

It was on that note in September 1936 that Rollo May returned to Manhattan to complete his degree work at Union Theological Seminary.[29]

9

"The Choice of a Mate"

If surveying the vast Colorado vista in the summer of 1936 inspired May to fantasize about a future as clear and limitless as the western sky, coming back to Manhattan and Union presented more sobering realities. "No ecstatic joy at being returned to the city," he reflected in his diary; "my purpose is too serious for that, and the city too ugly." A "thrilling evening" with Elma Pratt did allow him to relive "the creative, free, effervescent, genuine, dramatic, interesting" time he experienced in Europe. Life at Union seemed "drab" by comparison. Rollo complained of sitting too much in too many classes concerning matters about which he cared too little.[1]

In other ways, however, things were looking up. May had already gained a reputation in Y circles as an innovative counselor, so much so that he received an invitation to address the December 1936 meeting of the Triennial Conference of Church Workers in Universities. Published a few months later in *Christian Education* as "The Art of Student Counseling," his talk proffered an original and innovative form of therapeutic counseling within the realm of spiritual life. He defined the "central mystery" of counseling as *how* it transformed souls. He envisioned it as a kind of priesthood, with the priest/counselor possessed of "a certain grace operative in these deep realms of personality." May argued, "God accords us a grace by which we can achieve understanding of the problems of another." It was essentially a "religious" process beyond scientific analysis. When the practitioner became "'initiated' into the mysteries of counseling," he entered a realm of "complete empathy" in which he moved "behind those frightened eyes" and became "the person stuttering out those words." This "ecstatic" empathy was something akin to a religious experience. "You feel that you have mysteriously gone out of your body," he wrote, "that you are in this student. . . . You feel his pain and despair—when he tells how his father used to beat him when he was back on the farm, you feel every blow upon your own body; and when he describes how painfully shy he was in high school, you feel that shyness cutting like a burning knife through your nerves with as much grief as it used to bring him."[2]

Dr. Harry Bone was in the audience for the talk, was impressed by its bold-ness, and asked May to join him in a workshop sponsored by the Student Christian Council at Columbia University in March 1937. They gave a session entitled "The Resources of Religion for Personal Life." May had not encoun-tered Bone, ten years his senior, before, but they seemed almost fated to meet. Bone began his career in the 1920s as a liberal Christian participant in the broad public debates over sex, youth, and marriage. A specialist in marriage and sex counseling, he worked with Grace Loucks Elliott on projects for the YMCA-sponsored Commission on Relations between College Men and Women. They led discussion groups concerning all aspects of religion, mar-riage, and sexuality, and in 1929 they published their findings as *The Sex Life of Youth*. Much of what May learned at YMCA College came from this text and from Grace Loucks Elliott herself. The book featured such chapters as "Human Sex Hunger," "The Pre-Engagement Years," "Complicating Factors," "Petting," "Auto-Erotism," "The Choice of a Mate," "During Engagement," "When to Marry," and "Religion and Sex."[3]

Short on scripture but long on psychological, anthropological, and so-ciological theory, *The Sex Life of Youth* relativized virtually every aspect of gender relations and sexual behavior. It promoted mutuality and growth be-tween men and women through healthy sex within monogamous marriage. The book frowned upon masturbation but only on the grounds that it iso-lated the individual and bred unrealistic sexual expectations in marriage. As for homosexuality, Elliott and Bone endorsed "intense friendships" between members of the same sex but termed homosexuality an unfortunate learned behavior. They recommended unlearning homosexual desire to experience the full joys of heterosexual love and marriage. They also supported women's newly found freedoms with historicized theories of evolution: "What we know as 'masculine' and 'feminine' characteristics are not inborn, but al-most exclusively due to training and environmental influences."[4] Bone and Elliott listed not a single "religious" book in their bibliography, instead recommending the most significant authors of the modern literature on gender and sexology: Havelock Ellis, Margaret Sanger, Edward Carpenter, Mary Ware Dennett, and Judge Ben Lindsey.[5]

By the 1930s, Bone had expanded his view of "religious work" to incor-porate psychotherapy and studied with Otto Rank in Paris. Rank, an apos-tate from the Freud circle, advocated a therapy that featured a more freely dialogic relationship between analyst and patient and a firm concentration on the "here and now."[6] Unlike Freud, Rank was also something of a sexual radical. Indeed, at the time Bone was his student, Rank was having an extra-marital affair with Anaïs Nin, the lover of Henry Miller and a diarist of sexual passion in her circle of artists and writers. Learning from the master, Bone attempted to seduce Nin, but Rank warned him off, and despite her admiration for Bone's "high browed, laughing eyes, American poise" and her desire "to enslave Bone completely," they never became lovers.[7]

May's work with Bone was important on a number of counts. He learned more about Rank's theory of neurosis as repressed creativity, as well as his emphasis on dialogue in the "here and now" of the therapeutic session—all of which would become crucial aspects of May's mature approach to therapy. He also became a patient of Bone's during various crises in the late 1930s. Finally, the connection with Bone gave him a certain cachet in liberal religious circles even as he was finishing his degree at Union. and it was not long before he was being invited to lecture on student counseling, love, and marriage to church groups on the East Coast. In one case, the YWCA of Wilmington, Delaware, invited May to give the keynote address for a "young adults" course, "Thinking about Marriage." In most ways, Rollo proffered common-sense advice. As the local newspaper headline put it: "Young Men and Women in Y.W.C.A. Course Advised Not to Wed Just to Get Girl to Cook Meals or Man to Provide Support." Using *The Sex Life of Youth* as a guide, May warned against the romantic notion that the wedding made the marriage, noting instead that men and women built a successful marriage upon the everyday details of life.[8] His views mostly reflected those common in liberal Christian circles. He noted that many forms of marriage had existed in history but that until recently marriage had subordinated women to men.[9] Now, women were "in a different position than even in the last century. They have apparently been emancipated." They could vote, get an education nearly comparable to men, and were "in a position where real partnership in marriage is possible." May emphasized that emancipation and rough equality would not make women and men exactly alike. They differed in basic physiology, psychology, and temperament. "Women cannot go into many fields of the man and do as well," he pointed out, "nor can the man do as well in the women's fields." However, May asserted confidently, they would come to know each other more clearly as individuals.

The easy authority with which May explored marriage might have led audiences to assume that his own intimate life, married or single, reflected a similar rationality and confidence. It was, of course, hardly the case. Returning to New York in September 1936, he continued to obsess about sex, women, his own conduct, and the impact of a "marriage decision" (as he came to call it) on his mission to the world. Each month brought new varieties of romance, illusion, and panic. He encountered old loves and found them wanting. In the shadow of his imagined great mission, Martha caused "vacant disappointment," while Florence's "garbled account of the trivialities of her past summer" failed to "inspire" him. Had he matured beyond them? Disappointment did not prevent him, after a few drinks, from going on a "sexual splurge" (probably "heavy petting") with Florence, though he was "disgusted" with himself the next day. "That stuff is unnecessary," he reflected, "and probably accomplishes little beyond disintegrating my poise." So much for the Christian knight of sexuality. Sex now got in the way. Rollo had a world to conquer and vowed to live "the life which is autonomous, poised, and moves under the impulsion of its own creative urges."[10]

Passion, however, trumped his heroic vow. For the next two years, even as success in the professional realm bolstered his public confidence, Rollo remained tormented by romance. He sought the everyday rewards associated with married life—sexual intimacy, stability, companionship, and primary significance in the life of the other, elements of the very relationship he recommended to others from the speaker's rostrum, but with whom and at what price? One price he would not pay was being with a woman who would challenge him, no matter how magnetic such engagement felt. These common desires and fears among men were in Rollo's case exacerbated by the confusions of his relationships with the most powerful women in his life: his mother and sister Ruth. Ruth and Matie were also women whose lives had been wrecked by limitations imposed upon them by society. Sympathetic as he might have been even then, Rollo felt drawn to the familiar qualities of intellectual and emotionally engaging women but struggled with fear of an equally familiar entrapment in depression and despair.

This may explain Rollo's early attraction to and ultimate rejection of Martha. It also may have been at the root of his initially cool reaction to seeing Florence again. She was a woman of some formality and reserve, seemingly less needy of his presence. He felt safer with her, despite his fear of involvement and worry that she did not share his free and creative sense of the world. After the evening at Elma Pratt's home, he pondered whether sex alone drew him to Florence. He found her intellectually and emotionally "drab." Were his feelings for her "a certain sympathy for her as a child, a certain recognition of her 'cuteness,' and a great pity"? A few days later, a surprising source of hesitation surfaced. Something in Florence reminded

Florence

him of "the sloppy, courage-less habits of mother!" What if he should marry her and she actually turned out like his mother? "Ibsen's pen," he exclaimed, "would not be able to touch the quality of that tragedy!" He would "go slowly" and not let her discourage his "old, courageous, free self, regardless of tendencies to hesitate."[11]

May could resolve these conflicts in part by diminishing the importance of his choice of mate. He admitted that hovering "on the fringe of my consciousness" was the sense that his "calling in life [was] *work*," that marriage should be subservient to his calling, and "in such a case Florence would do."[12] Still, he submitted Florence to the sort of obsessive evaluation he usually reserved for himself. She passed "physically," as Rollo put it, "hands down." "Intellectually," he noted, she was "all I could ask." She shared "fields of interest and learning common with mine; my vocabulary, etc." As for her spiritual life, "she is excellent—has my idealism and high unselfishness, and would further my work immensely as much as anyone." For Rollo, a man with a mission, Florence seemed the perfect—perhaps all too perfect—pick.[13]

May's ever-vacillating view, of course, had more to do with his own inner conflicts than with the "real" Florence DeFrees. She was hardly the "drab" character that Rollo needed to make her. A Norfolk native from a prosperous Virginia family, she graduated Randolph-Macon Woman's College and moved to New York to get an MA at Columbia University's Teachers College. She took courses at both Columbia and Union in preparation for a career in religious education. Florence also involved herself in labor union activities and committees for interracial understanding. She presented to Rollo a mixture of beauty, intelligence, and vital activity, all filtered, almost masked, by a reserve and deference endemic to her southern upbringing. Unlike M., Florence allowed him a kind of dominance even as she struggled to retain her own will.

Love posed special challenges for such a woman. Florence confessed to a friend in February 1937 that she felt deeply confused since having "had the fortune or misfortune to fall in love." She felt that she was "doing violence" by calling it a "misfortune." It was more of a conflict between head and heart—"I have been living on an emotional plane and my intellectual life has suffered." She found herself paralyzed. "It is so hard for me to think and plan from here on with that possibility in the future," she complained. "It means that I can no longer think of a separate career for myself, and any job for next year or the next becomes a sort of stop-gap—a thing that is almost as intolerable to me as the idea of the two of us not sharing our lives." The conflict had been made clear that very afternoon. A minister from Albany, New York, wanted her to be director of religious education at his church. However, he also sought a two-year commitment. In love with Rollo and captivated by the idea of marriage, Florence withdrew from consideration. She made that and other sacrifices despite "difficulties and misunderstandings" between her and Rollo, since she sensed that after each estrangement they had emerged "on a better footing and deeper relationship."[14]

And how did she describe Rollo? He was "a lovely person, a charming person in many ways." He was "highly artistic," "intellectually my equal or better," and a "religious person, with a strong sense of a divine calling but a radical interpretation of what the ministry is and of what he as a minister would be and do." "I love him, dear," she wrote to a woman friend, "and I can say to you in all truth that in the thought of him I feel no more the frustrated longing, the heartache of which you know."[15]

Distance at times helped eased the stress of their relationship. In the summer of 1937, Rollo served as temporary pastor of a church in Stonington, Maine. He wrote ironic letters to Florence almost as if they were married, mostly heaping scorn on a congregation stone deaf to his heaven-storming ideas and "radical interpretation" of the ministry. He painted a series of watercolors depicting the ungodly nature of church life and penned a short "play" about the clergyman's life. It centered on a newly arrived congregational minister, one Reverend May (sporting a bright tie), who finds himself surrounded by two old women and a young girl. They ask him to sing and, when he protests, assure him that the mission people ("A Billy Sunday outfit in town, meeting in a barn on which is painted, 'Full Gospel Mission, Inc.'") always perform for them. He accedes but sings "Win Them One by One" instead of "Fighting for the Bleeding Jesus," the song they requested. He misses all the high notes and otherwise mangles the tune. The play ends with the Reverend May exiting and walking down to the sea. He "lights a cigarette and looks out over the ocean," the script reads, "as he reflects on the infinite variety, seriousness and silliness of life, and has a hell of a good smoke." Rollo's play was but a mild rendering of the contempt he felt for some of his parishioners. "And by heaven," he exclaimed to Florence, "if that is what the ministry consisted of, I should get out in a hurry!"[16]

Rollo's ambivalence toward Florence revived upon his return to New York. He stared at other women and even indulged in occasional flings. "I do not love Flo deeply," he confessed in December 1937, "otherwise all these little affairs would be obviated."[17] At the same time, he felt a compulsive need to possess her completely, to control her every thought. He raged at the idea of others influencing her. His greatest jealousies centered on Florence's commitment to labor and "inter-racial" causes. He hounded her about one particular relationship with a labor organizer which, her protests notwithstanding, he was sure had turned sexual. Despite his own socialist sympathies, he developed a "strange feeling of hostility against the labor movement" and realized that his jealousy and mixed feelings about her were inspiring a narcissistic paranoia that the Left was out to get him. "I have the feeling they will take her," he reflected, "yet I am not willing to take her myself." He imagined radicals inspiring "moral anarchy" and "*using*" Florence. He even became sick while reading *The Communist Manifesto*. First they would take Florence, and then they would "*get*" him because he wasted his time on "this individualism, this philosophy." If the revolution came, he worried, "I will be crushed."[18]

Rollo felt such volatile indecisiveness that he entered therapy for the first time since his seminar with Adler in 1932 and 1933, this time with Harry Bone. May's appointments with Bone centered ostensibly on the "marriage decision," but with the analyst's guidance he realized just how deep his conflicts ran. And he was vividly reminded of the reality of transference. First came the realization that he was tailoring his discussions to gain Bone's moral approval, hoping "to get a judgment *to marry*" from the analyst, even though he felt quite the opposite outside his office. As they delved deeper, Bone helped him to see that he was confusing Florence with his mother, "my imperialism regarding Flo—*jealousy*, unbased, even concerning her attitudes and interests, showing my demand that she be absorbed in me."[19]

Through the first weeks of January 1938, Rollo saw no way out of his jealous rage. Then he experienced what seemed like a breakthrough. One night, he dreamed that he met two girls who took him to a meeting, one of whom was part of a "crooked gang." The "crooked" one went home with him, and he laid her down to sleep, Rollo settling into a different bed. Suddenly she was in Rollo's bed, her body "heaving up and down fitfully" and her "vagina against me." She scared him. Rollo thought she had a venereal disease, and he had no condom. "The idea of having sexual relations with her," he remembered feeling, "seemed very ugly to me." He also recalled from the dream "that she had changed her name, and was of foreign extraction." Still, he felt an urgent sexual pull and thought about "going home (?)" to get a condom. Instead, he woke up having had a wet dream.[20]

The memory of the dream disturbed him all the next day. He couldn't interpret it and feared its implications. That evening, he prayed as earnestly as he had in years, pleading with God to show him "the right way." Then there came upon him, he recalled in the diary, "suddenly a feeling, a word from God, that I should have peace, that it was not necessary that I strive so, that my striving was really arrogance. He then took my burden; I felt peace, both about myself and Florence; no longer did that foolish jealousy trouble me and thru the night into the morning this peace has lasted."[21]

The "peace" soon vanished, however, as his inner debate over marriage returned with a vengeance. A variety of arguments in favor led the way. "Last night," he wrote on January 30, "I felt that I did want to marry her: 1) I want to get married to someone; 2) I can do my work much better in that case." Sometimes he felt romantic toward her, as when he and Florence lost themselves in the loud commotion of a Chinatown festival—"I have not had more fun in one afternoon in my whole life!" The next day he ripped up photographs of women whom he had loved (except those of Bets Hunner).[22] Ten days later, a day before his weekly appointment with Harry Bone, he began obsessing again about the labor organizer boyfriend: "Terrific emotion was excited in my mind at phantasies giving rise to jealousy!" After his session with Bone, Rollo fell into a deeper malaise. He vowed to conquer his neuroses before entering marriage, but these brave words disintegrated into a self-pitying wail:

> God, I did not ask to be born! It is not my fault I was born into that family. I am caught. It is not [out of] perversity that I make Florence suffer, nor get us so tangled. I wander thru life, lonely, wishing to live but not knowing how, sex throbbing, and at 28 still lonely. I find one to love, and it turns out crooked. Take the books and the art and everything and burn them, O God! I will give them up. I will not demand that I be great or different. I will give up everything. Let me be a simple man, who can love a wife.[23]

Sometime in the spring, however, he decided to jettison Florence from his life. "You are planning your future without reference to me, aren't you?" he casually let slip into a chatty letter. The next day, he wrote to her in appreciation of all that he had learned from her, as if their relationship was at a close.[24]

It was all driving Florence more than a little crazy. "I don't believe I am made to bear the kind of tension you would have me bear," she wrote. "I go round and round like a squirrel in a cage and come out nowhere." Unnerving to Rollo was Florence's increasingly colder acceptance of his judgment that the relationship was not right. "I am deeply thankful that this has happened," she wrote of the proposed separation; "I was blinded by the overpowering experience of physical mating and felt that we had achieved the same union on all levels. I see now that there is much lacking to that achievement."[25]

Flo's agreement seemed to work magic, the intimation that she might be judging him even as he was judging her. Within a month they had set their wedding date, and on June 5, 1938, they were married. May left no explanation for his mercurial reversal.

10

Paul Tillich

Rollo May needed a new model and guide, a mentor in every sense, one who might understand and shape his mission. By his own gleeful reckoning, he had long ago "grown" beyond E. T. and even beyond Buck Weaver and Charles Wager, his beloved teachers in college. He needed the love, the intimacy, and the example of a courageous new father. Paul Tillich became that person, though it took a while for their bond to develop. Tillich and May were drawn to each other by interests, personality, and a faintly erotic connection. They shared a passion for exploring the modern condition, for seeing it in its full artistic, scientific, philosophical, and theological dimensions. May's rapacious, untethered exploration of psyche and soul took effective shape for the first time in a dialogue with Tillich that continued until the theologian's death in 1965. So too Tillich and his wife modeled an experimental and sometimes tortured sexual risk-taking that guided—though did not resolve—Rollo's problematic relationships with women.

May and Tillich met by chance in January 1934. During Christmas break, as he was leaving his room in an empty Hastings Hall, Rollo saw a "bewildered" figure walking toward him and helped the man find his way. He was struck by the stranger's visage, "a large leonine head with a shock of bushy hair over a high forehead. High color, and a face constructed not in curves but in planes, like a portrait by Cézanne."[1] Soon after, he came upon a placard announcing a series of lectures by a Paul Tillich, who had just arrived from Germany to join the Union faculty. "His name meant nothing to me," Rollo wrote years later. "But the titles! 'The Spiritual Implications of Psychoanalysis,' 'The Religious Meaning of Modern Art,'—and the same with Karl Marx and communism and other crucial aspects of our then-contemporary culture."[2] May attended the lectures, along with seventeen or eighteen other students and an equal number of faculty. Much to his surprise, the man at the lectern was the one whom he had helped in the dorm. Meanwhile, Tillich had already noticed him among the students at the first lecture and remarked on his interesting face.[3]

Such sensory chemistry helped break down the deep gulf of status, age, and culture that separated them, as did Tillich's sometimes humbling awkwardness in his newly adopted language. Once, Tillich elicited howls from students when he said, "spice and tame," and then corrected the phrase to "tame and spice," when what he really meant was "time and space." The laughter turned Tillich's memorable face a deep red. Rollo wrote him a short note explaining American informality and assured him that the laughter was not meant as mockery. Tillich sought him out to tell him how much the note had helped.[4]

Tillich's intellectual impact on May was apparent from the time of these introductory discourses. His sense of an implicit conflict between psychology and religion dissolved, as Rollo noted in his diary in the spring of 1934, with Tillich's suggestion that one needed psychological insight to "find our true existence." And Rollo found a name for his deepest moments of transcendence in the "unconditioned" realm of which Tillich spoke. Such early attractions, kindnesses, and shared passions for redefining the transcendent prefigured what would become for both an essential bond.[5]

These instinctively shared proclivities bound Tillich and May despite vast contrasts in culture and generation. Tillich was twenty-three years May's senior, born in 1886 near Berlin, the son of a Lutheran village pastor. As his father rose in the hierarchy of the German church and the family moved to Berlin, young Paul's world became that of the Prussian aristocracy. Amid this world of privilege, Tillich showed an imagination, vulnerability, and compassion not normally associated with the word "Prussian." It was a sensibility tested by trauma. In 1903, the year after his confirmation, the death of his beloved mother so shattered Tillich that he repressed all mention of her until much later in life.[6]

Such angst reaffirmed a deep if troubled commitment to the church. Tillich studied theology at Berlin, Tübingen, and Halle and decided on a career as a theologian. He fell in love and married in September 28, 1914. However, Tillich's orderly building of a life was interrupted, as for millions of others, by World War I. Three days after his marriage, he enlisted in the German army as a chaplain. On the battlefield, he prayed over the dead and helped dig their graves. However, the war soon began to take its toll. In May 1916, after his division entered the battle at Verdun, he wrote to his father: "Hell rages around us. It's unimaginable."[7] Several times over the next months he collapsed from the strain. "I have constantly the most immediate and very strong feeling that I am no longer alive," he wrote to a friend. Only the discovery of Nietzsche's

Also Sprach Zarathustra brought him renewal of faith, albeit a radical departure from traditional Lutheranism. "I have long since come to the paradox of *faith without God*," he wrote, "by thinking through the idea of justification by faith to its logical conclusion."[8]

The dark chaos of Tillich's life continued as he returned home to an unfaithful wife and a homeland racked by the battlefield deaths of two million soldiers and the maiming of millions more, military defeat, and political revolution. Soon, however, both he and Germany set forth on new paths. He divorced his wife and embarked on new sexual adventures. A continuing atmosphere of cultural upheaval in Germany fostered in Tillich not only a vigorous, exploratory sexual life but also an embrace of the new modernist cultures in literature, music, painting, and dance. Aiding his engagement in this experimental world was the fact that he began his academic career as a *Privatdozent* at the University of Berlin, the epicenter of the Weimar Republic's romance with the avant-garde.

Tillich gathered a group around him known as the Kairos Circle, named for one of his most enduring theological and historical concepts and also one central to May's spiritual development. As opposed to *chronos*, linear time that is intrinsically meaningless, *kairos* in the original Greek signified a more qualitatively meaningful moment or opportunity. In Christianity, it came to denote a time of momentous divine intervention or fulfillment. Tillich's more historically colored usage deemed a *kairos* any period in which society had become so shaken that the power of the divine as well as the demonic could radically transform human consciousness and society. The concept summed up his sense of the postwar 1920s as that special moment of sacred renewal and defense against demoniacal catastrophe.

Such vast metahistorical concepts tended toward an abstraction not easily translatable into the events of this world, and even among theologians the exact meaning of Tillich's concept of *kairos* has been debated since the 1920s. However, a vivid sense of Tillich's intent can be found in his book *The Religious Situation*, a critique of society that located modern spiritual life in contemporary music, dance, literature, and painting. At its heart lay a search for spiritual unities capable of reenchanting a world that capitalism and crude science had made material and finite. Tillich celebrated Nietzsche, Strindberg, and Van Gogh as "three great warriors" in the cause. He argued that these and other writers and artists captured a "religious" vision far better than many "religious" writers or painters. "It is not an exaggeration," he noted, "to ascribe more of the quality of sacredness to a still-life by Cézanne or a tree by van Gogh than to a picture of Jesus by Uhde." German expressionist painters like Otto Dix and writers like Ernst Toller had "uncovered the demonism present in the social world" were moving toward a state of "a *belief-ful realism*."[9]

Tillich found sacred meaning in modern literature and performance as well. Some poets (in this case Rainer Maria Rilke) took "a directly religious turn" or mounted (in the case of Stefan George) "powerful protests against the spirit of capitalist society with its reduction of all things to a common level, a common shallowness and spiritual impoverishment." Modern dance, illustrated by the German dancer and choreographer Mary Wigman's expressionist borrowings from Asian and African culture, attacked individualism through group dances that sought "to give inner content and organization to space" and through "expressive gestures [that] try to reveal metaphysical meanings."[10]

In the personal dimensions of morality and ethics, especially love, sex, and marriage, Tillich again saw the need to revolutionize what had become hypocritical practice. Already stripped of its sacred character by the Protestant churches, civil marriage in the modern age reeked of hypocrisy, coldness, and infidelity. Authenticity in love, as in art, was crucial. However, love proved difficult to achieve in capitalist society. "This is one of the places," he remarked, "where the misery of a self-sufficient finitude reveals itself in the tragic fate of countless individuals and where it demands that breaking-through to the transcendent on which sex morality can be built anew."[11]

Tillich practiced what he preached. Free love was common enough among the Weimar avant-garde, with or without the high purposes Tillich attached to it, so it was unsurprising that his second marriage, to Hannah Werner in 1925, was forged in a commitment to freedom and experiment. From almost the day of their marriage, each engaged openly in affairs, testing the limits of free love and other rejections of bourgeois life. For Tillich, though, the search for physical intimacy and "break-through" seemed as much an obsession as a principle. With his conscious idealization of sexual and artistic freedom, Tillich masked the emotional devastation of the deaths of his mother and beloved sister, the war years, and the shock of his first wife's betrayal.[12]

Tillich spent his final years in Germany at the University of Frankfurt, befriending Max Horkheimer, Theodor Adorno, and others of the Frankfurt School. For Tillich and the Frankfurt School, Hitler's rise to power in the spring of 1933 posed an existential threat. It spelled instant disaster for Jewish academics and those, like Tillich, on the political left. Tillich was among 1,684 scholars suspended from university positions in the first year of the Nazi regime. On May 10, 1933, he watched helplessly as a Nazi mob in Frankfurt created a bonfire of books written by Jews, Communists, Socialists, and others despised by the new regime. His own works were among those burned.[13]

As the Nazis implemented their takeover of German universities, faculty and administrators at Union Theological Seminary and Columbia University took action. In the noblest of gestures, Union's faculty voted to contribute 5 percent of their salaries to hire Tillich. By early November he was in New York. Tillich accepted the offer with great trepidation, sharing the common European view of America as a land of vulgarity and anti-intellectualism. He had been forced into exile at the height of professional fame in his homeland. Yet, with a kind of Nietzschean zest, he began to re-create life, especially after discovering that liberal Protestants and America's more freewheeling religious culture would give his radical notions a hearing perhaps more open than in Germany. Hannah and Paul's personal proclivities, however, made those around them a bit uneasy. Much to the chagrin of his colleagues, the couple frequented burlesque shows downtown and more exotic sexual performances in Harlem, and hosted parties in the style of "Weimar" decadence.[14]

It was during the 1936–37 school year that an informal mentorship blossomed into a deeply congenial, intimate, and wide-ranging relationship. May and Tillich talked about art, psychology, and politics. Though Tillich remained the master, May's experiences and friendships with Adler (who died suddenly in 1937) and Binder (who had settled in New York), as well as his ardent Midwestern innocence, appealed to his sophisticated European mentor. Tillich introduced May to an extraordinary group of émigré intellectuals, including Max Horkheimer, Theodor Adorno, Kurt Goldstein, Ernst Schachtel, Herbert Marcuse, Erich Fromm, and Frieda Fromm-Reichmann. Whether members of the Frankfurt School, Gestalt psychologists, neo-Marxists, or scientists, they shared a critique of the modern era akin to Tillich's, one that emphasized the decay of a unified and humane vision of existence at the hands of capitalism and dominant strains of experimental science.

Not surprisingly, Tillich agreed to direct May's bachelor of divinity honors thesis, "A Comparison of Modern Psychotherapy and Christian Theology in Respect to Doctrine of Man."[15] Though written under Tillich's care and critique, the thesis reflected Rollo's own cumulative thoughts and experiences from classes at Union, his reading and thinking, and his counseling experience in Lansing. With clarity, precision, and originality, May juxtaposed psychotherapeutic theory and Christian theology, finding that "psychotherapy, in its analysis of human nature, uncovers the problems which are also basic in Christian theology, but is unable to solve these problems because of its inadequate understanding of man." Psychotherapy best analyzed the complexity of a human being's "existential" state, he argued, while Christianity established the conception of God so "essential" to describing the true state of being in the world: "the root tension of existence." It was the conflict between what Tillich called the "Unconditioned Command" and the finite, "existential" facts of human life.[16]

May prefigured his comparison of religion and psychology with a retrospective look at the "roots of psychotherapy," the awareness since the Greeks of the debilitating split between the objective and subjective in human beings. He moved quickly through Rousseau and Nietzsche and their celebration of both the irrational and the individual before positing the compartmentalization of life in the nineteenth century, especially as a result of science, the marketplace, and industrialization.[17] Enter the revolutionary insights of Freud, Jung, Adler, and Rank as they attempted to reinject the complexity and fullness of the irrational into understandings of human nature. May judged Freud's "discovery" of the unconscious and basic psychoanalytic theory as the most profound, though Freud's determinism and rejection of religion as an illusion seemed limiting.[18] Adler's contribution of a familial and social analytic framework proved more useful. At the same time, May found Freud's core idea of the inevitable conflict between instinct and culture more compelling than Adler's somewhat rosier view. Otto Rank, in his emphasis on creativity as well as his insights into the relationship between guilt and creativity, added a crucial dimension to a psychoanalytic description of human nature. Jung came close to a concept of God, but Jung's God, May concluded, was in the end only a function of the individual unconscious in relation to the collective unconscious.[19]

May argued that these partial readings of man's nature—"libido, "will to power," "freedom and guilt," and the "individual unconscious" as portal to a "collective unconscious"—were inadequate without the broadest conception of man and God, which only religion could provide. In Christianity, Adam's fall set in motion the basic tension of human existence. This was at the heart of the Christian doctrine of man. Humans sinned and yet yearned for salvation. Man did not deserve Grace, and yet, when present, it cured him of sin. It reconnected him to the infinitude of which he was a part before God commanded Adam and Eve to leave Eden and enter a finite world of work, pain, and death. Only grace, only religion, he argued, could provide true mental health.[20]

May's honors thesis, his first major statement of a developing sense of the relationship between religion and psychotherapy, broke new ground in its concepts, questions, and sources. For instance, he grappled with Kierkegaard—about whom he had learned in Tillich's lectures and whose works were only beginning to be published in English translation—in a manner quite original to American theology, especially in regard to psychoanalysis. May's readers at Union recognized his work's original contribution, and the seminary's library gave it the unusual distinction of being placed in the stacks alongside master's theses and doctoral dissertations. The honors thesis also foretold May's later interests. Such figures as Nietzsche and Kierkegaard would eventually undergird a very different life project for May—a weaning from Christianity per se in favor of existentialism. The thesis's central focus on the "doctrine of man" or "anthropology" would resurface as ontology. As such, "Comparison of Modern Psychotherapy and Christian Theology in Respect to Doctrine of Man" was both summary and prologue.

If the thesis contained concerns that would remain with May, it also revealed weak points predictive of his own eventual estrangement from the hegemony of Christian theology. An astute graduate student friend, E. M. Fleming, endorsed May's basic view that psychotherapy, as opposed to Christianity, had not developed a metaphysics and thus represented an incomplete "doctrine of man," but disagreed with the assumption that psychotherapy could never develop its own metaphysical stance. Nor did he see May's description of psychotherapy as offering an incomplete cure as anything but a priori assertion. "I think you assume too dogmatically," Fleming argued, "without sufficient demonstration, that this Christian conceptual framework is the only *operative* or effective one."[21] May would ultimately concur.

Work on the thesis immensely strengthened the intellectual bond between Tillich and May and in turn allowed their relationship to grow more intimate and inclusive. May's marriage to Florence, whom Tillich found quite attractive, thickened the connection. The Mays and Tillichs soon began socializing together, the older couple taking the lead and introducing them to New York's émigré community, as well as to some semblance of the sexual experimentation endemic to the city's artistic and intellectual societies and anathema to many at the seminary.

Steps in this direction began in the spring of 1938, when Tillich had his first "real" conversation with Florence after she attended one of his lectures at a nearby university. Tillich invited her to go for a walk on campus. Settled under the shade of a tree, he began to spin a web of fantasy around their meeting and invited her to contribute. Like the teller of a good German folk tale, he populated his story with elves, trolls, and sprites, all of which led to a grand finale. As May told the story after Tillich's death, the theologian asked Florence to supply an ending. "She—who was not one to suggest such things lightly—answered," May recounted, "We would lie together." The next day, each told their version of the story to Rollo, and he recalled feeling "glad both of them had had their delightful hour," emphasizing with pride that he had felt no jealousy. "Though nothing physical occurred," wrote May, "it was a kind of psychological reenactment of the old custom of the deflowering of the new bride by the Lord of the Estate." Whatever he felt at the time of this first encounter, Rollo would not always be so free of jealousy or so sure that later meetings were innocent. Indeed, sharing his wife in erotic play highlighted, if nothing else, the tangled depths of May's apprenticeship.[22]

11

"Life-Affirming Religion"

Since meeting Alfred Adler, May's sense of calling in "religious work" had rarely focused on the ministry per se and instead moved decisively toward a vigorous merger of religion and therapy. However, as he approached graduation from Union in the waning years of the Great Depression, having started a marriage and with family looming large, a ministerial position seemed the wisest course. When, in late 1937, the First Congregational Church of Verona, New Jersey, announced its need for a pastor, Rollo applied for the post. The success of his trial sermon—he recorded in his diary that an influential member of the congregation called it the "best" he had ever heard—encouraged him to put aside his doubts and fantasize about becoming "a great great preacher." It offered a security and community prominence not easily gained otherwise. Counseling, hardly established as a profession, promised far fewer rewards. Psychotherapy in general was in its infancy, and despite his precocity, May had no formal training in the field. If he wished to make his mark on religion by invigorating it with psychology, formally entering the ministry seemed the best route. He imagined, in addition to distinguishing himself as a preacher, that he would also create a "'Psychological Clinic,' possibly direct the local asylum, organizing the work—dishing it out to the others [and] making friends with the people."[1]

Such a vision was inspired by long-standing and deep ambivalence about the minister's role and its possibilities, the darker side of which had already surfaced in the humorous play he had written about the Reverend May in Maine. In 1938, he pondered the question with greater seriousness in an unpublished essay, "The Role of the Minister in a Small Town," again based on his brief experience as a pastor in Maine. May described how a thinking, feeling, fallible minister might be reduced to a one-dimensional symbol of "the town's holiness," just as a prostitute typified sin incarnate rather than a real human being. "No wonder so many ministers in small towns become indecisive chameleons," he complained. "The minister who aims to make a real contribution to his community in terms of real ethical action and genuine worship of God and true Christianity, will take arms against this role."[2]

Girding himself to do battle, he accepted the offer of the Verona church and was ordained on October 4, 1938. The star-studded ordination featured a scripture lesson by Herman Reissig, a sermon by Paul Tillich, and a charge to the minister by Henry Sloane Coffin. Yet in the months that followed, May's attempts to remake the church faltered. He felt suffocated by a politically conservative congregation and day-to-day administrative tasks. Years later, he joked that he saw little "genuine worship of God" except at funerals.[3] Such an atmosphere spurred him all the more to champion "real ethical action" in his sermons, an extraordinary number of which dealt with current events. He infuriated many in the congregation with his progressive politics, as when he embraced the Loyalist cause in Spain and drew the wrath of a church member who taught Spanish in the local high school.[4] In another sermon, "Suburban Christians," he charged congregations like his own with spiritual stagnation and coldness toward the needy.[5]

Perhaps his most controversial theme, however, was anti-Semitism. Schooled by Tillich and others in the evils of Nazism and quite cognizant of local anti-Jewish incidents, he forthrightly condemned enemies of the Jews, whether in Germany or the United States. In November 1938, a few weeks after Kristallnacht—the deadly, coordinated Nazi riot against German Jews—May devoted a sermon to the history of Jewish victimhood at the hands of Christians. He admitted that it was not the "most popular kind of sermon" but urged members of the church, when they felt prejudice toward a Jew or Negro, to say, "I dislike him because my people has persecuted his people." Through such self-understanding and contrition, one might "glimpse" the Kingdom of God.[6] Rollo also regularly visited the local synagogue and the B'nai B'rith Lodge in neighboring Union City. He became their Christian champion when anti-Semitic incidents occurred, their protector in the press and at city hall. In public addresses, he tied the fate of democracy to the defeat of American anti-Semitism and stressed the unity of Jewish and Christian faiths in the Old Testament. The Jewish community deeply appreciated his efforts and honored him with a special scroll celebrating his friendship to the Jewish people.[7]

In all, despite or perhaps because of the deep frustrations May faced, the Verona congregation had a way of eliciting the best from him. It allowed him to translate his dreams of a public presence into reality as he faced issues and powers in the local church with frankness and courage. It was one thing to write a play or essay on the quandaries of the "thinking" minister and another to meet that challenge head on. As a minister he could participate fully in the fellowship of liberal Christian and interfaith efforts for ameliorating race relations and promoting social justice. At age thirty, May had successfully moved from an extraordinarily promising apprenticeship to vital adulthood.

The ministry also enabled May to establish a presence before a wider audience as an innovator in counseling. May's early articles, lectures, and work with Harry Bone had already garnered him a growing reputation in Y circles and beyond when an editor from Abingdon Press, a major religious publisher, heard one of his talks. He suggested that May turn his lectures into a book. *The Art of Counseling* was published in the fall of 1939. It was a propitious moment in the fledgling romance of Protestantism and psychotherapy. Since the last decades of the nineteenth century, liberal Protestants had felt drawn to psychology as a window on the spiritual world, a scientific map of the soul that might replace, in modernity, the biblical literalism against which they fought. Boston's short-lived, turn-of-the-century Emmanuel Movement combined medical care with psychologically informed spiritual conversation to treat various disorders. But otherwise, the interface of religion and psychology mainly involved debates over the nature of transcendent experience or modernizing the Christian tradition's vocabularies and frames of reference. These ponderings enlisted such luminaries of American psychology as William James and G. Stanley Hall, among many others.[8]

In the first three decades of the century, however, even as academic psychology moved decidedly away from questions of spirit and religion, psychological vocabulary and approaches began to penetrate the worlds of pastoral care. Closest to May in this realm were YMCA professionals Harry Bone as well as Harrison and Grace Loucks Elliott, whose progressive use of psychotherapy May had experienced at the YMCA College and again at Union Theological Seminary, where both taught in the 1930s. Moreover, a generation earlier, other key figures who had sought to recruit psychology as a helpmate to religion had contact with Union. Anton Boisen, whose work was informed by his own and others' record of psychotic episodes, graduated from the seminary in 1911 and proceeded to do various kinds of church work, including a stint with the YMCA during World War I. Bouts of severe mental illness and institutionalization that involved revelatory religious awakenings inspired him to propose spiritually infused methods of treatment. The Reverend John Sutherland Bonnell, whose *Pastoral Psychiatry* (1938) became a standard text in seminaries, approached matters in a unique way. He redefined the common usage of "psychiatry" as "the healing of the soul of man" and proceeded to make Christianity a tool of medicine. Sutherland was inspired by his father, a nurse at a Canadian mental hospital who imbued his work with patients with spiritual love and teachings, and his first professional experience involved following in his father's footsteps.[9]

Psychology was thus alive in the religious world, promising both a new tool for understanding human nature and the possibility of more efficacious pastoral care. May's *Art of Counseling* was perhaps the first work to merge a spiritualized, psychotherapeutic vision of human personality with an intimate account of the encounter between counselor and client. It contained the seed of May's later existential vision and exhibited some of the breadth of his later books. Its uniqueness becomes even more apparent by comparison with Harrison and Grace Loucks Elliott's *Solving Personal Problems: A Counseling Manual* (1936). The Elliotts offered a comprehensive introduction to the field and its theories, methods, and treatment aims. They argued, as May had in his honors thesis, that spiritually informed psychological counseling could be far more effective than traditional pastoral work. Yet not one case history graced their text, even in their discussion of "the counselor and the counseling situation." *Solving Personal Problems* offered a view distanced from the emotional grit of the counseling hour, long on rules and frameworks but short on the "feel."[10]

The Art of Counseling, by contrast, presented both a hands-on picture and an innovative interpretation of human nature. Dutifully accepting counseling's modest status compared to psychiatry or analytic psychotherapy, May nonetheless couched its drama in such vivid terms that one would hardly have known that he was writing about an endeavor at the bottom of the therapeutic professions. He made the counselor a heroic figure capable of synthesizing "psychotherapeutic techniques" as he conducted his "own adventure in the understanding of people." As if to validate its importance, May prefaced his entire discussion with epigraphs from Spinoza, Socrates, and Nietzsche that implicitly argued for the profundity of counseling and the spiritual company its practitioners kept.[11]

Instead of opening the main body of the book with a philosophical discussion, May moved immediately into the consulting room with a case history: "George B. made an excellent impression upon me when he came into my office. He must have been over six feet in height, and his physique was unusually well proportioned and handsome. He shook my hand warmly, though a little too violently, and looked at me fixedly as he spoke in a slow, carefully controlled voice." George was a campus rebel who sought to reform institutions and people and, not incidentally, to bolster his own sense of greatness. Now, however, he was experiencing an emotional crisis, swinging from mania to depression and deep loneliness. College health officials suggested he leave school. May responded with his own regimen: "the deeper approach of psychological understanding."[12]

May focused on George's passion for fame and "his tremendous ambition" to dominate everyone and everything around him. He noted that "second children often manifest an exaggerated ambition because of their early striving to keep up with or overtake the older child. This is particularly true of a boy following a girl, for the girl develops more rapidly in the early years." So it was with George (and May), whose sister had preceded him at the same college and had excelled.[13] He was struggling unconsciously with a sense of inferiority. At first, he rejected May's theories but ultimately saw the light. He became friendlier, turned to religious work, and within a year was elected president of the Christian Association on campus and recognized as one of the "outstanding student leaders."[14]

Despite its sweet Adlerian ring of adjustment, for May the lesson of George's case involved the more difficult and important task of moving George's genius from inner destructiveness to outwardly directed creativity. "The very powers which had led him to the brink of neurosis," May noted, "now worked to increase his genuine leadership and prestige." "The more sensitive the inward balance of tensions," he argued, "the greater the creativity." Thus Dostoevsky, Nietzsche, and Van Gogh had experienced psychoses but when on this side of madness had unleashed their creative powers in order to enrich humankind. George's genius too might flower to the benefit to those around him.[15]

May elaborated his argument in the chapter-length overview, "A Picture of Personality." It expanded a major point in his honors thesis: the need for a rich view of human existence as the basis for psychotherapy. Its first sentence asked, "What is a man?"[16] May's kaleidoscopic answer emphasized, far more than in his honors essay, the capability of psychology—especially Freud, Jung, Rank, and Adler—to describe human nature. He celebrated Freud as the greatest of these theorists, the master who had discovered "the profound and powerful realms of the unconscious" and disabused the Victorians of their views on sexuality. Most of all, he had revealed in his theory of drives an essential part of human nature. May faulted Freud for discounting the power of free will and highlighting only the "ugly" aspects of human nature. He did admit that psychoanalysis as a therapy sought to free a margin of autonomy for the patient but also noted that one could too easily interpret Freud as a biological determinist.[17]

May turned to Otto Rank, the champion of creativity, for a more convincing vision of freedom. Rank's theories rejected a simple "freedom of the will" and instead described "freedom as a quality of [man's] total being." "We must admit that the individual creates his own personality by creative willing," May summarized, "and that neurosis is due precisely to the fact that the patient cannot will constructively." For Rank as for May, freedom and responsibility for the shaping of self lay at the cornerstone of successful living. May highlighted another important dimension of human identity by describing the Jungian road to selfhood. The process of "individuation" linked a person's development to humankind through what the Swiss analyst called the "collective unconscious" of endlessly varied combinations of character types. He completed the picture with Adlerian insights that emphasized the drive for power and significance, and theorized that unwarranted feelings of inferiority perverted this striving into antisocial or isolating behavior.[18]

May concluded his portrait with a discussion of religion's role in human consciousness, which in this rendering appeared more open-ended and creative than before. Rejecting common shorthand that equated psychological health and inner harmony, he argued that the most creative lives were marked by continuous struggle. "We do not wish to wipe conflict away altogether," May argued; "that would be stagnation—but rather to transform destructive conflicts into constructive ones." Here he agreed with Freud that inner conflict undergirded human nature and produced both neuroses and civilization. Unlike Freud, he saw religion as a primary element of being. May used guilt as an example, which by May's definition arose with the perception of the gap between what was and what should be, between "perfection and man's imperfect state." And, in a brief passage, May concluded that guilt proved "the presence of God in human nature. . . . It is the manifestation of God's continual impingement upon man's temporal life."[19]

The Art of Counseling then returned to the consulting room. Refining a point made in an earlier article, May highlighted "empathy" as the "key process" occurring between counselor and client. He defined "empathy" as "a much deeper [compared to sympathy] state of identification of personalities in which one person so feels himself into the other as temporarily to lose his own identity." Only the empathic counselor could truly effect understanding and influence. Employing the same example of the boy beaten in his youth as he had in "The Art of Student Counseling," he again emphasized the almost physical identification that empathy produced. However, whereas in the earlier piece he had described empathy as a religious mystery, in *The Art of Counseling* it became a state in which the counselor's "ego or psychic state . . . had temporarily become merged with that of the counselee; he and I were one psychic unity."[20]

Such empathy did not depend, as in today's common usage of the term, on similar experience. He argued that "reminiscences of the counselor" had no place in counseling, since such relating of memory "comes out of egocentricity, and empathy is precisely the opposite of egocentricity." Rather, empathy involved an opening of communication between two people similar to what some described as "mental telepathy." This broad entry of one person into the mind of another left little room to hide one's thoughts. That was the point. "There is no more cleansing experience in the world," he wrote, "than psychological nakedness." Such nakedness also carried with it an "ethical side" in its principle of honesty. One acted as if each could truly read the mind of the other, making deception "impossible."[21]

Empathy, nakedness, and the intrusion of the counselor's life all hovered around an elusive fact about *The Art of Counseling*: the case histories were in many significant ways autobiographical. The story of second-born George B. bore an uncanny similarity to Rollo's struggles with Ruth and his collegiate experience at Michigan and Oberlin. "Mr. Bronson," the prime actor in a later chapter on confession, resembled May in other ways. A professor of religious philosophy, Bronson had a problem with overwork. Interestingly, he too was second born with an older sister. Bronson's father was a minister, a telling parallel to Earl Tuttle May. Moreover, Rollo commented on one of Bronson's dreams as if he were analyzing his own traumatic experience with Ruth's aborted fetus: "I was climbing up into the attic of our house on a ladder. When I got to the top rung a monkey jumped out of a green box in the attic and scared me, and I fell down the ladder." May might well have been consoling himself about one of his own nightmares when he wrote, "All ended well, for Bronson understood that he need not compete with his sister nor be afraid of the strange monkey."[22]

Autobiographical inflections also played a role in the final section of the book, "Ultimate Considerations," though less directly factual and more as a reflection of May's growing sense of religious experimentation. In three fascinating chapters—"Personality of the Counselor," "Morals and Counseling," and "Religion and Mental Health"—he made radical departures from his prior views on the relation of religion to psychology. His honors thesis emphasized that only Christian theology could give final meaning to psychological insight. *The Art of Counseling* emphasized instead the role of false religion (as expressed in egocentric perfectionism and moralistic strictures), which "cramps and impoverishes life, thus destroying the possibility of living abundantly." Nor did true religion refer to Christianity per se but to "a fundamental affirmation of the meaning of life" possible in a Christianity purged of its neurotic tendencies. Thus, psychotherapy and religion traveled parallel courses and together produced a new unity: "Such is the transformation from neurosis to personality health. And such is what it means, likewise, to experience religion."[23]

May made it clear such an approach might lead to revision of commonly accepted views of personal morality. Interestingly, May was writing this chapter at the moment of final crisis in his premarital relationship to Florence, and its ideas took form even as he was recommending that she put their relationship on hold and plan life without him. He declared to her that the "morals" chapter was "the best thing I've ever written" and sure to create "a bit of talk." His idea: "*Libido* thru *structure*, the structure being eventually *logos* and God (or one aspect)." He claimed that Florence had inspired it, having taught him the true meaning of emotional integrity. "You have given me a new appreciation of purity and chastity," he noted, "things which mother used to stand for, but which I reacted against superficially."[24]

In that chapter, "Morals and Counseling," Matie May's concept of "purity and chastity" were hardly in sight. The experience of courtship with Florence within Paul Tillich's social circle and under Paul and Hannah Tillich's personal influence might well have helped May reject "a specific set of moral standards" and endorse "Creative Individuality in Morals" based upon self-expression and the personal translation of instinctual urges (Freud's id, Bergson's "élan vital," Nietzsche's "Will," or simply the "creative impulse"). Anticipating his later conception of the "daemonic," he argued that one could transform these drives for good or evil through creative confrontation of their power. May identified such moral creativity with courage and maturity.[25] One might even need to rebel forthrightly from the old codes, as one counselee named "Janice" did by going to a bar and treating herself to a "big drunk." No simple fling, it led her to a "life-affirming religion," a new major in college, and eventually a satisfying career. A talented but repressed and dissatisfied young woman thus transformed her life into one of "spontaneity," "genuineness," "originality," and "courage."[26]

Nor did May worry that such episodes might lead to personal anarchy, for he believed that broad social structures molded limits on expression and moral archetypes, much as Jung's "collective unconscious" shaped the deepest consciousness of each individual. It was, according to May, "humanity's psychic depository of morality, consisting of various moral patterns that have their seat in the very roots of man's being." Thus, one could "look into his own depths and there discover the faint outlines of a moral structure." Most of all, beyond the changing mores of society and the indistinct influence of archetypes lay the genius of universal religion. The creators of that faith—"Jesus, St. Francis, and the long line of them"—could "penetrate through the depths of their own unconsciousness into the collective unconsciousness of mankind." They had translated them into moral principles as applicable in Asia and Africa as in Europe. May summed up his vision: "This, then, is our solution to the moral problem: *instinctual self-expression through universal structure.*"[27]

The Art of Counseling was a great success. Abingdon Press advertised it with lavish praise from, among others, Reinhold Niebuhr and Anton Boisen. One reviewer declared that May's "penetration behind the usual moral standards to the religious basis of life, or 'morality of grace' [was] a rich contribution to Christian literature." Others touted the book's practical value to counselors. However, some cautioned that May's suggestions, especially about empathy, might be misunderstood by fledgling counselors all too ready to unleash their own emotions in a counseling session.[28]

Whether in its descriptions of the counseling situation or in its theory of meaning emerging from a struggle between instinct and various forms of internal and external order, *The Art of Counseling* began to set the agenda for May's future work. Creativity and its powerful but ambiguous relation to the instincts, the central importance of the experiential moment in every detail and dimension, the rejection of simple moral dicta—these became his characteristic themes. Less obvious but equally enduring was his employment of autobiographical material in disguised third-person case histories. One might rightly view such use as narcissistic and limiting, a conflation of May's subjective experience with the realities of others. Yet, for better or worse, he managed to turn an almost obsessive telling and retelling of his life story into an ever-evolving interpretation of the human condition. Freud, James, and others had already set firm precedents for the use of self as case history. May's relentless concern for self-holiness paradoxically led to an ongoing, creative grappling with the universal human question: "How Shall I Live?" No matter the authoritative tone of his first book, events soon revealed that he had not found a definitive answer.

12

"Therapist for Humanity"

Some months after publishing *The Art of Counseling*, Rollo received a letter from a young Methodist minister in North Carolina. "Your book," he declared, "has stimulated me to a new determination to relieve myself, if it is any way possible, of personality difficulties . . . before they become so fastened upon me that only a complete breakdown can result." In his first year at the church, married for two years, and blessed with an eight-month-old son, the clergyman had already seen a counselor but still felt that his "marriage was all but a failure for no other reason than that of my own confused and abnormal motives before and after the marriage." His distress was "almost paralyzing," but he hoped May could help him.[1]

The minister's letter was one of a great many Rollo received in the months after his book began to reach the public. A number of his readers wrote long and desperate descriptions of their personal problems. Some in the greater New York area sought counseling appointments, and fellow ministers referred their knottiest pastoral cases to him. Having tended his church for little more than a year, May was swept up in a second calling as public minister and therapist. Living in a "house by the side of the road" for the good of the world, to communicate new visions of the spiritual life through books—this role might fulfill the hope of significance he dreamed of only a few years before on a mountaintop in Colorado. It added one more flourish to an ever more impressive launch of May's life and career—ministry, marriage, and now authorship.

In late 1939, Rollo received the most thrilling news of all, that Florence was pregnant with their first child. Over forty years later, he remembered the moment of his son Robert's birth in 1940 as a great turning point of his life. "I had a kind of absence of real connection with the universe," he explained later. "I was a foreigner in the world, until my first child was born. . . . And from that time on, my real and deep connection with the universe was made." It was hardly an unusual reaction for a first-time parent, but in Rollo's case it was particularly profound. He had been driven by a quest bound in a protective narcissism. He had explored the world and his own consciousness with few commitments beyond those to his family in Michigan, and even those he viewed largely within a frame of personal triumph and martyrdom. Now he had gained that most elemental responsibility of parenthood. He had suddenly reached full adulthood.[2]

The richness of marriage, fatherhood, and professional success all encouraged a triumphal view of life. May had become a wise counselor in person and in print. However, deep conflict lurked behind this persona of confident prose and public bearing. It had become in some sense hidden to himself. One could not have easily guessed that he stood, like the minister and others who sought his advice, on the brink of physical and spiritual collapse. Signs soon began to appear that not all was well. Having two callings and a family to support stoked May's unquenchable, compulsive appetite for work. Parenthood brought new dimensions to May's marriage but also an unmistakable sense of being trapped. Florence experienced the shock of settling into marriage with a man who had continually expressed doubts about their love virtually until their wedding day and went on to spend much of his time with his congregation or on lecture tours. Isolation and general insecurity only increased as she became less a sexual partner for the ever-desirous Rollo. She had forsaken a career for the companionship of marriage, yet she often found herself alone in the parsonage, increasingly incapacitated by pregnancy and then totally immersed in the care of her infant son.

At the same time, Rollo ministered to a congregation that included adoring young women, moved by his sermons and dashing good looks—they compared him to film star Raymond Massey. He received similar adulation on the lecture circuit. His continued ambivalence about Florence, a sense of being trapped in a marriage he wasn't sure he wanted, the pressures put on an active libido by Florence's pregnancy, and an overweening belief in his singular destiny—all drove him to an affair with a church worker. For May, who had carefully worked out his own system of morality in *The Art of Counseling* and who in print asked the question, "How, then, shall we live?" it was an event of some import.

May might have returned to therapy of his own or grappled directly in some other way with the issues he faced. Instead, he wrote another book. *The Springs of Creative Living* interwove two strands—a striking merger of Christianity with psychology and, hidden in case histories and commentary, a spiritual autobiography alive with personal contradiction, denial, and palpable wish. The new book moved from the practical psychotherapeutic focus of *The Art of Counseling* to a specifically religious statement concerning the sources of human creativity and happiness. As a book for a more general audience, it naturally dealt in bolder and more certain statements. However, given its content and the moment in which it was written, it also revealed the soul of an author literally working through the incongruities in his own life.

The audacious theme of the new book revealed itself in the subtitle: *A Study of Human Nature and God.* May underlined these concerns with an epigraph by Nicolas Berdyaev: "Man is the dominating idea of my life—man's image, his creative freedom and his creative predestination. . . . At the present time it is imperative to understand once more that the rediscovery of man will also be the rediscovery of God."[3] May argued for "Christianity" rather than simply religion (as in *The Art of Counseling*) as the overarching source of meaning for humankind and introduced the usefulness of psychotherapeutic and psychological concepts in the search for personal spiritual truth within the Christian tradition. It was no less than an attempt to define the meaning of life in modernity through the reassertion and revaluation of central Christian ideas and values in the light of psychological insight. He assured his readers that *Springs of Creative Living* was, despite its upbeat title, no " 'pep' book" or a "how to" manual. Rather, it was an "endeavor to understand the meaning of being a person." Echoing Niebuhr, May made a special point of rejecting the easy optimism of liberal Christianity or the severely prescriptive moralizing of conservative versions of the faith. He offered instead a psychologically informed view of the darkness and light of life's spiritual complexities.[4]

May thus joined the ranks of authors in the 1920s and 1930s who recognized the public's "thirst for meaning" in the wake of modernity's great cultural upheaval, not to mention the Great Depression and the portent of America's entry into a new war. He entered a marketplace that later would be dubbed "middlebrow," aided and abetted by new techniques of advertising, an increasing dominance of reasonably priced books, and the taste-making presence of bestseller lists and such entities as the Book of the Month Club and the Religious Book Club. Sometimes denigrated for its supposed dilution and vulgarization of literary and intellectual standards, this "middlebrow" book in fact addressed a mass, mostly white, middle-class audience hungry for ideas and literary experience.[5]

In a market filled with bestsellers attempting to frame the stakes of life and spirit in relatively traditional terms, May sought a new approach by marrying the insights of psychoanalysis with the eternal quests of religion in a manner meaningful to the modern reader. He defined his own approach by contrasting it to a few of the most popular recent books that attempted to frame the "meaning of life" in one form or another—Lin Yutang's "epicurean" *The Importance of Living*, Henry C. Link's bestselling *The Return to Religion*, which recommended a concentration on "behaving oneself," and Walter Lippmann's *Preface to Morals*, which, "like the courageous Stoics of old," recommended a humanitarian attitude borne of "a self-made security." In a class of its own was Joseph Wood Krutch's *The Modern Temper* and its "gospel of meaninglessness." Even Krutch, May argued, might provide an individual with meaning for a little while, but the truly creative life required a philosophy both enduring and capable of growth.[6]

May began by positing the central issue: "Many modern persons have been unable to quench their thirst for meaning in the stream of organized religion." He offered a number of possible reasons—"the stagnation that results from any large organization, the preaching of dry forms in which the vitality has run dry, the fact that 'every institution ends by strangling the truth it was formed to perpetuate,' the great upheavals in our Western culture of the last century, and so forth." Citing alarming statistics concerning the rise of psychological illness, he saw its "great source" as the "mental unrest" created in an age of transition—"from farm to city, from shop to factory, from romantic love to casual marriage, from individualism to collectivism, and from confidence in peace to almost continuous warfare." "Forced to live 'on the margin . . . ,'" he argued, "we must continually make basic decisions; we are forced to live on the knife-blade edge of insecurity." Quoting Lippmann's *Preface to Morals* (1929), May noted that even the "flux" and "giddiness" of the 1920s could not cure a pervasive sense of emptiness and dissatisfaction.[7]

The onset of the Great Depression, he asserted, using Karen Horney's "expert discussion" in *The Neurotic Personality of Our Time* (1937) as his guide, triggered a basic sense of anxiety rooted in material insecurity that complemented and made unavoidable the confrontation of deeper spiritual issues already alive in the culture. By merging the psychoanalytic insights of Freud, Horney, Adler, and others with the spiritual and ethical ideals of religion and philosophy, May hoped to define "what kind of meaning makes for most successful and satisfactory living for ourselves and is most contributive to our fellow-men. To find this adequate meaning is to find creativity—the joie de vivre, the enthusiasm, the buoyancy and resilience that come from the health of the whole personality." May sought a route to the profoundest "kind of meaning" for modern human beings through a combination of religious and psychotherapeutic exploration.[8]

In this sense, *The Springs of Creative Living* returned to the concerns of May's honors thesis and those of his formal Christian ministry. However, in his definition of religion he marked a major turn, one that outstripped in its breadth the view of liberal Christianity even as it honored its basic approach. "Call it confidence in the universe, trust in God, belief in one's fellow-men, or what not," he argued, "the essence of religion is the belief that something matters—the *presupposition that life has meaning*." The function of religion, he continued, was "to aid the human being to affirm himself, affirm his fellow-men, and affirm the universe in which he lives." Atheism became "the denial of meaning in life." Interestingly, though, the choice of paths for imbuing life with meaning seemed limited either to Christianity or nonspecific, psychological attitudes that nonetheless emerged from Christian culture. If other religious traditions were an option for finding meaning, they were not mentioned.[9]

May moved from this general appreciation of the problem to case histories layered with psychological or theological meditations, each complementing the other as they moved toward a psychospiritual solution to the question of meaning. As in *The Art of Counseling*, he plunged into a clinical encounter, this time with a young man named Charles D. whose spiritual search replicated to a large degree his own. Charles D. sought a counselor, as May told it, because "he could not make the marriage decision." May's client was "prepossessing in appearance, blond, tall, and well-built, though somewhat thin." He seemed calm and collected, and identified himself as the product of a solid midwestern upbringing. Charles told May that his parents were intelligent, hardworking, and devout. They continually concerned themselves with building "strong character" in their son, which meant in part encouraging an aversion to sex. Their "facts of life" lectures consisted largely of warnings against "doing bad things." Despite or because of their strong character, the parents had a stormy marriage and eventually divorced.[10]

Charles shared personal diaries and letters demonstrating that the young man "was highly moral in the authoritarian sense." Throughout college, he had been a devout Christian. He spent much time praying but not much time making friends. In fact, he was quite lonely and aloof. He did have girlfriends but never became entangled. "The petting parties in which he participated on college dates, during which he occasionally had orgasms," May related, "left him with poignant guilt feelings." Charles was also plagued by the urge to masturbate, "the act always being followed by a cutting experience of guilt and resolutions never to commit it again."

Charles's response to sexual anxiety echoed his parents' rigid moral rules and approach to building "character." He filled his college diaries with plans for mental and physical health, fulfillment of high ideals, and moral purity. In one entry he drew a diagrammatic plan for "keeping my body at its best, giving attention only to what is right, controlling my will." In another entry, "Tentative Purposes for Senior College Year," he set forth rules and methods through which he might become "free and genuine," "work hard but not with a strain," and "keep close to God as my living power." To combat his shyness, he made "rules to be friendly, which he would repeat to himself in a social gathering." None of these strategies worked, and some backfired. Indeed, "his resolutions concerning masturbation not only did not help him to conquer the habit but even increased his temptation."

Upon graduating college, Charles taught at an American missionary college in Egypt, and on the voyage fell in love with a fellow American, a young woman who was going to teach at a "near-by" school. He saw her often but failed to express his true feelings. He lost her to another man. Charles then threw himself into teaching and continued to dissect every minute of his day in his diary. Such introspection led to continued loneliness and crisis. Even his students mocked his stiff reserve and moral punctiliousness. They rightly saw that he and the other teachers didn't really care about them except as objects of missionary goals. "This knocked the pillars out from under me," he reported to May. "My life had not been real, solid, genuine. No wonder I had not made friends, and no wonder I had been unhappy and lonely."

These feelings only made Charles apply himself more intently, and so when he suffered a "nervous breakdown," he and those around him attributed it to "exhaustion because of his hard work." He tried a rest cure. May, however, noted that "the breakdown occurred simultaneously with the realization that the meaning by which he had been living was destroyed." Thus, the real cause was a crisis of meaning: "His expression 'knocked the pillars out from under me' is psychologically accurate. His scheme of life had collapsed. A breakdown is the crisis at which the individual stops, retreats, and in the cure finds new meaning and a new path down which he can move." Nor was May surprised at Charles's redoubled commitment to work just before he fell ill. "The human being fights hardest for his psychological pattern," he asserted, "just before it collapses."

May's thinly veiled recounting of his own life through the time of his collapse in Greece inspired a more general analysis, one that focused on the unhealthy nature of submission to "authoritarian" religion, to the subjection of self to an entirely external set of rules, "ten or one hundred commandments," and to honoring blind "determination" over "freedom." "Such a viewpoint is found typically among individuals who are afraid of life." May emphasized, "afraid of their instinctual tendencies and erotic urges." The "drying up" of these urges led to "illness of the soul."

Of course, the term "authoritarianism" resonated for May not only with ongoing struggles within the church between liberals and conservatives but also in a world plagued by Hitler, Stalin, and Franco. The healthy individual was one resistant to totalitarian seduction, whether in church or in politics and society. As if to underline these commonalities in both religious and secular worlds, May mixed sources in waging war against "authoritarianism." He cited the "parable of the talents" from Matthew, which honored the taking of risk and creative activity over a closed and defensive mind, the lesson to May being that "nature's instinctual coin . . . must be spent." He invoked the "Pharisaism" of the New Testament as a "classic example" of authoritarian religion in its seeking "to reduce all living to rules and maxims." "It was the central task of Jesus, and later Paul," he noted in the traditional Christian formulation, "to point out that this great concern for external rules is really a sign of lack of faith in God. The law, indeed, kills the spirit." But he also invoked Alfred Adler's characterization of "Men of Principle," who "feel themselves so insecure that they must squeeze all of life and living into a few rules and formulae, lest they become too frightened of it."[11]

May's fidelity to his own evolution continued with a fictionalized account and assessment of his own crucial encounter with Adler and staff, one in which Charles gained new but ultimately limited insight into his life from an anonymous therapist. The therapist convinced him that "his moralism had been really a technique for bolstering up his own prestige," that he had been pampering himself, and that he needed to forget himself and to turn unself-consciously to others. The therapist had "set him free," and Charles's response was to lose himself by "worshipping experience." He immediately joined a group of musicians and traveled with them across Europe in uninhibited enjoyment of art, music, and women. It was "gloriously romantic," and his "senses came to life." He fell in love with one of the musicians, and after the group broke up they enjoyed an idyllic time alone, camping by the sea. In the year that ensued, he had affairs with five women.

Therapy also imbued Charles D.'s social philosophy, and while he continued to consider himself religious, he gave up prayer and for moral inspiration turned to "the poems of the exuberant Walt Whitman." He sang "the body electric" and thought "general understanding" was the cure for world tensions: "Let the French understand the Germans and vice versa and they would feel the ties of brotherhood of which Walt Whitman wrote." However, being in Europe at the time and experiencing the deep divisions among peoples, he almost immediately gave up such notions for the "masses." Still, he thought the Whitmanesque life of experience was possible for "the aristocracy of mind and spirit who have the courage to live abundantly."

He returned to America possessed by this newfound hedonism and his own membership in that "aristocracy of mind and spirit." But picking up the pieces of his family in the wake of his parent's divorce and watching friends go through painful breakups began to undo his faith in "experience." Having bolted forever from the hold of authoritarian moralism, he despaired of living in pure, sensual, and unthinking freedom. He veered toward another breakdown and only slowly came to realize that "libertinism" was no better than "authoritarianism" and that "the only healthy self-expression [was] expression through structure." Charles's experience before treatment illustrated the dilemma of modern consciousness. He found himself caught between "freedom and determination" and searched for some way of living in the tension between his inner creativity and the demands of the world and God.[12]

Charles decided that it was time to settle down to a life of marriage and family. He soon fell in love with Helen R. and hoped to marry her. Yet he noticed that he desired her most when she "was only mildly responsive to his ardor." When she finally warmed to his advances, "his passion cooled." She herself began to act boldly toward him, throwing him "into a fright." At the same time, he became intensely jealous of any attention she paid to other men. He would often list good reasons for marrying Helen R. but then create an equivalent list of reasons for not marrying her, framing the question in an almost mathematical fashion that yielded no answer. It was this paralysis that led him to seek counseling with the author, Rollo May.

In their sessions, Charles told May that his problem was really that Helen was not a "sufficiently 'high type' for him" despite her fine education, unusual attractiveness, and family's high social standing. It turned out that what Charles really meant was that she did not seem "strong" enough to withstand his dominant personality and that he would soon tire of her. Then he would be faced with endless boredom or divorce, neither of which seemed to be agreeable choices. "The divorce of [Charles's] own parents had convinced him," May wrote, "that nothing of that sort must occur in his marriage and hence that he must keep his ideals high and be very careful about the selection of a wife."

One episode underlined the highly emotional stakes of the relationship. Charles and Helen had begun to talk about marriage, but about a month after this discussion began, Charles indicated to her that he had his doubts about their future together. Shocked and disturbed, Helen took up (platonically, she said) with a radical labor organizer, "whose zeal challenged and fascinated her and with whom she liked to talk at great length." This threw Charles into a jealous frenzy. After a sleepless night, he treated her to his rage, coercing her into admitting that she had mistreated him despite the facts of the case. Of course, he was disgusted that she could be so weak as to give into his rage.

Charles avoided contemplation of his own complicity in this sadomasochistic marathon by embracing a delusional martyrdom. The question, he wrote in his diary, was really whether he ought to marry her, given the fact that they had slept together and had made tentative vows. After all, he reasoned, "at least one person would be happy" because she loved him so completely. He hoped that he could help her develop strength after marriage and that someday she could be a person he could love.

This strategy also failed. Charles moved toward a resolution of the problem only after initiating an agonizing separation. He believed it would help Helen grow stronger. Of course, it also had the effect of forcing him to be less dependent on her as an object of his "kindness." At first he could not resist bombarding her with letters filled with advice on career and caution about other men. Soon each recognized the need to break their cycle of emotional dependency and therefore to recognize themselves and each other as individuals with unique characteristics and responsibilities. In the end, they married and lived realistically ever after. Moreover, happily, if we are to credit what Charles told May a year after the wedding: "It turned out to be an excellent marriage. We are happier than we imagined possible before marriage. . . . Our marriage is certainly worth the neurotic agonies I went through at the time of my consultations."

Interestingly, May envisioned Charles's case not as a triumph of therapy but as the successful outcome of a personal religious drama. "What was the real flaw in Charles D.'s personality," he asked, "which had kept him from making a successful marriage decision?" After rejecting a variety of psychological propositions, May concluded: "Charles D. was trying to play God—that is the way we should express it from the religious point of view. . . . This meant that he really did not have faith in his own freedom; he hung on to it tightly, ere it escaped him. So he judged the girl minutely as God would.... In striving to make himself God, Charles D. gave evidence of his own lack of trust in any true God outside himself." Charles's surrender to marital bliss demonstrated that "the norm for human living is to have a God outside one-self and therefore be able to accept one's own imperfections" and those of others. Clarification of this point led to grace and made Charles D.'s story one not only of a decision for marriage but also of religious conversion.[13]

May drew a broader lesson from Charles D.'s case, one that demon-strated how firmly he had moved toward the neo-Orthodoxy epitomized by the theology of Tillich and Reinhold Niebuhr. Specifically addressing the Christian dimensions of "freedom and determination," he argued that the "modernist revolt against fundamentalism was a necessary step" but that the "liberal gospel" had gone too far in its declaration of "individual autonomy" and a one-dimensional "goodness of creation." No wonder, then, that many turned to the psychotherapist instead of the minister and his church. By re-envisioning the "age-old doctrines" of Christianity within the compelling insights of psychotherapy, May argued, "we find ourselves rediscovering the orthodox Christian ideas about human nature in a 'liberal orthodoxy,' which, unlike fundamentalism, springs up out of the soil of real experience."[14]

May spent the rest of the book highlighting details of the argument through pointedly titled chapters—"Too Much Freedom Makes Us Mad," "Creativity and Sin," "What Is Healthy Religion?," "Happiness," "A Theology of Life," and "Grace and Clarification"—at all points hammering home the compatibility of psychology's insights and yet its need for the structure afforded by a faith in God that preserved the wisdom and faith of the Christian tradition. "Only by having an 'Other' who is not ourselves," he asserted at one point, "can we be freed sufficiently from subjectivity to be ourselves."[15]

May emphasized the creative value of living within the tension be-tween self and God as well as the insufficiency of life that did not appre-ciate the richness of both. He followed Adler in underlining the sickness of perfectionism and the "courage of imperfection," and played off of G. K. Chesterton's "good news of original sin." "We are not what we should be," May argued; "it is indeed sin that we are not, but that is the human situ-ation." Human creativity involved the attempt to reach toward the ideal, knowing the futility of the quest and accepting the feelings of guilt and remorse involved. He especially highlighted the acute sense of transgres-sion and failure that accompanied artistic creativity: "So Degas says, 'A pic-ture must be painted with the same feeling as that with which a criminal commits his crime,' and so Thomas Mann speaks of the 'precious and guilty secret' which the artist keeps." In sex, lust, and desire, as in art—all the things that fundamentalists and moralists in general railed against—sin rightly seen was as much the key to bold creativity as it was to evil. "The healthy personality is one who creates courageously but who admits the imperfections of all his deeds," May concluded, "and who asks forgiveness for his successes as well as his failures."[16]

May revealed in the final chapters of the book what would become a hall-mark of his work—the broad and sometimes dazzling synthesis of Western culture as he brought together strands of philosophy, religion, and psychology. May's definition of a "healthy religion" was one that encouraged personal re-sponsibility, choice, and courage in spite of imperfection, one that "lets the individual know there is purpose in his standing in his autonomous human position" even when that might mean standing alone in society. However, it was also one that, like Calvinism, affirmed God "without demanding that God affirm oneself." And, in the final chapter, "Grace and Clarification," he imagined the ultimate merger of psychology and Christianity: "This, then, is the function of Christ. He is the therapist for humanity."[17]

The Springs of Creative Living thus advocated a radical fusion of religion and psychology in the cause of enriching lives and saving souls. It was, in its sphere, a critical and commercial success. "Among many helpful books dealing with psychotherapy and religion," *Publishers Weekly* declared, "this is outstanding." The religious press raved, and the Religious Book Club made it the November 1940 main selection. The *Christian-Evangelist* called it "a valid and valuable work in a field that is crowded with charlatan stuff." *Church Management* proclaimed: "This book is one in a thousand. Many chapters in themselves are worth the price of the book." The highly influential *Christian Century* noted it as a significant exploration that expanded the scope of *The Art of Counseling* and dubbed it "an important contribution" to the literature on religion and psychology.[18]

Personal correspondence reinforced these judgments. In a letter to May, Reinhold Niebuhr declared that *The Springs of Creative Living* had "opened up a field of thought for the Protestant Church which has not been touched in any significant way before." Lewis Mumford, whom May had never met but to whom he sent a copy of the book, exclaimed: "I rejoice to have become acquainted with a mind as vigorous as yours—and as morally acute—capable of bringing together the old dispensation of theology and the new dispensa-tion of science, without loss or betrayal."[19]

This moment of triumph, however, was cut short by profound tensions in May's own life, contradictions that were revealed in the subtext of the book. Internal evidence illuminates May's own turmoil in his assessment that Charles, while teaching in Egypt, "had thrown himself into his work with increasing vigor during the year preceding the breakdown," and in May's declaration that "the human being fights hardest for his psychological pattern just before it collapses."[20]

It was for May as it had been for Charles. He wrote *The Springs of Creative Living* as part of a hard fight against personal realities. The book's assertions of eventual clarity and faith stood in stark contrast to the conflicts and confusions that were growing around him. Most obviously, the denouement of Charles D.'s quest for Helen R. had a parallel in May's own defenses concerning marriage, but not so much in its final reality. Like Charles, May had struggled with jealousy, domination, and deep doubts about marrying Florence before and after their wedding. Unlike Charles D., however, he could not report marital bliss by the end of the first or ensuing years. Whether due to unresolved neurotic tendencies, a basic mismatch, or a combination of the two, May's marriage rarely attained a semblance of harmony. Within a year, he confided to Tillich that it was a disaster.[21]

His ministerial role was also replete with a bundle of contradictions. May's day-to-day responsibilities, the politics of the church laity, and the smug anti-intellectualism of his congregation made for a sobering contrast with the world of ideas he had enjoyed at Union Theological Seminary. Indeed, he preferred the more comfortable intellectual and spiritual company of those in a local Jewish congregation, whom he periodically defended as waves of anti-Semitism rattled the town and the nation. Perhaps, then, it was not so surprising that the very first chapter of *The Springs of Creative Living* began with these sentences: "People suffer personality breakdowns because they do not have meaning in their lives. The struggle is not 'worth the candle,' they often frankly say, so why shouldn't one give up?" He followed these remarks with ones even more prescient: "That is the significance of a personality crisis—it is the symptom that the meaning of a particular style of life has broken down, and the individual finds he must retreat and start over again in a new direction."[22]

In this sense, the book could be read as May's last-ditch attempt to defend a shaky faith in his personal and professional choices and, given the commitments of his career, in a specifically Christian God. "About six months after it was published," he admitted years later, "I realized I didn't believe what I had written. You might say that I had a deconversion."[23] He didn't mean that he rejected the values of Christianity, some of the deepest questions it sought to answer, or the value of its presence in the broader culture. He meant simply and profoundly that his faith in the divinity of Jesus and the doctrines of transcendence, afterlife, and other theological tenets that comprised the central part of Christianity and its many traditions had begun to fade.

13

"The More Difficult War Within"

On the first few pages of *The Springs of Creative Living*, May described an everyman, "John Jones," undergoing a "personality breakdown" when he discovers that the "meaning" he lived within was "false or inadequate." Rather than facing that fact, Jones "throws himself" into meaninglessness until a state of "nervous exhaustion" or collapse brings him down and, in the end, he stops and looks for new meaning. Significantly for 1940, May used the metaphor of combat to assert that it was "not in the slightest surprising" that such individuals "welcome a war between nations as a relief from the more difficult war within."[1]

When, much later, May looked back to the early 1940s, he rarely mentioned the world war that raged all around him and that ultimately cost the lives of over fifty million human beings. Married, a father, over thirty when the draft was reinstated in 1940, and plagued by episodes of tachycardia and malaria, he was hardly army material. Looking back and at the time, he could not help but focus on his own "war within." May's war comprised no simple crisis of meaning like the plight of "John Jones," one explicitly resolved with new and more certain beliefs and goals. Rather, he faced ambiguities and new choices, a life with too many available meanings, all of which he pursued to the point of exhaustion.

One source of overwork in May's life came as a natural consequence of the successes of *Art of Counseling* and *Springs of Creative Living*. Writing popular advice articles was a temptation made attractive not only by recognition from colleagues and readers but also by the fees paid by magazines. A father and provider, May's financial needs outdistanced the meager salary of a minister. When religious magazines sought him out for practical pieces combining the wisdom of Christianity and therapy, he eagerly answered the call. Topics varied widely. An early piece argued against moralistic attitudes toward alcoholism and, through short case histories, demonstrated the effectiveness of counseling in ameliorating the personality problems that drove men and women to drink.[2] Between 1939 and 1942, May produced numerous pieces for *Pilgrim Highroad*, a popular Congregational youth magazine. A nine-part series, "Understanding and Managing Ourselves," which may well have orig-inated in talks at the Verona church, confronted common questions: "What is Personality?" "The Courage to Grow Up," "The Marks of a Friend," "Making Friends," "The 'Gas' that Makes Us Go," "Boy and Girl Friendships," "Getting Along with Family," "When Is Your Conscience Healthy?," and "A Grown-Up Religion." Each amounted to a small sermon, complete with Bible verse, and intermixed wisdom from the New Testament and psychology concerning the self and one's relations with others.[3]

As in his earlier work, May celebrated such therapeutic and Christian virtues as courage, faith, self-acceptance, and love. He emphasized the ways in which psychotherapy and liberal Christianity coincided in their focus on individual personality. As he concluded in a later article, "The interesting fact is that reverence for personality is the central Christian attitude to-ward people. The deeper the discussion of social life goes, then, the closer it comes to the attitude toward people which Jesus taught." In another piece, May identified the "central pilgrimage of our lives" as the need and search for Christ. "Counseling," he concluded, "helps each person make that pilgrimage in the way God has chosen for him."[4] Through counseling, one might rec-ognize and shape "the core of one's self so that the powers of God, like radio waves, come through one's self."[5]

May also expanded his role as lecturer and teacher, in part because it pro-vided more income and also because it kept him from confronting his inner conflicts concerning marriage and career. He spoke at summer institutes and workshops, traveling as far as Dallas to participate as keynote speaker or panelist. During the summer of 1941, he taught a course called Student Movements and Counseling at the Garrett Biblical Institute (now part of Northwestern University) in Evanston, Illinois, the first of a series of vis-iting teaching appointments at Garrett that lasted through the mid-1940s. After America's entry into World War II in December 1941, May served in the best way he knew how, contributing popular pieces directly related to the effect of the war on soul and psyche. One suggested how to overcome "war-time jitters," while another addressed the question "Does the War Destroy Our Values?" Without denying the corrosive effect of massive death and de-struction and the challenge to everyday morality that the war brought, he reminded the reader of the ways in which the war situation promoted coop-eration instead of extreme individualism.[6]

Even though he remained tied to organized Christianity through lectures, teaching, and popular writing, he decided to leave the ministry in order to train formally for a career in psychotherapy. He found that the two aspects of being a minister he loved best—pastoral counseling and the public pulpit—could be combined more effectively and authoritatively as a therapist. He also sensed that American society had only just commenced a love affair with psychotherapy, while the organized church was struggling to hold on to a loyal audience. Tillich agreed and urged him to change careers. May negotiated a half-time commitment at the church in early 1941, moved to New York in March, and by 1942 had resigned his duties completely. He enrolled for the fall 1941 term in the new counseling PhD program at Teachers College of Columbia University.[7]

While a major "professional" shift in many ways, May's switch to psychotherapy from the ministry displayed deep continuity with his lifelong strivings. After all, his new commitment was built on a devotion to healing in the liberal Christian tradition of growth in grace and maturity in personality, a mission that transcended the particulars of both theology and psychological theory. A poignantly revealing example of the overlap came as he wound down his life in New Jersey. He agreed to counsel a parishioner of a fellow clergyman, one who thought she would benefit from May's merging of religious and psychological insight. He saw her for a few sessions from July to early September 1941.

Edith Hammond described herself as single, thirty-eight years old, a teacher, artist, and musician, weighing 210 pounds and "confronted for a long time by stop-lights in all directions." Her minister, from whom she had in vain sought help on several occasions, finally handed her a copy of *The Springs of Creative Living*. Upon finishing it, she immediately wrote to May for an appointment, hoping he could help her vanquish the "unhappiness and ill health" that had been "festering" for years. "I am eager to find normality and health of personality," she declared, "and to release abilities that are now more or less dormant, and especially to be purged of fear and resentment."[8]

Rollo helped crack Hammond's emotional paralysis in the very first session. Somehow, his "exquisite casualness," she wrote in appreciation a few days later, allowed her to "confess" her shame and fear without his showing "the tiniest sign of being shocked." She now knew "*something* of how the woman-taken-in-adultery must have felt when she was brought before Jesus, and found understanding instead of judgment." He had shone light on her "inner-most hiding-places," and even after the session she felt as though she were "still being led, by your hand (and mind), closer and closer to the sunlight at the edge of a dark wilderness." She experienced this unfreezing physically—no more gagging throat, better posture, a relaxed mouth—and wondered whether perhaps all the ailments she had experienced, as well as her weight problem, were hysterical symptoms, as May had explained them.[9]

With insight and release, however, came ambivalent senses of the future in part set off by May's own writings, which promised the unleashing of the creative spirit. That very morning she had broken out in "spontaneous self-less prayer" and in the evening felt "such relaxation as I had forgotten could be" after painting a watercolor. And his assurance that masturbation was universal and perfectly natural helped to free her from compulsion and in-hibition in regard to love. However, she knew that masturbation was no sub-stitute for "true mating." She wanted the real love that May had described in his books, "a love that releases 'great creative potentialities,' in an enriching completion of personality." Yet she recognized that, whatever her new attitudes, for her it might be too late. The "dearth of unmarried men of my generation, and my ignorance of where and how to meet them, and my phys-ical state" cast long shadows on her prospects.[10]

Hammond wrote to May again in early August, requesting a follow-up appointment even as she continued a chronicle of "unfold[ing] and bloom[ing]," of acquiring "fragrance under [his] touch." She enclosed a sep-arate report detailing visits to old friends, an after-dinner smoke with a new bachelor teacher—commonplace human contacts that were revelations and sure signs that "inhibitions [were] giving way." She proudly listed "physical" gains: no more fatigue, no more aches and pains, no more insomnia, "a new spring in my step and swing in my whole body when I walk,—a buoyance, it might even be called an 'abandon,'" and three pounds lost without even trying. And, she confessed a "persistent tendency to feel an "in-love-ness" for each man, in turn, who has given me help during my life," most of all May. The exquisite delirium of therapist love underlined an incipient problem, one that she needed to discuss with May. "My old scale of values has been changed by your perspective," she observed, "and a new sense of proportion hasn't crystallized yet."[11]

May responded by gently warning that beyond this burst of emotional re-lease lay the hard work of forging a new life. He suggested an appointment in early September. Hammond wrote that she had already begun to feel the waning of the initial "blaze of light" and "realized that transformation must be more than merely an instantaneous miracle" but rather "a steady courageous development." She felt more urgently than ever the need for a new approach to life. "You see, your calm tolerance of actions which I had been unable to affirm has disrupted my sense of values," she wrote. "I think I need help in formulating a new one."[12] They seem to have had just one more meeting, the very day Hammond began a new school year and just a few days before May moved from Verona back to New York to start a new professional life.

Teachers College was across the street from Union Theological Seminary and shared some faculty and facilities, but in terms of professional future, the two schools led mostly to radically different places. The curriculum indicated as much. In his first semester, May took courses in cultural dynamics, casework, theory of personality adjustment, and psychotherapy. The second semester included more casework, more theory, and an introduction to the use of the Rorschach test. Of course, May was a special sort of student. He had already studied with Adler, published two major books in a related field, lectured widely on counseling, and actually practiced counseling at Michigan State and for parishioners at his church in Verona. Yet he never had received formal training or supervised clinical hours, nor had his approach been scrutinized by counseling professionals. He possessed no demonstrable skills in the experimental scientific methods that were the backbone of academic psychology.

If May entered the field of psychotherapy at the right time, he also did so in just the right place. May's special access through Tillich to the world of New York's émigré community, and especially to its psychologists and psychoanalysts, made his move to a career in psychotherapy far more profound an experience than one of simply obtaining a degree. By the late 1930s, New York had become the center of psychoanalytic practice and discussion thanks to Hitler's progressively draconian policies toward German and Austrian Jews. A number of the most significant voices in the Freudian and other psychoanalytic persuasions had emigrated either to England or the United States. As in the case of émigrés in the arts, humanities, and sciences, the analysts enriched and sometimes revolutionized their chosen fields in America. One need name only a few of the neurologists, psychiatrists, psychologists, and psychoanalysts who made New York their new home— Alfred Adler, Erik Erikson, Otto Fenichel, Erich Fromm, Frieda Fromm-Reichmann, Kurt Goldstein, Kurt Lewin, Otto Rank, Theodor Reik, Ernest Schachtel—to imagine their collective impact.

May's first contacts with those who would become refugee intellectuals were made while he was in Europe, the most important being Alfred Adler and Joseph Binder, but his relationship with Tillich opened him to a much wider circle. Since their arrival in 1934, the Tillichs had actively aided and befriended the growing community of German and Austrian exiles. They helped them find jobs, introduced them to influential Americans, and created a lively social world in which the Tillichs' New York apartment, for all intents and purposes, at times might have seemed to be in Berlin. Their dinner parties and cocktail hours included vigorous debates, sexual flirtations, and the forging of professional alliances. At first, Tillich tried to bring the Union Seminary community into the orbit of these entertainments, but awkwardness abounded. In the end, Rollo and Florence May were among the few Americans to participate regularly in these soirées.[13]

For May, the direct intellectual impact of the émigrés in the Tillich circle began in 1937, when Tillich introduced him to neurologist Kurt Goldstein. From then on the scientist's thinking gradually but deeply enriched important dimensions of the young American's thinking about psychology and the meaning of human existence. The most visible link between the two would emerge much later in May's use of Goldstein's notion of "self-actualization," whose appearance in popular culture actually owed more to Abraham Maslow than to May himself. However, Goldstein helped to shape May's conception of a more profound and pervasive value, what one of the most perceptive students of Goldstein's work has termed an "ethic" of "courage of action in the service of personal meaningfulness." It was a vision that connected Tillich and Goldstein as friends and colleagues despite their different backgrounds and fields of endeavor.[14]

Born in 1878, Goldstein was Silesian Jew with a broad intellectual curiosity that led him first to philosophy and literature and then to neurology. During World War I, Goldstein organized the Institute for Research into the Consequences of Brain Injuries in Frankfurt to find ways of rehabilitating soldiers who had suffered brain damage in combat. He and his colleague Adhémar Gelb developed a number of successful therapies and soon formulated a radical conception of mental activity. Rejecting the prevailing wisdom that treated various brain functions as discrete activities of particular brain areas, they came to see a more integrative picture of consciousness. Impairment in one area could trigger an adaptive strategy utilizing or limiting function in other areas. In short, the whole organism reacted and adapted strategically to particular damage. Goldstein argued that this reaction was an instinctual survival mechanism that might allow the neurologist to construct therapeutic strategies that coaxed and guided adaptation.[15]

Goldstein's vision of the organism within contributed to the general intellectual and scientific ferment of Weimar Germany, expanding on themes that had been alive since the late nineteenth century. As the historian of science Anne Harrington has argued, in the 1920s Goldstein was "increasingly active in an effort within medicine to overcome Cartesian dualism and articulate a psychosomatic approach to medical diagnosis and therapy." This more general movement was part of a wide mixture of ideas and disciplines. Existentialists, gestalt psychologists, theologians (like Tillich) who sought a rebirth of essential religious spirit, and such influential philosophers as Max Scheler felt drawn by the need to mend a world ruptured by what they saw as intellectual dehumanization.[16]

The Nazi seizure of power in 1933 redrew lines in German holistic thought by excluding Jews and socialists and severing lifelong personal and professional relationships. The great existential philosopher Martin Heidegger became an ardent Nazi even as his Jewish students endured exile or worse. Tillich left Germany, while Emmanuel Hirsch, a member of Tillich's Kairos Circle and one of the foremost Kierkegaard scholars, sided with the Nazis as Germany's saviors. Alfred Adler sought refuge in New York, while his assistant Leonhard Seif (who had analyzed May) became a member of Nazi Germany's psychotherapeutic establishment.[17]

As for Goldstein, after the Nazi takeover he was arrested in his examining room, imprisoned, and severely beaten. Only the intervention of Matthias Göring, a cousin of Hermann Göring and himself an Adlerian psychotherapist, saved Goldstein's life on the promise that he would leave and never return to Germany. He took immediate refuge in Amsterdam but in 1935 came to New York under a visa arranged by the Rockefeller Foundation.[18] While in Amsterdam, under the most trying of conditions, he dictated and published *Der Aufbau des Organismus*, a comprehensive elaboration of his thesis concerning the intentionality of biological drives and especially of the "self-actualizing" function of the brain. Its publication in English in 1939 as *The Organism*, followed in 1940 by a shorter book of lectures, *Human Nature in the Light of Psychopathology*, established his work among a growing circle of American psychologists and others concerned with placing study of the person in the broadest philosophical and scientific contexts.[19]

Goldstein was just one of the émigrés whose life and influence would be crucial to May's transformation from pastoral counselor to psychotherapist. As luck would have it, while he was working out the cultural and religious meanings of psychoanalysis and the terms of possible merger, some American psychiatrists and recent arrivals from Germany were seeking a psychoanalytic approach widened by the insights of sociology, anthropology, and politics. Another central, substantive, and bitterly contested issue, on both sides of the Atlantic, was the place of non-medical psychoanalytic training and practice.

May's professional future was shaped in important ways by the nature and resolution of these creative and often hurtful professional fissures, which birthed new institutes, new approaches, and new freedom to practice. A key figure in this series of schisms was Karen Horney, who had come from Germany in 1932. She was of the first generation of women in Germany to have full access to the university system. She became a member of the Berlin Psychoanalytic Institute in 1926, accepted a position at the Chicago Institute of Psychoanalysis in 1932, and two years later joined the New York Psychoanalytic Society and Institute as a training analyst and instructor.[20]

Almost from her arrival in New York, Horney sought out compatriots with whom to work out new visions of analysis. Especially important were her friendships with Clara Thompson, Harry Stack Sullivan, William Silverberg, Abram Kardiner, and Harold Lasswell, who, within the traditions of American psychiatry and social science, had begun to seek ways of integrating psychoanalysis and a broader study of human society and individuals. Of the émigrés who began to arrive in 1933 and 1934, no one was more important to May and central to the integration of sociological, humanistic, and psychoanalytic perspectives than Erich Fromm, who became in America an influential and widely read popular philosopher. He was born in 1900 and grew up in an Orthodox Jewish family in Frankfurt. Early on, he became enamored of Talmudic study and, in 1919–20, helped Martin Buber and Franz Rosenzweig to found Frankfurt's Freie Jüdische Lehrhaus, an institution devoted to Jewish adult education that sought to revivify Jewish culture in Germany. Fromm then moved to Heidelberg and wrote a comparative study of different Jewish approaches to Torah interpretation for his doctoral dissertation in sociology. Remaining in Heidelberg to study Talmud, he entered psychoanalysis with Frieda Reichmann, but within a year they had ended treatment in order to pursue a romantic relationship. They married in 1926. Fromm also began psychoanalytic training, attending classes and analysis in Munich and Berlin.[21]

In a sense, Fromm carved out a German Jewish parallel to May's migration from religious to psychological concerns. Steeped in religious orthodoxy but increasingly drawn to Freud's rejection of religion, Fromm and Fromm-Reichmann moved toward a Judaism without God and an enlightenment humanism imbued with Talmudic wisdom. Their work together in the late

1920s also contributed to the holistic strand of German scientific thought. Indeed, Fromm-Reichmann did a residency in neurology under Goldstein, whose influence remained throughout her career. While their professional lives flourished, Fromm and Fromm-Reichman's marriage dwindled to one of convenience as each sought asylum from the Nazis in the United States. Fromm left Germany in early 1933 to lecture at the Chicago Institute of Psychoanalysis and, after a brief return to Germany, was in New York by May 1934. Once a member of the University of Frankfurt's pioneering faculty group that sought to integrate psychoanalysis and Marxism (Institut fur Sozialforschung), Fromm helped to reestablish the so-called Frankfurt School at Columbia University. Fromm-Reichmann escaped Germany and in 1935 joined Harry Stack Sullivan's staff at Chestnut Lodge, a pioneering psychiatric clinic in Rockville, Maryland.

It was in America that Karen Horney and Erich Fromm became enmeshed in each other's lives. Soon they became lovers and commenced an intense, decade-long personal and intellectual relationship. A circle that included Sullivan and his American colleagues, as well as Fromm, Fromm-Reichmann, and Horney, began to challenge Freudian orthodoxies. Horney published new views in scholarly articles as well as publicly acclaimed books such as *The Neurotic Personality of Our Time* (1937) and *New Ways in Psychoanalysis* (1939). She downplayed the significance of the Oedipal complex in favor of tracing "Oedipal" symptoms to a wide range of dysfunctional family relations. She also challenged Freud on the psychology of women, especially explaining "penis envy" as a result of powerlessness in the world rather than an innate biopsychological reaction to gender difference.

Horney came to be seen as an enemy within by some in the leadership of the New York Psychoanalytic Society. Personal matters as well as theoretical heresies came to the fore. Her peers became troubled by Horney's sexual compulsions (though they seemed little disturbed by those of the male members of the institute), which she sometimes directed toward those in training with her. Nor did it help matters that in a largely Jewish and male profession, she was a non-Jew and a woman. Other émigrés may have resented the fact that she had come to America just before the Nazis took over and had established herself professionally and financially, experiencing few of the problems that plagued them.

Some combination of these factors inspired an internal campaign against her and her allies. The final blow came in April 1941, when the New York Psychoanalytic Society officially demoted Horney from instructor to lecturer, thus stripping her of equal status with the group's other analysts and of the right to act as training analyst. The vote was twenty-four to seven, with ten or more abstentions. She and four other analysts walked out of the meeting. Two days later, they submitted a letter of resignation. "We are interested only in the scientific advancement of psychoanalysis in keeping with the courageous spirit of its founder, Sigmund Freud," they wrote. "This obviously cannot be achieved within the framework of the New York Psychoanalytic Society as it is now constituted." Meanwhile, Fromm began to deviate not only from strict Freudianism but also from the Marxist approach of the Institute for Social Research. Merging understandings of various members of the Zodiac Group and insights from his own intellectual journey, he began to publish in English. His first two pieces, "The Social Philosophy of Will Therapy" and "Selfishness and Self Love," elicited stinging rebukes from more traditional Freudians.[22]

In December 1941, Horney, Thompson, Fromm, and Sullivan, among others, founded their own institute, the Association for the Advancement of Psychoanalysis. However, new problems arose. Horney jealously grasped the reins of the new institute and, in an unanticipated move certainly related to their deteriorating personal relationship, refused to allow Fromm—by then enjoying budding fame due to the publication of *Escape from Freedom* (1941)—to train analysts. The official reason was that Fromm was not a doctor. Fromm, Thompson, and others resigned from the AAP to form the William Alanson White Institute in 1943. By the late 1940s, Fromm, a lay analyst, had become head of the White Institute's training program.

This was the renegade world of psychoanalysis that May entered about the same time as beginning his formal program at Teachers College. He began to attend classes at the Association for the Advancement of Psychoanalysis, taking Clara Thompson's Fundamentals of Psychoanalysis and, in the spring of 1942, Erich Fromm's Society and Psychoanalysis at the New School. The effect of this plunge into the study of psychoanalysis immediately appeared in May's own continuing counseling practice, where evidence of grappling with "transference" and peculiarly psychoanalytic notions of "guilt" began to appear even before his course with Thompson began. At some point in late 1940 or early 1941, he began a training analysis with Fromm.[23]

Accelerating May's entry into this exciting and unsettling world of New York psychoanalysis was his participation in a rather unusual experiment, a private seminar known as the New York Psychology Group. While the nature of religion and religious experience had been of central concern to

William James, G. Stanley Hall, and other pioneers of American psychology, most psychologists and psychoanalysts were wary of connecting a nascent profession in need of scientific grounding to the speculative realm of the spirit. Yet since the late nineteenth century, liberal Christian theologians—taken with personalism and individual growth in grace as the heart of Christianity—saw great possibilities in psychology's exploration of the inner workings of mind and soul.

Important among them was one of May's professors at Union, Harry Emerson Fosdick, who sought the advice of a psychoanalyst to improve the effectiveness of his grappling with parishioners' problems and eventually incorporated psychotherapeutic thinking into his sermons and popular books. Anton Boisen, after being hospitalized for a bout of mental illness and finding a cure in religious experience and renewed faith, became chaplain at Worcester State Hospital in Massachusetts and began to experiment with a combination of psychological insight and religious quest in the treatment of schizophrenia and other debilitating mental diseases. May himself contributed to the field with his lectures, articles, and books on religiously oriented counseling.[24]

The New York Psychology Group owed its existence in part to another pioneer of pastoral psychology, Seward Hiltner. Hiltner had been working within church organizations to promote pastoral clinical training when in 1940 he and some others had invigorating discussions on psychology and religion with Erich Fromm at meetings of the National Council on Religion in Higher Education. Hiltner and Fromm sought an ongoing dialogue, and from that idea grew the New York Psychology Group, which brought together an extraordinary array of persons from varied backgrounds, generations, and points of view.[25] The group met mostly in the homes of its senior members and attempted to foster personal relations across institutional and theoretical lines.

In an era when rival schools of psychological, political, and religious thought mostly ignored or condemned each other, the seminar was unusual in bringing together Jungians and Freudians (or at least neo-Freudians), Christians and Jews, believers and atheists, psychologists and social scientists, native-born Americans and émigrés. The first few meetings, in late 1941 and early 1942, grappled with the nature of faith and featured Martha Glickman, Elined Kotschnig, and Frances G. Wickes, all Jungian analysts, presenting clinical evidence that argued for the "validity of the inner experience." In discussion, Tillich, Fromm, and others asked questions: Could faith exist without God? Without religion? Were different forms of faith equivalent? The dialog continued in February and March, with Harry Bone and Erich Fromm presenting a vision of faith as autonomous, individual well-being shorn of sacred connection. May questioned their vision of faith without external authority and argued that a human being could exist only in relation "to a structure of meaning which is greater than himself, which takes in his fellow men," and which moves one to the realm "where in religious faith we use the word God." May added that "the dynamic individuals in religion (Socrates, Jeremiah, Job, Isaiah) have stood on their own spontaneity against a crystallized form of God" but not against the authority of God. It was his major contribution to a debate that resulted in few compromises.

This religious emphasis returned in April with Tillich's discussion of faith in Judaism and the various Christian churches. He sharply dissented from both the intrapsychic views of the psychologists and the moralistic religious visions of traditional churchgoers. "Faith is union, adherence which includes the promises which contradict our real sinful state cannot but fail," he asserted. "The object of faith is *the paradoxical acting of God* which is especially visible in the character of Christ." To Tillich the "*only* sin" was "*unbelief.*"[26] Ruth Benedict approached the topic from an anthropological perspective. Referring to the unselfconscious religious practices of the "primitive" societies that she and her fellow anthropologists had studied, she noted that faith could exist as a rational rather than paradoxical phenomenon (Fromm over Tillich) but that it very much referred to external powers (Tillich over Fromm). "Faith, in primitive societies," she stated simply, "is just a part of living." The final meeting on the subject was devoted to a general discussion of the meaning of faith and the positions that had been taken in prior meetings.[27]

In the end, these discussions on faith seemed to change no one's mind; each remained basically committed to his or her way of viewing the phenomenon and the implications of that position for religion and culture. Yet the very need to discuss a common set of terms with which to describe otherwise highly specialized theological, psychological, or anthropological positions tended to relativize what in other settings might have appeared to be more rigid positions. The phenomenon of faith became more generically religious, cultural, and psychological than in any of the participants' personal view. In this sense, the discussions of the group modeled a vital phenomenon of a pluralistic society and the need for cross-communication among groups.

One became aware of others' beliefs, speaking to them of one's own faith in a common language.

Having examined the topic of faith from these various perspectives, the group adjourned for the summer and decided to devote its fall 1942 meetings to an exploration of the psychology of love. Love, too, presented myriad problems of definition. Fromm charted the psychoanalytic dimensions of love but also emphasized its ethical dimension. Tillich thought Fromm's ethical humanism excluded "the power of being in reality," the irrational and divine force of Eros as the essence of love, its "saving element," which acted beyond the realm of ethics. It provided the individual with the "possibility of reuniting with the elements of the cosmos from which one is separated." Love became "the will to union," with the cosmos or with another. "In every kind of sex, even perverted forms," he concluded, "there is an element of this will to union which is love. There is an ontological element of identity. Even hate or sadism are perverted forms of love."

May remained mostly silent on the topic of love, even more so than during the discussion of faith. Perhaps he was muted by the intimidating presence of his more famous elders. Perhaps he also felt unsettled enough about both faith and love in his own life to wonder what he might have to contribute in conversations that pitted one firm worldview against another.

14

"Such a Blow Just Now"

May's engagement in school and the invigorating discussions of the New York Psychology Group enriched his life immeasurably but also contributed to a gnawing fatigue and irritability. A man of almost boundless energy, he wavered near the edge of his limits. "Irritable, weary, limping from this place to that, coming home only to fall on the bed, drinking coffee to stimulate tense nerves into some sensibility, taking thyroid to keep at work"—that was how he described himself at the time.[1] He did almost nothing but work— as student, counselor, lecturer, and writer—leaving to Florence the tasks of managing household and child. He did try to keep up with the Tillichs and others around him in the salon culture of arts and flirtations, but this brought as much strain as relief. Whether from exhaustion alone or in combination with guilt and an even more desperate sense of entrapment in marriage, he admitted to Florence that he had, at times, been a "snarling rattlesnake."[2]

Then came the happy news in the fall of 1942 that Florence was pregnant again—though this too increased pressure on Rollo to work still harder as the family's provider. Luckily, he had agreed to teach a course, Religion as a Factor in Personality Adjustment, at Garrett Biblical Institute in the spring of 1943. Teaching at Garrett brought in much-needed financial support and strengthened a budding connection with one of the important seminaries in the nation. Rollo had not been in Evanston long, however, before he came down with a harsh cold, fever, and night sweats. Bed rest didn't help, his symptoms got worse, and doctors at Northwestern insisted that he go to Methodist Hospital in Chicago for diagnosis and care. The doctors tested his sputum and, despite a negative test, suspected tuberculosis. His fever reached a peak in the first nights, and after it receded, they sent him to a local sanatorium for rest and further testing.

The very possibility of tuberculosis left Rollo in a daze. The disease was universally dreaded for its deadly power. Despite modern medicine's attempts at treatment, it remained a major threat. In 1909, the year of May's birth, the disease was first among causes of death in the United States and accounted for more than 10 percent of total fatalities. Improvements in prevention and treatment helped matters, but even in the year of Rollo's diagnosis, nearly sixty thousand Americans died of TB.[3]

Florence consoled him on the telephone but stayed in New York. Pregnant, caring for their son, and facing the difficulties of wartime travel, she knew joining him would have been difficult and possibly dangerous. The only family member in the area was Ruth, who proved to be no help at all. She had come to Chicago for psychotherapy after leaving her husband and adopted child and suffering a mental breakdown. Rollo had lunch with her, and when he told her that he had tuberculosis, she just laughed and joked that she was the one in the family who was supposed to get TB (from her immoral life). She then chattered on about her own problems.[4]

Opinion differed on TB's cause and cure, but all agreed that rest helped enormously. With just a few weeks' break from his busy life, Rollo quickly recovered, finished his teaching, and returned to New York. He suspected a misdiagnosis and by April had advanced to doctoral candidacy, accepted a counseling position at City College of New York, and rejoined the Psychology Group, while Florence entered her eighth month of pregnancy. The pall cast by tuberculosis had begun to lift, but not the whirlwind of work.[5]

The month of April also brought a new dimension of darkness to May's consciousness. His prior counseling experience had been with college students and parishioners at a middle-class church. He had seen poverty and its effects only from a safe distance, among refugees in Greece and in New York during the 1930s. For required degree work, Rollo spent a month counseling indigent, pregnant young women at Inwood House, a charitable agency on West Fifteenth Street in Manhattan. One purpose of this assignment was to employ qualitative and quantitative assessment tools and to create and test psychological hypotheses. Toward that end, May was schooled in the use of various diagnostic tests and scales. For his direct therapeutic supervision, he secured the services of Erich Fromm. May's work at Inwood House met course requirements and also supplied him with case studies for his doctoral dissertation. However, perhaps the most lasting impact of these sessions was a deepening of May's intimate sense of the effects of poverty and perverse family situations and the depths of personal tragedy.[6]

Inwood House was a venerable and forward-looking institution that had been founded in 1830 as a rescue home for prostitutes who wished to reform their lives, and it later expanded into a residence for pregnant and otherwise wayward girls. By the early twentieth century, it had become a progressive force in dealing with sexually related problems among the poor, at first treating venereal disease and by the 1940s adopting modern social work approaches to the problems of its teenage clientele. Starting in the Depression, Inwood House took in girls of all religions and races, in contrast to the denominational and racial segregation practiced at most other social agencies. It was a model of enlightened treatment, and the link with the psychology program at Teachers College signaled its modern outlook. It afforded professional, non-moralistic care to its wards and gave fledgling therapists the most challenging sorts of problems to solve.[7]

May's assignment consisted of assessing and counseling new arrivals. He interviewed individuals, gave them tests, and engaged each in a series of counseling sessions. Most were pregnant, unmarried, and from families in dire straits, and many were victims of incest. Pregnancy out of wedlock was nothing new to the May family, but Rollo had never imagined cases like these. There was Lulu, for instance, a young woman who stood for many and about whom May wrote this in his internal report:

> Lulu is from a waterfront family. She and the large family have lived on a barge on the Jersey shore. It is an incest pregnancy; several of them slept together in one bed, and when the brother would go up on deck the father would have intercourse with Lulu. This happened about three times. The father said he would kill her if she told. The father was in Sing Sing for raping the older sister. . . . Indications that Lulu did not take initiative with father, perhaps tried to resist, but was helpless because of father's threat to kill her. When the mother found out about the pregnancy, she beat Lulu. Mother (who "identifies" with the father, apparently took his side) insists Lulu should bring her baby home and take care of it. The [social workers] have stood by Lulu, indicating that if she does not want to see the baby (as she doesn't), she need not. They are helping her to move out of the family after the pregnancy. Some indication of epilepsy in father, which would be the one thing to make difficulty in the baby's adoptability.[8]

Although Lulu had no time for in-depth psychotherapy before her child was born, her talks with May restored a modicum of trust in the world. He mostly asked her how she was, gently suggested options, and let the social workers of Inwood House try to create opportunities for at least a marginally better future.

The contrast with Florence's pregnancy was vivid. While Rollo worked with victims of incest, Florence took their three-year-old son, Bob, to Lynnhaven,

Virginia (near Norfolk), in order to have her family by her side for the final stretch before she gave birth on May 8 to twin girls, Allegra and Carolyn. Rollo joined the family just in time for the delivery. The next month was an idyll. The DeFrees family was comfortably situated, and being in Virginia provided a striking contrast to the bare-bones life Rollo and Florence could manage in New York. May rested and enjoyed the new infants. He also helped Florence by being a companion to Bob during what was surely a difficult time for his son. In the wake of physical collapse in Chicago and entry into the harsher realities of society at Inwood House, Rollo felt a deep sense of renewal in his marriage. However, the need to support a significantly larger family as they looked toward a return to New York, as well as an itch to get on with things, convinced May that he was well enough to fulfill a commitment he had made to teach in Garrett's summer program, this time giving a course titled Counseling Procedures, Programs, and Plans.

Each night from Chicago, he typed a letter to Florence and in one declared that he had conquered his own worst habits: "I have become convinced that what actually ailed me was that I have been tired for a full two years! It is such a relief to begin to get rested. . . . Now I feel like a new man." He apologized for his prior nastiness, pleading that he had been "just played out." He remembered his prior summer sojourn to teach at Garrett. "Always as I got up before my class I was weary," he wrote, "so weary I was doubtful whether words would emerge when I opened my mouth; always when I came to see you and Bobbie on the beach it was to collapse and smoke to draw frayed nerves together." Now, he assured her, he strode into class "as tho' on spring stilts, leap[ing] into the fray with a licking of chops." He even found it possible to relax. "I work only till noon," reported. "I rest after lunch, then take to the beach where I gather sun among the shapely legs of Northwestern Co-eds, swim a bit and laze the rest of the afternoon." True, he often heard a little voice whispering, "Too much leisure—you better map out some new work to do." Yet he was "fighting the bastard" and was sure that this time he would "lick him." With rest came desire. "I *will* laze away half my days all summer," he promised, "and be brown and fit (and full of libido) when I see you again."[9]

With desire also came a reformed vision for the future. "In accord with the new plan of not killing one's self," he promised to turn down a teaching position at Teachers College and instead concentrate on his dissertation. That was just his first of "many ideas on being a more considerate husband to wife and children." Desire also brought the titillation of jealousy: "Do take care of everyone, Sweetheart, and sleep with yourself a few nights for me." And, as if uneasy about this closing, he added a handwritten line: "I am still very lonely for you, darling. That's the one lack here. But I'll try to bear up!"[10]

Florence continued their oblique and uncomfortable discussion of desire. She had been helping her family with its summer room rentals in the mountains of Virginia and told Rollo a story that proved to her that, in his absence, she had not lost "all feminine allure (is it by any chance increased, I wonder?)." A shy college professor from Kentucky had rented rooms for himself and his two daughters. One morning in the parlor, he asked Florence about Randolph-Macon College for one of his girls. They talked a bit, and when Florence got up, he took her hand. "He mumbled something," she continued, "and began to draw me into his arms! I resisted and looked at him very hard and said, 'What *is* this?'" She pulled away and vowed not to rent to any more lone men. "Well, heigh-ho," she concluded, "it gave me something of interest on which to speculate a while. And I suppose a little inflation to my ego."[11]

This clever sparring lasted until late July, when suddenly Rollo succumbed again to coughing, fever, and sweats. This time there was no mistake—it was tuberculosis. He was rushed to a Chicago hospital, and his condition was so bad, his coughing so intense, he couldn't hope to telephone her. Instead, he scribbled her a simple note to announce the crushing news. She immediately wrote back: "I am still in the first shock of grief—and I suppose—fear. It is so hard to be separated from you—I only want to be with you, to comfort you." She reassured him that "it will be all right in the end," since he had written that the disease seemed only in its earliest stages. She asked for details of the diagnosis and treatment and wondered whether, if he had to spend time in a sanatorium, it could not be one closer to her, in Charlottesville or Lynchburg.[12]

Most crushing to them both was that he should have "such a blow just now when, as you say, everything looked so beautiful for us." She vowed to wait: "If it is possible that you can be back in N.Y. this fall, then truly the short interim is very little time to wait. But even if it takes much longer, we can wait that long. I will send you lots of pictures and daily diaries of the children. I hate so much for you to miss the lovely babyhood of the little girls." She urged him to "do all as they tell you and come back to us soon."[13]

Rollo finally called from the hospital. A doctor had held out hope for a quick and effective treatment. Florence's mind raced from one possibility to the next. She wanted to come to Chicago but worried about overburdening her mother with the children and spending money they did not have. Besides, she imagined Rollo would be in the hospital only a few days longer and then perhaps rest elsewhere for some weeks. Then, she hoped, they could meet in the mountains of Virginia or Pennsylvania. "Have they suggested that six months or so of rest would be the best thing for you?" she asked. "You know I would *dread* such a separation, and you too would hate *it*, but now is the time to do exactly as the doctors advise." And she reiterated her dream for the future, that she might have "a husband who works from 9–5 and then comes home, like other husbands, to relax! I suppose we should have known that nature would take a hand in settling those Olympian tendencies."[14]

As it turned out, the doctors advised a stay at Edward Sanitorium in Napierville, Illinois, where May was admitted on August 18, 1943, with the diagnosis of "moderately advanced fibrotic tuberculosis in the right upper lung field." His sputum test read positive, as did the blood sedimentation test. X-rays confirmed the diagnosis. The doctors performed a pneumothorax— a collapsing of the lung—and tracked its slow healing. At first, Rollo had predicted that he would be back in New York by October. Now, the doctors told him December, possibly January or February. Florence was crushed. She had been reading the letter when Seward Hiltner came by to help construct the twins' new crib. She broke down in tears as she told him the news. Hiltner sat her down, gave her a cigarette, and tried calm her. "There's no getting around the fact that it's damned hard," she complained to Rollo. Despite praising him as "calm and courageous," she couldn't help but be angry with the doctors and, she hinted, at Rollo himself. "I wonder why they haven't already drawn the fluid from your chest, if that is one method of treatment," she asked. "One would think that you, as well as they, expected to make a life-work of T.B. cure." But she closed with love: "I think of you all the time and dream of happy days when all of this will be a long-past trauma like the birth of a baby—the pain forgotten and only the happy results remembered."[15]

May's colleagues and teachers took the news more calmly. Fromm, who himself had contracted and recovered from tuberculosis while still living in Germany, asked to be kept abreast of his progress and noted from his own experience years before that "this kind of enforced rest can be a great blessing in a life which otherwise is so hurried and rushed as that of most of us." Tillich, for his part, thought that it might give him the "Creative Pause" that he needed and hoped that Rollo wouldn't "interrupt the pause too early." The theologian recommended that he "learn in the meantime the art of non-action and meditation with reality *as it is*! There is strength in the unchangeable 'ground of being' and its manifestation in everything that *is*."[16]

Their wisdom did not prevent a sinking feeling of doom and despair. On his first night at Edward Sanitorium, Rollo cried from sheer loneliness and frustration. He knew now there would be no quick cures. He faced the prospect of death or long months, even years, in treatment. Most of all, he missed his children and dreaded the possibility of not seeing them grow up. Rollo finally rejoined his family in November, traveling directly from the sanatorium to Florence's family home in Virginia. It was excruciating. Fear of contagion ruled. He couldn't touch the twins, much less kiss or hug them. Indeed, doctors recommended they always be in different rooms. He could play with Bob, but "not too intimately," which in practice meant at more than arm's length. He returned to New York in late December 1943 and had actually gained twenty pounds during treatment. Nonetheless, the superintendent at Edward Sanitorium and his doctor in Norfolk cautioned against undue optimism and recommended "close observation" of his lungs and periodic testing. The doctor told him that he could continue with his studies but with much reduced activity.[17]

However, May could not curb his compulsion to work. Well before his return, he began to plot out the immediate future. He expected to begin his dissertation in January and was already learning the requirements for graduation. He had been home only a few days before agreeing to give a five-lecture course at McCormick Theological Seminary in Chicago in July and August 1944. By April, he had accepted an invitation to teach a summer course for the Baltimore Conference of the Methodist Church as well. In April and May 1944, he again returned to Inwood House to counsel pregnant girls.[18]

And then, sometime in late May, Rollo's lung cavity began to fill with fluid again.

15

Saranac

The summer of 1944 saw no improvement in May's condition despite a canceled schedule and much rest. In the fall, after further tests and consultations as well as unanimous recommendations from friends and doctors, May sought and secured admission to Trudeau Sanatorium at Saranac Lake, in New York's Adirondack Mountains. He could have chosen no better place to fight for his life. Founded in the late nineteenth century by Dr. Edward Trudeau, the sanatorium grew into a complex of research labs, rest cottages, and a hospital, and by the mid-1940s it had become the country's premier tuberculosis treatment center.

The institution's origins set its personal and humane tone. Trudeau had witnessed his brother's agonizing death from TB and, after contracting it himself, made it his life's mission to find a cure using his own body as a test case. When he noticed that a peaceful trip to the mountains had improved his health, Trudeau experimented and found that a combination of fresh air, peaceful rest, good food, and a modicum of exercise brought him significant recovery.[1] This was in 1874, just as Dr. Hermann Brehmer began to institute a more organized version of the fresh air and rest cure at Görbersdorf, Germany. Robert Koch's discovery of the tubercle bacillus in 1882 paved the way for greater knowledge about how the disease spread. While Trudeau continued his personal struggle against the disease, he and a colleague combined Brehmer's experiment and Koch's breakthrough with his own experience to create the Adirondack Cottage Sanitarium, which admitted its first two patients in 1884.[2]

Adirondack Cottage almost immediately began to expand and spawned the growth of more private cure colonies. This explosion transformed the small village of Saranac Lake, with the nearest railroad stop forty-two miles away in the 1870s, into a bustling health spa with two railroad lines and a population of four thousand by 1903. By 1907, local doctors saw that its popularity might be a health hazard and founded the Saranac Lake Society for the Control of Tuberculosis (better known as the TB Society) to act as a clearing house for information and registration and to aid the Board of Health in enforcement of proper sanitary measures so that the thousands seeking a cure at Saranac Lake did not turn it into a breeding place for the disease.[3]

Although Trudeau Sanatorium served notable patients like writers Robert Louis Stevenson, Stephen Crane, and Walker Percy over the years, it mostly admitted more anonymous souls. Cottages ranged widely in price and level of care, but what counted most was proper attitude and doctors' judgment that the patient's disease was not so advanced that little hope remained. A stay at Trudeau promised more personalized and humane treatment than Edward Sanitorium or the various hospitals at which Rollo had been treated. Neither the institution nor the community stigmatized patients. As the lucky ones regained strength, they mixed freely with townspeople and often returned after they were cured to vacation in the area. The doctors and staff combined a variety of approaches to the disease, treating it surgically as best they could but also relying on the curative powers of rest. Knowing that a patient's attitude and understanding might win victories in cases where the bacillus had not advanced very far, doctors encouraged patients to read, ponder, and write about their experience even as they faced the dark prospect of death.[4]

Rollo thus entered a supportive community and partook of a standard regimen that sought to bolster his will for survival. Arriving from the train station, he was observed for twenty-four hours or more at the reception center and assigned a room based on his physical state. May first spent time in the infirmary but soon moved to a cure cottage where he was restricted mostly to bed rest. As he recovered, he found new lodgings in an "up cottage," among those whom the doctors allowed modest exercise. Rollo passed most days adhering to variations on a schedule implemented by Dr. Lawrason Brown, whose *Rules for Recovery from Pulmonary Tuberculosis* (1916) became a bible for sanatoria across the country. The key principle, of course, was exposure to fresh air, but Brown also believed in a daily plan open to variation depending upon the patient and the severity of the disease.

7:30	Awake. Take temperature. Milk (hot if desired) if necessary. Warm water for washing. Cold sponge.
8:00	Breakfast
8:30	Out of doors in chair or in bed
10:30	Lunch when ordered
11–1	Exercise or rest as ordered
1–2	Dinner. Indoors not over one hour, less if possible.
2–4	Rest in reclining position. Reading, but no talking allowed.

3:30   Lunch when ordered.

4–6   Exercise in prescribed amount.

6:00   Supper.

7:00   Out on good nights.

8:00   Take temperature.

9:00   Lunch and bed.[5]

In all seasons, May and others lay still for hours on a "curing porch," sometimes in the most extreme weather. In the dead of winter, they braved the porch under electric blankets, dressed in fur parkas and mittens, sometimes in temperatures as low as twenty degrees below zero. Such endless repose inspired new and acute sensory knowledge. Rollo learned to tell the temperature by listening to the snow crunch under the feet of the orderlies bringing breakfast—the louder the crunch, the colder the air. Boredom, anxiety, a searing sense of aloneness, appreciation mixed with anger at the calm demeanor of the medical staff, and the desperation of seemingly endless, motionless rest broken only by a slowly increasing modicum of exercise motivated many patients toward self-reflection, spiritual quest, and the creation of myths of causation and cure.[6]

May engaged in all three. Later, in various references to the significance of his stay at Trudeau, sometimes written in the third person, he turned his cure into a striking psychological drama of accepting responsibility for one's life. He observed the habits of those around him who survived and those who died, and the rhythms of his own body as it responded or did not respond to treatment. He decided that he must take control of the tuberculosis as his own and make himself responsible for recovery. Only he could "listen" to his body and "sense when it is strong enough to exercise, to walk . . . what I had to do was take the responsibility myself for the disease."[7]

These retrospective descriptions emphasized taking personal responsibility for one's life—to the extent possible, choosing to live or to die. In one version, he reported "a considerable increase of guilt feeling, because I was the one not only who had the disease but who got it. . . . I had simply run my body into a frazzle." He noted that his "own way of life [was] wrong." He recognized it as an "old pattern," one that first brought him to collapse in Greece. This time he had to accept "the fact that I was not listening to my body . . . that I was living apart from a human society which might have cushioned me against these problems." He knew that he could not depend on medicine and doctors pure and simple, that he faced "struggle within myself." But the facing of self also brought hope. "If I had had some responsibility for getting the disease," he noted, "I then also could have some hope for getting over it." May very much emphasized that passivity had an unfortunate appeal and dire consequences. He remembered a patient at Trudeau, "a very nice girl," perhaps age twenty, who was "sweet to everybody" and seemed quite optimistic. It turned out to be a pretense. One night she overdosed on Seconal and drowned herself in the lake.[8]

May's later focus on the notion of a patient "taking responsibility" made much sense in light of the existential psychologist he would become. His struggle at Trudeau involved profound spiritual and religious experimentation as well as self-analysis and will. Despite the essential loneliness of his situation, his isolation was not as complete as he later depicted it. He enjoyed the close intellectual and emotional companionship of Cyril Richardson, professor of church history at Union and a fellow victim of tuberculosis. Richardson had begun treatment a little over a year before, and by the time May arrived in September 1944, he had graduated to a kind of maintenance rest home just outside the sanatorium proper on Saranac Lake's ritzy Park Avenue. He and Rollo were the same age and had known each other slightly in New York. At Saranac Lake, they became intimate friends.[9]

Cyril Richardson was one of the most beloved faculty members on the Union campus.[10] Born in England in 1909, educated first at the University of Saskatchewan and then Union Seminary, he was brilliant and quirky, the consummate individualist. One admirer who heard Richardson preach in the 1960s and 1970s, described him as having the look of "a proper English gentleman, and you could imagine him with a bowler and a cutaway on his way down Bond Street in London." He spoke with a "thick English accent." He was a student of the early church, and his translation of representative patristic documents, *Early Christian Fathers*, remains a standard text in the field. Richardson's work on Gnosticism provided the groundwork for the later exploration of homosexuality in the early church. Late in life, Richardson wrote about Christianity and ecology.[11]

In all, he was a deeply affecting, charismatic, and inventive Christian, one who sought out the mystical and the miraculous in his own religious experience and strove to expand religious dialogue to include intimations of and experiments with the transcendent. May's residency at Trudeau allowed Richardson to share his experiences, discuss ideas, and try to help May conquer his disease. Richardson was especially anxious for May to try spiritual healing. He credited most of his own "recent progress" to the "faith and intercessions" of one healer in particular, Rufus Moseley, and had already asked Moseley to include May in his prayers. Richardson's embrace of the healer marked a fascinating intertwining of American spiritual odysseys. Moseley studied on a graduate level under William James at Harvard while James was writing his epochal work on psychology and religion, *The Varieties of Religious Experience*. James exposed him to mind cure and in particular to the healing practices of Christian Science. Moseley felt deeply drawn to the curative aspects of "positive thinking" and prayer but remained committed to biblical Christianity. He spent the rest of his life working out what seemed to most an embrace of opposites. After some involvement with Christian Science, he accepted the Holy Spirit in a spiritual vision and converted to Pentecostalism in 1910. By the 1940s, he had already become an important part of Camps Farthest Out, a Pentecostal retreat movement that sought to combine Christian fellowship and experiential, curative prayer.[12]

Richardson countered May's initial skepticism by arguing that one did not have to "believe" in Moseley's method to be helped. "One of the things known about telepathy and clairvoyance is that conscious doubts do not interfere with it," he assured May, "if one approaches the problem with an inner sincerity—with the will, let us say, the will to enquire truthfully and make an effort." He himself was "in an honest quandary about it—believing and disbelieving." Richardson rejected only the "*will* to disbelieve." Thinking of himself and Rollo, he noted that the more highly trained the intellect, the less likely one is to remain connected to the world of spirit. However, he thought Moseley was capable of bringing a curative spirit to both of them.[13] Rollo had reservations but, like Jung, Freud, James, and others, did not reject the possibility of telepathy and other invisible communications. Indeed, May employed not only Moseley but also a second spiritual communicator. At that moment, like Richardson, he drew few boundaries in his search for physical and, ultimately, spiritual well-being. He explored, systematized, explored again.[14]

May and Richardson engaged in a constant dialogue despite the logistics of Trudeau Sanatorium and Rollo's health. Sometimes, once a week at most and only after he could muster the energy and gain permission from his doctors, May traveled the short distance to Richardson's abode for a few hours of conversation. Mostly they engaged in an unusually brisk correspondence, exchanging letters while living only a mile apart. Although May's letters do not survive, the enthusiastic discourses from "Cy" reflect some of the urgency and substance of their views. One clear disagreement emerged in Richardson's valuation of religious and psychic experience over psycho-logical cure. Early in their correspondence, he speculated at length about "psychosomatic [Christian] medicine" and what his battle with a common cold taught him—"all disease is *providential*: it is the bodily expression of *inner conflict*, and rightly used brings health of soul *first*, and then of body." He then worked out a "study plan on the hierarchy of healing" that included four roads to health: "mechanical-biological," "psychological," "psychical," and "religious." Each worked autonomously though in harmony. Like May, Richardson sought the proper boundaries between these kinds of phe-nomena. Thus he noted that the "bath at Lourdes" was not an "analytical couch."[15]

May shared Richardson's sense of the close interactions of mind and body and accepted the efficacy of ritual and prayer. He did protest, however, Richardson's touting of psychical cures and the value of séances. Rollo espe-cially objected to his friend's favorable impression of Edgar Cayce, the famous medium and faith healer. When Richardson got word (through his fiancée, who was a nurse at Trudeau and acted as courier for the correspondents) of May's "by no means enthusiastic" opinion of Cayce, he fired back a four-page response in which he confessed that he had already asked Cayce to assess his own case. He even noted that he was thinking of giving a course on par-apsychology at Union but feared he would be "skinned alive" for doing so. "Why shouldn't a Christian try to understand the miracles of the Bible," he protested, "instead of wasting time fooling with E, P, D and Q!" (The letters are references to the way modern biblical scholars ascribe authorship for var-ious parts of Scripture.)[16]

The pair also discussed psychoanalysis. Richardson had been analyzed by Harry Bone and hoped to gain even more from self-analysis. May gave him some tips on the subject during one of their talks, and psychological self-understanding began to rival psychic experience as one of Cyril's passions. He admitted to Rollo that he had made himself "a bit of a wreck" after dig-ging deep and weathering "the worst analytic storm of my career." Part of the storm was drug-related, for he had taken Seconal as a sleeping pill and soon discovered it had other effects. "I let myself *see things* under its influence," he reported, "which I hid from myself when sober."

In particular, he had worked an entire afternoon on one longstanding emotional conflict. He became deeply anxious, took Seconal that night, and "got a very clear picture of what I had purposely confused for years." He supposed the drug gave him the "inner, subconscious confidence" to grapple with tough issues, "in much the same way a drink gives you the confidence to smash the boss on the nose instead of being his doormat!" Richardson admitted that drug-induced insights might be "exaggerated and distorted" yet praised Seconal for shortening the time needed for self-discovery. "I think I shall write [Karen] Horney a letter on *Sekonal* [sic] *as a short-cut to self-analysis*," he joked to May, "for in truth, this Experience rates in intensity and advance only with two crises during my years with Harry [Bone]."[17]

Rollo tried to help his friend view his drug-induced visions through a lens of psychoanalytic theory. For instance, after a conversation with Rollo about the nature of Seconal, Cyril worked out a system to differentiate the revelations by noting their relation to Freudian concepts of free association and dissociation. Richardson's remarks are noteworthy not only within the context of his dialogue with May but also as a nascent exploration of hallucinatory drugs, religious experience, and psychological insight that became more common in the 1960s and 1970s.[18] Richardson was sure that Seconal had helped him go beyond the valuable but limited state of free association ("you *look out* the window" and report everything) to his own ecstatic state ("In D[issociation] you *are out* of the window"). In "F.A. you 'will' to *record* the 'madman'" whereas in "D. you will *to be* the 'madman.'" And so on. Richardson exulted in the complete loss of rational consciousness, called it true ecstasy ("being 'out' quite literally—'out' of Freud's window"), and saw great similarities between such moments and the trance states within which parapsychologists worked.[19]

Richardson most often responded excitedly to May's suggestions, though not always. Rollo once sent him a copy of Karl R. Stolz's *The Church and Psychotherapy*, which had been published the year before and had made a splash in the pastoral counseling world. May recommended it to his friend and was no doubt unprepared ready for his friend's nasty condemnation of the work. Richardson blasted it as "uninformative and uninspiring," "downright Methodist balderdash," and "typical of the Abingdon Press." "[Stolz] has about him," Richardson wrote, plunging in the dagger, "something of the Methodist—YMCA—'extrovert' (in the bad sense) counselor, who thinks neuroses can be cured by a trick of prayer and calisthenics. . . . His book is ample evidence of the danger of ministers getting a smattering of psychiatry." It is unclear whether Cyril knew of May's YMCA background, Methodist upbringing, or previous work with Abingdon Press. Perhaps so, because, realizing what this rant might sound like to Rollo, he added that he was "devoutly thankful that you and a few others are in a favoured position by training and experience eventually to produce something decent along this line."[20]

Richardson's combativeness barely hid the turbulence of his conflicted attraction to May, feelings most often ignited by May's visits to his house. "So strongly does my subconscious have to protect itself against you," he confessed, "that what seems to happen on my part is a sort of bellicose strategy of defense—a kind of Maginot Line tactic of security." He disputed every point Rollo tried to make and all because, he admitted, what he really wanted was "to put a dragon in your warm, sunny garden. But I have a hell of a time to get 'in.'" Recounting a parable in "symbols," Richardson juxtaposed "Mimi" and "Horseflesh," the feminine and masculine in him, and realized that Mimi needed to turn herself into a dragon in order to brave any sort of surrender to May. Nor did he doubt that his friend "might resent having a fucking dragon turn up in this warm and sunny spot." "I want to get into your garden but can only do so by turning myself into a dragon," he repeated. "The result is we make little progress while we are together. Only afterwards, by reflecting on much you have said, do I see and feel things I had to prevent myself from seeing and feeling while you were here."[21]

Now, however, Mimi was ready to show herself. Richardson suggested that he be invited to Rollo's room at Trudeau:

> and you would put on your black eye-shade [standard issue for a TB patient] and take me into your garden where it is warm and sunny. Fix it up just as you would like with prayers or Bible reading or whatever you prefer. But nothing would give me greater joy than to have you take me there, when I don't have to wear a dragon's disguise of which I have now disposed. Will you set a date for my pilgrimage?[22]

Pilgrimage. That is surely what it would have been, because aside from his plainly sexual passion for Rollo, Cyril felt the pull of Christian love in the profoundest sense, a joining of souls in the spirit of Cyril's beloved early Christian community. Their discussions of Christianity and psychotherapy, he assured Rollo, were "touching on the most vital parts of our being." He needed forgiveness for "all the tumult and shouting" but was sure that it would be granted because their spirits needed each other. "There is a part of me which is you, just as there is a part of you which is me," he wrote. "That is the mystery of friendship. And only when the part of you which is identical with me tells me you forgive me will the harmony be complete." He realized that Rollo the analyst might view such a declaration as mere projection. "But here I am more Christian than analytical. I feel you have borne my sins, and you owe me either a forgiveness or a resentment. If only the latter emerges there is no harmony, and the best I can do is to forgive myself. But if the former entails we are both closer to the Ground of Being."[23]

Cyril longed for a soul mate and perhaps a lover but had to settle for what Rollo himself had found in Cy, an exciting if sometimes exasperating intellectual companion. In this sense, their friendship was reminiscent of Rollo's relationship with Oberlin's Charles Wager. In both cases, May would go only so far in meeting the yearnings of his male companions.

May's less effusive tone in dialogue with Richardson no doubt had to do with fears of his friend's intimate designs, not just sexual but spiritual. If Richardson's creative expansion of Christian faith and psyche were flowering in powerful but quirky ways, May's commitment to a specific Christian vision was quickly receding. Paradoxically, the influence shaping his retreat was that most passionately Christian of philosophers, Søren Kierkegaard. Even as Richardson recommended books on psychics and parapsychology routes to spiritual rejuvenation, Rollo returned the favor by suggesting that Cy read Walter Lowrie's biography of the dour Dane.[24]

Kierkegaard stood at the very center of a transformation in May's thinking—indeed, his whole concept of human consciousness—as well as his change in calling. May's reading of Kierkegaard not only aided in his recovery from tuberculosis but also provided the inner foundation for the doctoral dissertation that he had begun to research and that would become his next book, *The Meaning of Anxiety*. Years later, May discussed reading Freud and Kierkegaard at Saranac, and especially his reactions to the views of each on the anxious state. Freud's approach distinguished realistic fear—caused by conscious awareness of inner conflict or external threat—from the more unconscious, "neurotic" anxiety that pervaded consciousness and seemed to spring from no specific source. "Kierkegaard, on the other hand," May noted, "described anxiety as the struggle of the living being against non-being, and went on to point out that the real terror in anxiety is not death as such (with which we T.B. patients were daily confronted) but the fact that each of us within himself is on both sides of the fight," that "anxiety is a desire for what one dreads." Like an "alien power it lays hold of an individual, and yet one cannot tear one's self away." In short, the philosopher described while the analyst diagnosed, and the former's description reflected May's own desperate searching at Saranac.[25]

May found most compelling Kierkegaard's concept of the "leap of faith," and particularly the role of will in life and in combating disease. These questions he discussed with Richardson, who agreed with May that, knowing what was "right," one willed that state by "letting all the fears and demons and ambivalence emerge, and by fighting them in terror and faith." In the case of TB, Richardson argued that one "must first find the *reason* for being sick, psychologically, and *will* the new 'gestalt' which will bring mental health—then physical." Unlike Rollo, however, Richardson felt that "a final resolution comes by grace—the 'lights' all suddenly go on. It is the repeated and repeatable experience of conversion. By willing a new 'gestalt' one finally *becomes* it."[26]

We do not know exactly when May embraced Kierkegaard's vision of anxiety, but it was most certainly during his convalescence. While he could understand Richardson's idea of willing despite terror, he came to reject the dramatic denouement—"the lights go all on" and one is made new. Cyril's vision represented one sort of Christianity, Kierkegaard's another. May embraced the latter's idea that only with death does the battle with terror end, and at the same time, only with the terror of anxiety can the individual truly become himself. One passage from Kierkegaard's journals seemed to sum up May's feelings at the time:

> Deep within every man there lies the dread of being alone in the world, forgotten by God, overlooked among the tremendous household of millions upon millions. That fear is kept away by looking upon all those about one who are bound to one as friends or family; but the dread is nevertheless there and one hardly dares think of what would happen to one if all the rest were taken away.[27]

Facing death stripped Rollo of his defenses against that dread, even the fear of losing those bound to him as friends and family. This was especially true in the case of Florence, mostly in Virginia grappling alone with the demands of parenting three young children. His extended stay at Saranac Lake devastated her. The once vital dream of a new Rollo, who finally saw the dangers in his impossibly busy life, a husband who came home each day and relaxed with family, and, perhaps, a spouse whose sexual life had become more focused on his wife—that dream had been crushed.

Nor did she withhold her feelings. When Rollo reported some happier moments in his convalescence (perhaps his discussions with Cyril) and worried about her tendency to overwork, she snapped back: "I am compelled by the needs of three little children and my situation differs from yours in that my body is tough enough not to get T.B., but I suffer all the fatigue and enervation of a depleted physical state." To his suggestion that they rent a house in the Saranac area for the following summer (assuming he was well enough), she pointed out the work involved in maintaining a house. "No, thanks," she demurred, "I don't want any vacation like that." Rollo scribbled on the note: "Resentful letter after I wrote her of my good times—I have heretofore wrote her my unhappy aspects so that she would not resent—If I get along well, her resentment increases. . . . Conclusion: I must write merely objective letters. . . . I have to get well on my own—regardless of her."[28]

Things seemed a little better when Florence visited him later in the fall, leaving the children with her mother in Virginia and taking the long train ride from Norfolk to Saranac Lake. She wrote soon after that she had "finally" come to see the bleakness of his life as a patient. "I thought I understood before," she admitted, "but no one can who has not been there; and now, because of better understanding of myself as well, I honor you where before I sometimes blamed you." She resigned herself to his long-term convalescence. Still, she lived a harried life, "surrounded and distracted by the myriad demands of children, the home situation," all of which were compounded by her mother's complaints about their son's behavior while she was away.[29]

By January 1945, May had recovered to the degree that his family could visit him. On the surface and in the company of others, all was jolly. Rollo rented a place near Cyril (who had just married), and the couples visited each other. Cyril wrote later that the twins "stole [his] heart" and that Louise, his new wife, now "has to have twins!" Still, his doctor ordered May to stay far enough from Florence and his children so that no droplet of tubercular bacilli could reach them. No kisses, no hugs.[30]

More searing still was Florence's revelation that she had been having an affair with Harry Bone. Hints punctuated letters here and there—she and Harry went to the movies together or Harry lent her a book—all things that good friends might do in innocence. Later, Rollo claimed he felt some relief that, while he was convalescing, she might be paid such attention, and that only when the affair continued after his return to New York did he feel hurt. In fact, he kept such feelings well hidden, perhaps even speaking only obliquely about them with Florence. After all, he had had his own affairs before TB, so he had little ground upon which to stand when facing his wife. Twenty-five years later, in a correspondence that Harry Bone initiated to clarify his friendship with May, one of Bone's letters revealed just how bottled up May's feelings had become and, perhaps, how conveniently obtuse were Bone's own perceptions. "I was totally unaware of your feelings of vulnerability after [Saranac]," Bone wrote. "If you had expressed your self to me you could have ended what bothered you promptly. I thought you didn't mind but even welcomed it as a convenience for your own adventures. How wrong, apparently, I was." Harry also reminded him of his ambivalence about Florence from the very beginning, implying how easy it was to misread his feelings.[31]

Before Florence informed him of the affair with Bone, May's attitude toward Florence and infidelity had been a mixture of jealousy and a rationalizing paternalism concerning the proper forms her adultery should take. In correspondence with Florence after his first relapse, Rollo admitted that a string of jealous letters following a trip she had made to New York from Virginia was inspired by her staying with the Tillichs. He had not wanted to mention it specifically, since he wanted her to live her own life while he was gone. Florence wrote about the trip, saying she hoped he hadn't "lost any sleep, with 'jealous pictures,'" but added, "or do I hope so?" Rollo responded, "Yes, I did have jealous pictures, not one night, Miss, but *two*. . . . But apparently you had some ideas yourself—hoping I would be jealous . . . ? And possibly some phantasies (meaning 'hope?') yourself?" Rollo had figured that when she did sleep at the Tillichs', "there was more than a 50-50 chance of . . . his not coming into your room at some nice hour like 2:00 AM." Hannah, he thought, "would have connived nicely, seeing that you and Paul had plenty of privacy. Now, I knew you were carrying around a fairly good-sized *yen* for a man on that trip. So, I ask you, what should I think?"[32]

Rollo confessed to great jealousy but insisted that it was far less "possessive" than before. He had decided that he hadn't treated her "enuf as a responsible, autonomous human being." He also had realized the unfairness of "allowing myself more liberty in dating others, having women friends, etc., than I was permitting you." What if Tillich *had* made an early morning conquest? He couldn't imagine being "rabidly angry" at either of them. "One thing, however," he explained, "which I could *not* have stood was your subsequent explaining it in terms of, 'he came in, I just couldn't send him away,' or 'I so much wanted a man,' etc.—any of those rationalizations on the basis of *weakness* would have blown me up." Rather, if it came, he hoped Florence would embrace such an encounter "as a strong, responsible, autonomous person." In all, he anticipated that "my permitting you responsible freedom, and being willing to take the adjustment if it did lead to relationships with someone else—might make you appreciate me more. (!!! Is that male conceit?) Actually, conceit or not, it might make us appreciate each other more." And he signed off with an "all my love" to "the most desirable woman in all the world."[33]

In the affair with Harry Bone, Florence played by her own rules, not Rollo's paternalistic permissions. It hurt his vanity no end and, even after she gave up her lover, further poisoned their marriage with mutual resentment and icy disillusion.

16

"The Most Important Thing"

May's return to New York City—and to a scarred marriage that had settled into a routinized détente—marked a quiet rebuilding of his professional life. For the next five years, until doctors declared him totally free of tuberculosis, May lectured little, traveled less, and concentrated on finishing his doctoral dissertation. His plans to become a psychoanalyst and continue writing for the public had not changed. Nor was he a slacker. In addition to researching and writing what would become his third book, *The Meaning of Anxiety*, he also started a counseling practice and, late in the decade, resumed his training analysis with Erich Fromm at the William Alanson White Institute. Yet he approached the world more aware of its darkness and with even greater commitment to affirming the worth of individuals. May took his brush with tuberculosis and marital comeuppance as twin reminders of life's contingencies. He rushed into life with breathless ambition and a brittle surety that he had mastered its truths, but he could deny neither mortality nor the possibility of shame and loss.

These lessons greatly deepened May's sense of the stakes of existence. A famous quotation from Spinoza that he first used as an epigraph for *The Art of Counseling* perhaps brought solace and insight to him in 1945: "I saw that all the things I feared had nothing good or bad in them save as the mind was affected by them. He who understands himself and his emotions loves God, and the more so the more he understands himself and his emotions." Tuberculosis and sexual humbling became, among other things, grist for the mill.[1] They also seemed to inspire an empathy distinct from that of his pastoral counseling days. Rather than emulating Christ in striving to completely identify with the patient, he mixed a warm empathy with analytic distance as he started his practice in 1946.

Some cases from the first few years of his new practice reflected May's developing therapeutic style, as well as his approach to issues of will, courage, and the relationship of individual authenticity to meaning. In at least one case, he proffered rather advanced sexual advice for a therapist of his time. Thirty-year-old Elver Barker entered therapy with what he thought was a simple problem of will. Although he was gay, Barker desperately wanted to marry a woman and have a family—to be "normal." As a teenager, he had felt comfortable with his sexual orientation but at age twenty-four "became converted" to the notion that homosexuality was "a mental illness to be 'cured.'" He abstained from sex with men for six years "in a futile endeavor to become heterosexual" and saw two therapists who promised they could make him change. Neither abstention nor therapy did the trick but rather nearly caused him to have a "nervous breakdown." "It was when I was fighting my nature," he recalled, that he read one of May's books (probably *The Springs of Creative Living*) and set up an appointment. "He was very kind," Barker noted of May, "and helped me to understand that my problem was not homosexuality but fear." Such insight and acceptance took hold over time. Within three or four years, Barker gave up his quest and fully accepted his sexual orientation, developing a career as an artist and teacher and eventually becoming a gay rights activist in Colorado.[2]

That May could defy psychoanalytic orthodoxy concerning homosexuality at such an early date spoke not only to his training—a mix of neo-Freudian influence at the White Institute, rather open sexual boundaries honored by his mentor, and the broad valuation of love implicit in liberal Christianity— but also to the fact that, though he was clearly heterosexual, many of his most intimate and rewarding relationships were with plausibly gay men like Charles Wager, Buck Weaver, and Cyril Richardson. May seemed never to give their sexuality a second thought unless they wished to be too intimate, as in the case of Richardson, and the value he placed on being authentic to one's own inner self trumped even social taboo.[3]

The same might be said of his attitude toward his women clients. While Matie and Ruth shaped his fear of entanglements with women, they also made him deeply aware of the problems women faced in society and relationships—as did his own marriage. All three in some way inspired in him a commitment to support and comfort, to be a "knight," which often translated well in the therapeutic hour. For instance, a young woman in college emphasized the reassuring aspects of May's presence. Plagued by a dominating father and "psychotic alcoholic" mother, she suffered disturbing symptoms—writer's block, constriction in the chest, and colitis. She had tried various therapists without success. One told her that the real problem was her father and "that's basically all you need to know." Another began with a variation on Freud's cardinal rule of analysis: "Now just lie down and tell me anything that comes into your mind, even if it's a little obscene." A third declared himself an "orthodox Freudian" and insisted that she would have to give up her strong religious beliefs. These were all men. She tried a woman doctor, who repeatedly interrupted her mid-sentence "with aggressive snap judgments" and called her "a very sick girl" when she protested. She tried one last psychiatrist, whose first question was whether she could pay for treatment.[4]

No wonder, then, that with May she felt she "hit gold." She had heard him speak on the subject of psychology and religion and felt drawn to him. She called him from a church phone booth after a debilitating panic over school exams and asked whether he could help. May responded, "I think I can help you help yourself," and arranged to see her the next morning. They met four times a week for several years, and after the first session her panic attacks vanished, never to return. Rollo's response to her effusive gratitude for helping to transform her life was that she was "worth it." She became a successful academic in an age that put myriad roadblocks in the way of women pursuing such a career. That May felt she was "worth it"—that her individual, meaningful goals were worth preserving in the face of resistance—had much to do with her ultimate triumph.[5]

Both patients suffered at least in part from symptoms of what we would now call anxiety. They experienced them during decades when use of the word in English—*Angst* in German—was moving from the simple denotation of a generalized fearful feeling or affect to one that referred to a metaforce of individual and cultural existence. May's woman patient had, in retrospect, actually labeled her malaise an "anxiety attack," though she may not have called it this in the 1940s. Elver Barker's brush with what he called a "nervous breakdown" over his homosexuality was a variety of what therapists now classify as "generalized anxiety" or "panic disorder." Both of his patients came to understand their symptoms as created in part by broader social and cultural forces at work around them.

One oft-cited reason for this transformation of anxiety from symptom to cultural "problem" in the postwar period was that cataclysmic events—the Great Depression, two world wars, state-sponsored genocide, and the atomic bomb—had in little more than three decades pulverized a sense of everyday security and introduced the possibility of humanly engineered global suicide. Yet anxious symptoms had plagued bodies and minds for millennia before the twentieth century. Shamans, witches, doctors, philosophers, theologians, biologists, and poets had all strained to describe, explain, and cure anxiety's manifestations, which without warning might paralyze the mightiest in nameless terror. Most in the distant past had credited the onset of symptoms to direct intervention of God, the Devil, or multiplicities of invisible spirits from without, while others, especially early doctors and scientists, traced its origins to physical disorders.

However, by the nineteenth century, an intertwining of scientific, theological, and literary forces began to underline, isolate, and define the anxious state in increasingly comprehensive ways. Some saw anxiety's mood of pervasive unease develop as a reaction to various disorienting aspects of modernity—the rationalizing tendencies of the market, the rise of nation-states, the decline of ecclesiastical power and questioning of theological traditions in the wake of scientific developments and the continuing corrosive effect of the Reformation. The anxious fear that religious faith and, indeed, civilization were slowly crumbling expressed itself as a vivid theme in philosophy and theology as well as in literature and music. Some of May's favorite romantic poets gave it powerful voice, none more so than William Wordsworth and Matthew Arnold (May's college favorites) and such later writers as William Butler Yeats and T. S. Eliot.

In addition, the once obscure Kierkegaard, who had made angst central to his sense of human existence, caught the imagination of such thinkers as Tillich and Martin Heidegger during the first third of the twentieth century. Translation of Kierkegaard's works into English, which began in earnest in the 1930s, led to an intense interest in and popularization of his thought in seminaries, universities, popular magazines, and even the Roosevelt White House. W. H. Auden read Kierkegaard during World War II and gave a name to the postwar epoch in his long, six-part poem of 1947, *The Age of Anxiety: A Baroque Eclogue*. Auden's poem inspired Leonard Bernstein's Symphony no. 2, *The Age of Anxiety*, which premiered in 1949 and in turn became the musical backdrop for Jerome Robbins's ballet of the same name. Even Alan Watts, who had already become a popularizer of Zen Buddhism, borrowed the phrase for a chapter title in his 1951 volume *The Wisdom of Insecurity*. "Anxiety" had become a keyword of the culture.[6]

Even as poets, philosophers, and theologians explored the world of anxiety, doctors, biologists, neurologists, and psychologists were broadening their own definition of anxious symptoms. Nineteenth-century psychiatrists and psychologists began to redefine such symptoms as having their origins at least partially in mental distress, especially where there otherwise seemed to be no obvious organic problem. In complicating the question of mind-and-body interactions, they opened one of the most fruitful and endlessly complicated scientific questions, one that remains unresolved.[7]

A crucial shift for psychiatric medicine's understanding of anxiety came with Freud's invention of psychoanalysis. In his *Introductory Lectures in Psychoanalysis* (1917), Freud described the "problem of anxiety" as "a nodal point at which the most various and important questions converge, a riddle whose solution would be bound to throw a flood of light on our whole mental existence." He did not claim that he had a "complete solution" but assured his readers that traditional anatomical approaches were a dead end. "I know nothing that could be of less interest to me for the psychological understanding of anxiety," he declared, "than a knowledge of the path of the nerves along which its excitations pass." By the 1920s, Freud came to see anxiety more as the result of generalized unconscious conflict within the ego. However, this less mechanical explanation in some ways only deepened anxiety's mysteries. Indeed, in his detailed rethinking of the phenomenon, *Hemming, Symptom und Angst* (1926, translated as *The Problem of Anxiety* in 1936), Freud admitted that in confronting the "riddle" of anxiety, "after decades of analytic effort this problem rises up before us, as untouched as at the beginning."[8]

May was becoming familiar with these various new views of anxiety from the mid-1930s onward, largely through Tillich, who first exposed the young American to Kierkegaard and Heidegger, as well as to the work of Kurt Goldstein. However, some indication that even in the late 1930s the word itself had not yet attained its vivid cultural power was its absence from both *The Art of Counseling* and *Springs of Creative Living*. These works focused on the physical and mental effects of fear, melancholy, and "the abyss of meaninglessness" and described "being forced by an invisible nemesis to do battle but being able to find nothing to fight" as "the most paralyzing of all horrors." Yet May never called these conditions anxiety.[9]

However, several books published between 1939 and 1941 helped May and others frame anxiety in ever-broader terms. Most publicly visible was Erich Fromm's pathbreaking *Escape from Freedom* (1940), a psychosocial explanation of fascism's appeal that became a bestseller even as America edged closer to entering the war against Hitler. Fromm avoided the word "anxiety" but nonetheless laid the basis for its expanded meaning. He argued that modern capitalism, built upon freedom within a world of competitive individualism, engendered a sense of alienation from one's fellow citizens and led to a profound loneliness that might be relieved by giving up one's freedom in favor of identification with a disciplined movement or authoritarian nation. Fromm applied his analysis to its most extreme case—the German surrender of freedom to the Nazi state—as well as to the less politically explicit but still powerful surrender of autonomy evident even in "democratic" mass societies. For Fromm, loneliness and the feeling of powerlessness in modern forms of freedom led inevitably to a wish to escape: "Aloneness, fear, and bewilderment remain; people cannot stand it for ever." Interestingly, Fromm mentioned Kierkegaard, a prophet of this modern condition, but eschewed his theological understandings in favor of Freud and Marx.[10]

Less visible but just as influential on May was Kurt Goldstein, whom May had interviewed on the question of anxiety in 1937. At the core was a theory of self-actualization rooted in biological survival and reproduction, but crucial to the more speculative realms of consciousness and creativity. Like Fromm, Goldstein posited that modernity encouraged a sense of isolation that individuals experienced as an unbearable threat to the self. However, Goldstein emphasized intellectual rather than socioeconomic causes. In his view, the nineteenth-century explosion of scientific knowledge, aided and abetted by disciplinary specialization and materialist narrowing of data and theory, had paradoxically shattered an older and more unitary view of human existence. Implicitly and sometimes explicitly, he posited a continuum between the brain-damaged veterans he treated after World War I and the modern everyman. The veterans struggled to recover in a world made strange by injury, while modern humankind uneasily tried to make sense of a world crippled by the splintering effects of science and materialism.[11]

In that theory, anxiety played a central but ambiguous role. It was the result of what Goldstein called the "catastrophic condition," in which an organism feels its very existence endangered. Perception of possible destruction from a particular and objectively dangerous cause creates fear. "Anxiety is the subjective experience of that danger to existence," Goldstein noted. The catastrophic shock that created such anxiety might have been rooted in a real event. However, anxiety was experienced as a more diffuse and objectless feeling: "It is the inner experience of being faced with nothingness." Panic Anxiety arose when facing new circumstances or challenges, a condition endemic to modernity. To face a nameless threat and conquer it, in short to live uneasily but successfully with anxiety, was the gateway to creativity and self-actualization. Goldstein even made reference to Kierkegaard, paraphrasing him to the effect that "the more original a human being is, the deeper his anxiety is."[12]

Exposure to these visions and personal contact with Fromm and Goldstein inspired May to propose the "meaning of anxiety" as the topic of his doctoral dissertation. It appealed to May not only because of its central importance but also because of his urge toward critical juxtaposition and synthesis. Tuberculosis precipitated both a break in his research and a profound insight concerning anxiety. Hovering on the brink of death as he read Kierkegaard's *The Concept of Dread* made profound what might have been an academic exercise and reinforced his commitment to placing an ontological frame around Freudian theory. We do not know the original scope of his dissertation proposal, except that as part of a degree program in psychology it would have at its core a project in experimental psychology. Returning to the dissertation in 1946, he planned to weave together strands of science, theology, philosophy, social science, and psychology to understand anxiety's significance as comprehensively as possible.

May was aided in this process by members of his doctoral committee and others with whom he consulted while writing. His official chair was P. M. Symonds, a central figure in educational psychology whose own interest in anxiety can be gauged by the fact that he devoted an unprecedented two major chapters to the topic in his 1946 book *The Dynamics of Human Adjustment*.[13] Symonds in turn had learned much from the University of Illinois behaviorist O. H. Mowrer, who did pioneering work on anxiety in the late 1930s and early 1940s.[14] Symonds contacted Mowrer, who consulted with Rollo as he was writing his chapters. In addition, May shared his draft chapters with Goldstein and, as always, with Tillich.

May received his PhD in 1949, and the dissertation was published virtually unchanged as *The Meaning of Anxiety* in 1950. It helped to revitalize psychological research on and general interest in the significance and origins of the anxious state. The book summarized and critically evaluated the presuppositions, theories, and implications of modern experimental psychology, interpreted May's own data from Inwood House, and put the concept of anxiety in a broadly humanistic context. It shared with May's earlier books a syncretic spirit, one that summarized the range and substance of prior thinking. Despite the formalistic infelicities of a dissertation, it moved beyond any one theory in order to understand anxiety in its fullest human dimensions.

May structured the study in two parts: "Modern Interpretations of Anxiety" and "Clinical Analysis of Anxiety." The first part provided a comprehensive cross-disciplinary review of the modern scientific and social science literature on the subject within the cultural contexts of Western literature, theology, and philosophy. The second presented empirical evidence from his work at Inwood House and a case study of an analytic patient. May held in tension a view of the contemporary era and the postwar moment as peculiarly prone to anxiety, while at the same time emphasizing a more religio-psychological view of anxiety as an ever-present fact of the human condition. As important, he argued that the concept prevalent in psychology—anxiety as pathology—was incomplete in its dismissal of the role of anxiety as the inevitable source and handmaiden of growth, creativity, and wisdom.

First, May established a philosophical pedigree for anxiety. He noted that Spinoza and Pascal had each identified anxious shifts of consciousness brought about by the rationalist revolution of the Enlightenment and beyond. Spinoza attempted to conquer fear and anxiety with reason, while Pascal took on the lonely task of highlighting the anxiety of human lostness and the insufficiency of reason alone to cure it. By the nineteenth century, even as society increasingly turned to science, markets, and technology, a sense of nameless, irrational unease seemed endemic. Enter Søren Kierkegaard, who recognized the alienation inherent in the commercial age but also posited a more timeless theory of anxiety. In tortured meditations that relived his own vivid existential struggles, Kierkegaard argued that angst (imperfectly translated as anxiety) was the natural partner of human freedom, the daunting recognition of the aloneness that freedom bred. Indeed, for Kierkegaard the devout Christian, angst originated in Adam's aloneness before God's creation of Eve and remained the ultimate mark of human consciousness. Indeed, the dreadful pain of existential loneliness spurred an anxious attempt to embrace not only God but also one's own self—in Kierkegaard's words, "a leap of faith." Kierkegaard's conceptualization of angst, of its stakes and significance, became for May the master frame for his exploration of modern psychology's theories of anxiety. "What is amazing in Kierkegaard," May noted, "is that despite his lack of the tools for interpreting unconscious material . . . he so keenly and profoundly anticipated modern psychoanalytic insight into anxiety; and that at the same time he placed these insights in the broad context of a poetic and philosophical understanding of human experience." Kierkegaard placed anxiety at the center of existence:

> I would say that learning to know anxiety is an adventure which every man has to affront if he would not go to perdition either by not having known anxiety or by sinking under it. He therefore who has learned rightly to be anxious has learned the most important thing.[15]

In fact, as he surveyed various neurological, psychoanalytic, and psychological theories, May often seemed to treat them as modern, scientific elaborations of Kierkegaard. Goldstein's theory of anxiety as "catastrophic reaction" when an organism cannot cope w ith its environment and "feels a threat to its existence (or to values it holds essential for its existence)" fit very well into Kierkegaard's sense of human isolation. Largely agreeing with Goldstein's focus on a threat to existence, May also endorsed the neurologist's emphasis on a breakdown in "the awareness of the relationship between the self and objects" as a key aspect of anxiety. Anxiety is thus experienced "as a disintegration of the self, a 'dissolution of the existence of his personality.'" In reviewing research that grappled with physiological change and psychosomatic conditions in the anxious state—for instance, ulcers and susceptibility to infection—he emphasized that most symptoms were intimately related to culturally generated anxiety-producing situations.[16] *self-object?*

May then tracked the evolution of anxiety as a concept in O. H. Mowrer's work, in part to illustrate the possibility of moving from traditional empirical studies to more philosophically and socially inflected concepts. Mowrer had begun with a simple behavioral definition of anxiety as "the conditioned form of the pain reaction," a response to the signal of possible pain and the goad to pain reduction. Thus anxiety became a gateway to primitive learning. However, he became deeply dissatisfied with this approach and sought a conceptual framework that considered human intelligence and the ability to transcend immediate circumstance—those characteristics that gave human beings the freedom to move beyond the pain reflex. He instead constructed a theory of "anxiety" as a product of the "social dilemma."[17]

May was particularly taken with a central aspect of this new position, one that had arisen not just out of the behaviorist's recognition of methodological limits but also from Mowrer's own life experience. He had re-embraced Christianity, and that produced both a reaction to behaviorism and a new twist that stood Freudian theory on its head. Rather than blaming an overly severe superego for "repudiated moral urgings," he blamed bad psychotherapy. He argued, in May's words, that "the endeavor of many psychoanalysts to dilute and 'analyze away' the superego (and concomitantly the individual's sense of responsibility and guilt) only too often result[ed] in a 'deep narcissistic depression' rather than in the growth in personal maturity, social adequacy, and happiness which one has a right to expect from a really competent therapy." May confirmed that his own patients exhibited such "repression of guilt feelings" and that this was a "prevalent characteristic of certain groups in our culture and in some ways [was] pervasive of our culture as a whole." Especially among "defiant, aggressive types of patients," he found that many felt guilt and anxiety "because they have become 'autonomous' without becoming 'responsible.'" "When aggressive, sexual, or other behavior in egocentric form emerged in the analysis," he noted, "these patients showed no anxiety. But when the opposite needs and desires emerged—i.e., to have responsible and constructive social relations—there appeared much anxiety, accompanied by the typical reactions of patients who feel a crucial psychological strategy to be threatened."[18]

May did fault Mowrer on two crucial points. He found his seemingly blanket endorsement of the superego prone to precisely the same criticism—though in reverse—that Mowrer had made of Freud. That is, while some associated the superego with strictly negative forces in the unconscious, many who felt sympathetic to Mowrer's view might well ignore the "destructive, negative aspects of our cultural tradition." Furthermore, May argued, Mowrer recognized the concept of an *Urangst* as a primal force but limited his use of the term "anxiety" to the neurotic variety, leaving unexplored the very important hypothesis of what May termed "normal anxiety."[19]

Turning from Mowrer to the psychoanalytic tradition, May noted a similar progression from the biological to a more complicated cultural and sociological approach. May reviewed Freud's ever-evolving sense of the concept of anxiety but concentrated more on heretical figures. He underlined Otto Rank's connection of anxiety to individuation and creativity, while rejecting Adler's emphasis on the ways in which individuals used anxiety to dominate others or to paralyze their own ability to act. Of much greater consequence to May's concept of anxiety were the "neo-Freudian" explorations of Karen Horney, whose greatest contribution was to link neurotic anxiety to perceived attacks on the adult's psychological defenses. Thus, while the narcissist might feel threatened in a situation in which he is unrecognized and ignored, the person who has used unobtrusiveness as a defense will feel anxious when "thrust into the limelight." Furthermore, she argued that at the heart of most neurotic anxiety lay hostility born of culture's conflicting demands on issues of independence and dependency and the need to repress anger toward individuals upon whom one feels dependent. May's only major qualm with Horney revolved around her commitment to constructing the origins of adult neuroses entirely within the interpersonal relations of everyday life. In her reforming zeal, she was too eager to reject wholesale the Freudian concentration on early childhood."[20]

Finally, May grappled with the related theories of Horney's colleague Harry Stack Sullivan, whose psychosocial interpretation of anxiety revolved around the individual's quest for approval from others. Sullivan envisioned human tasks in two categories. The first involved satisfying basic bodily needs—eating, drinking, sleeping, and the like. The second focused on issues of security within society and among other individuals. Anxiety, according to Sullivan, arose originally from the first social relationship—parent and child—and the helplessness felt by the infant, including the "apprehension of the disapproval of the significant persons in his interpersonal world." As the infant matures into childhood, adolescence, and adulthood, his or her fear of not securing the necessary approval from significant others provides the filter through which desire, creativity, and motivation pass. Those activities or feelings deemed capable of putting one's security at risk are repressed, despite their possibly life-giving qualities. May summarized Sullivan's position and its relation to therapy: "Anxiety restricts growth and awareness, shrinking the area of effective living; emotional health is equal to the degree of personal awareness; hence clarification of anxiety makes possible expanded awareness and an expansion of the self, which means the achieving of emotional health."[21]

In a final theoretical section, "The Historical Dimensions of Anxiety-Creating Cultural Patterns," May discussed the work of Abram Kardiner, Karen Horney, Erich Fromm, R. H. Tawney, Karl Mannheim, and others. All shared the notion that the West had evolved from a traditional society with collective duties and security but little freedom to one dominated by personal freedom in the form of competitive individualism. Some scholars emphasized the impossible, anxiety-producing binds in which common citizens found themselves. Kardiner, for instance, underlined the tensions of believing in limitless social and economic mobility in an economy with few opportunities for advancement. Horney described the common citizen's emotions as "wavering between a feeling of boundless power in determining his own fate and a feeling of entire helplessness."[22]

May summed up the contemporary situation as one in which "contradictions and inconsistencies" in social values heightened the sense of anxiety already present from the contrast between individualist dreams and hard realities. "The threat the individual experiences is therefore not just to his possibility of attaining his goal," he argued, "but almost any threat may likewise raise doubts as to whether the goal is worth attaining." May thus upped the ante, posing one anxious drama within another. The very individualism that bred anxiety also eroded the sense of community that might offset its worst excesses. Freedom was in turn threatened by the insidious totalitarian temptation described by Fromm, which promised community but delivered only an enslaving and aggressive collectivism. May's solution for free society was heartfelt if unexceptional: "One of the central requirements for the constructive overcoming of anxiety in our society is the development of adequate forms of community."[23]

After almost two hundred pages of detailed and careful consideration of virtually everything that had been written about anxiety by scientists, philosophers, social scientists, and theologians, May was ready to offer an interpretive synthesis. He found general agreement on certain matters. Anxiety was a "*diffuse* apprehension" rather than a fear directed at a specific object, and it provoked equally diffuse if sometimes overwhelming "feelings of *uncertainty* and *helplessness*" in the face of a danger perceived to be "*a threat to some value which the individual holds essential to his existence as a personality.*" The threat might be to one's literal or psychological life, or to key aspects of meaning felt to be essential to one's personality. In this basic sense, one could draw a direct line from Kierkegaard's sense of anxiety as the "fear of nothingness" to the latest constructions of Kardiner, Fromm, and even Mowrer.[24]

May's most important contribution to psychological theory was his elucidation and differentiation of two kinds of anxiety, "normal" and "neurotic." The term "normal" referred to anxious states endemic to human existence, ones that in a particular individual could be "managed constructively" rather than through "panic" or other symptoms of neurotic anxiety. "Normal" anxiety also included those states of *Urangst* or *Angst der Kreatur* in the philosophical and theological literature—the vulnerability to nature and sickness and, ultimately, the certainty of death. When faced with courage, this awareness of human contingency—of the inevitable disappearance of ourselves and our worlds—often inspired profoundly creative moments and deep feelings of human solidarity.[25]

Having outlined and evaluated the vast array of approaches, May moved to the heart of his own research, the clinical studies that tested the interpretations he had already offered and, not incidentally, that qualified *Meaning of Anxiety* as a dissertation. Although he had administered rough-hewn questionnaires for his study of student religious life at Michigan State and had reported statistical evidence, never before had he subjected his psychological investigations to stringent quantitative and testable research methods. He found the transformation of human experience into "data" both intriguing and frustrating. Never again did he attempt to engage in standard methods of psychological experiment, in part because they seemed a mismatch for the subjective and qualitative aspects of consciousness that interested him most. However, he did come away with an appreciation of the importance of empiricism. Like William James, he sought some broader concept of the empirical, one that included not just easily quantifiable aspects of experience but the full range of realities experienced by human beings, including the emotional and ideational, with a holistic and complex sense of cause and effect—an empiricism that reflected the uniqueness and intricacy of human consciousness. Within a few years, May was calling explicitly for just such a "science of man," though in truth it served more as an aspiration than a concrete goal.

The concerns that led to such a quest revealed themselves in the design of May's six research categories: "The Nature of Anxiety and Its Relation to Fear," "Anxiety and Conflict," "Anxiety and Culture," "Anxiety and Hostility," "Methods of Dealing with Anxiety," and "Anxiety and the Development of Self." He would use this framework to interpret the data from fourteen cases. The first was that of a thirty-two-year-old psychoanalytic patient called "Brown" whom May saw in the late 1940s. The other thirteen were unwed mothers with whom he had worked at Inwood House (Walnut House in the book) in 1943 and 1944. His findings confirmed a variety of the hypotheses.

May made clear from the outset that, given anxiety's pervasiveness and the difficulties of isolating it from other disorders, qualitative study of human case histories was problematic at best. Its "inner locus" demanded a combination of psychoanalytic and behavioral methods in order to approach full description.[26] Addressing these problems meant designing simultaneous angles of vision, including numerous tests and the independent judgment of others connected to the study sites. For the Inwood House data, May had conducted hour-long interviews with each unwed mother four to eight times and compared findings with a resident social worker who met twenty to forty times with each girl. He also administered three checklist questionnaires focused on different aspects of the subjects' experience and history of anxiety, as well as a Rorschach test (where individuals are asked what they see in the shapes of abstract inkblots) to each of the young women both before and after childbirth. The scoring of the Rorschach was checked by a specialist for the accuracy of May's interpretation. In addition to these tools, May collected as much background as possible on the social and familial lives of the girls.

For the psychoanalysis of Brown, May worked with his supervising an
William Alanson White (in this case, Erich Fromm).

The results were mostly predictable. Brown's psychoanalysis provided the
most detailed evidence of the direct relation of "neurotic fears" to "underlying anxiety." Those among the unwed mothers who exhibited measurable
anxiety offered more limited evidence of the interplay between manifestation of anxiety and its source. However, both Brown and the anxious young
women demonstrated a sense of being "trapped," with every option available
threatening their "vital value," their basic sense of self. It was the ultimate
trigger of anxiety.[27] More surprising were May's findings that, in the case of
the unmarried mothers, parental condemnation and rejection caused anxiety for most but not all of the girls. May hypothesized that those girls who
objectively accepted the parental attitude as a fact of life experienced the least
anxiety from being condemned. Furthermore, on the basis of an admittedly
limited sample, he speculated about a class basis for his findings: the middle-
class girls lived in a cultural environment where parents hid their hostilities
and resentments toward their children behind "*pretenses of love and concern.*" Much less anxious were the girls from "proletarian" families, whose
environments of open parental hostility allowed no illusions.[28]

May returned to the paradoxical nature of anxiety already discussed in
the "theoretical" section of the book—the anxious state could lead both to
the "impoverishment of personality" and to its opposite, the encouragement
of "creative personalities." Brown's psychoanalysis demonstrated that when
highly anxious, the patient "exhibited a low degree of productivity, no originality, very little use of either feeling or thinking capacities, a predominance
of vagueness of response, and a lack of capacity for relating to concrete realities." Some of the unwed mothers displayed similar correlations; one even
retreated "into periods of vacant silence." May thus confirmed Goldstein's
theory that anxiety produced "dissolution of the self." Perhaps a more disturbing mirror of this process appeared in some of the other women, who
avoided anxiety at all costs in exchange for a creatively impoverished life. This
brought May back to the enlivening inner arc of the book, the Kierkegaardian
and Goldsteinian paradox—anxiety had the potential not only to cripple
the individual but also to foster the creative actualization of one's finite but
unique self. Indeed, his work with the Inwood girls inspired in him still another formulation of anxiety's paradoxical dimension. His original observation that the disparity between expectation and reality created high anxiety
in the middle-class white girls focused on neurotic anxiety. He added, in a

last sentence, that such a distance also had a key role to play in "all creative activity." Artists, scientists, and philosophers all placed a creative shape or form on the anarchy of existence. "Thus man's power to resolve the conflict between expectation and reality—his *creative* power—is at the same time his power to overcome neurotic anxiety."[29]

It was a curiously hopeful conclusion to May's excursion into the murky world of anxiety. His recognition of its darkness and despair, his own ordeal at the hands of tuberculosis, and his personal knowledge of the persistence of anxiety after the creative act notwithstanding, May chose to end with a firm and triumphant assertion of the creative *over* the anxious. Furthermore, May the psychotherapist recommended creative struggle rather than therapy as the antidote for anxiety, incorporating a value above symptom reduction and indeed preferring a route that he saw as inducing, rather than reducing, at least one kind of anxious state. In a work whose main task was to advance psychological understandings of anxiety, he clearly found the tools of the craft inadequate and struggled to move beyond them. Yet unlike Freud or even Kierkegaard, neither of whom declared victory in their struggles with anxiety, May felt it necessary to end on a note of triumph.

The Meaning of Anxiety displayed both continuity and progress in May's writing. A decade before in *The Springs of Creative Living*, he had disguised a deeply troubled autobiographical narrative, complex in its origins and consequences, to explore issues of meaning and faith in modernity. Yet he sacrificed real-life irresolution to the happy ending of a psycho-religious conversion. *The Meaning of Anxiety* was a great leap forward in breadth and careful analysis, one that featured little specific autobiographical material and creatively expanded upon key understandings of anxiety to forge a new, comprehensive view that, while rooted in psychology, pushed the discipline back toward its philosophical roots. It trafficked boldly in the basic ambiguities of psychological discomfort, arguing that both "neurotic anxiety" and the single-minded quest for the anxiety-free life were debilitating conditions, no matter their contrasting symptoms. Most of all, he highlighted the creative possibilities of "normal anxiety" in ways that countered common understandings, folding the insights of Kierkegaard and Goldstein into the mix of mainstream psychology. In that sense, *The Meaning of Anxiety* set forth an implicit agenda not only for May's future work but for the profession as well.

The ambition and accomplishments of *The Meaning of Anxiety* guaranteed wide notice. Most reviewers praised its boldly inclusive approach, yet its range invited criticism from some specialized journals. Rudolf Ekstein, in the *Bulletin of the Menninger Clinic*, called it "very often excellent" in its "thorough" coverage and synthesis of various theorists. However, Ekstein was disappointed that in the end May could only conclude about "neurotic anxiety" that it resulted "from a cleavage or contradiction between expectations and reality." Qualified praise came from the *Journal of Nervous and Mental Diseases*, which called the first part "refreshing" and of great service in sorting out what had become, in its words, a "confusion of voices." It found the case studies less impressive, avoiding "the basic dynamic understanding of why the neurotic is unable to make the necessary convergence of reality and hopes." The most damning reviews were from Freudian circles—unsurprising given the fact that May had been trained by such heretics as Fromm and Sullivan. One scoffed at what he read as May's dismissal of Freud and endorsement of the cultural school and concluded that *Meaning of Anxiety* "hardly fulfils the prefatory promise of enlightening any intelligent citizen who feels the 'anxiety-creating conflicts of our day.'" He also questioned May's case study method—"On the basis of four cases he tentatively suggests that anxiety is less frequently experienced among the proletariat than in the middle class."[30]

Others were heartier in their praise. Psychologist George F. J. Lehner assured the readers of *Scientific American* that *The Meaning of Anxiety* "should be of value not only to psychologists and psychiatrists, but also to any person interested in a psychological understanding of modern problems." The *American Anthropologist* called it "definitive" and "ahead of its time." *Pulpit Digest* applauded May's "successful attempt to present anxiety consistently . . . of as great interest to us as to the scientists." *Religion in Life* called it "one of the most significant books for a clergyman to read that has been published in a long time." Perhaps more important, references to *The Meaning of Anxiety* began to appear in a wide variety of psychological articles in both its philosophical and experimental aspects, and in lay discussions especially because of its discussion of "normal anxiety."[31]

Beyond the reviews, a particularly poignant example of *The Meaning of Anxiety*'s influence can be seen in the work of none other than O. H. Mowrer. In publishing a collection of his important papers in 1950, *Learning Theory and Personality Dynamics*, Mowrer revised a key 1947 paper on anxiety in light of May's work and dwelled at length on Kierkegaard's contribution. He credited May with "bringing the problem of normal anxiety to my attention with the emphasis which it deserves, first in conversations and later in . . . *The*

Meaning of Anxiety," from which he then quoted several pages. Mowrer also commissioned May to write the lead article in an influential introductory volume to the study and practice of psychotherapy published in 1953.[32]

* * *

In July 1949, with his dissertation finished and its publication assured, May took his family to Nantucket for a vacation. He swam and played with Bob and the twins and painted bright watercolors of Florence on the beach. Intruding into this idyll, however, came news of his father's death. Rollo reacted with outward calm and walked down the beach, alone and silent. He had seen E. T. only eight or nine times since his parents' divorce, in awkward encounters tinctured with mostly unspoken hurt. Occasionally, his brothers and sisters would pass along news.[33] Yet so unresolved were his feelings that Rollo refused to attend the funeral in Ohio. Forty years later he explained simply: "I thought as the family goes he'd done a bad job. . . . I had picked up the pieces and held it together. I didn't think that he deserved my going."[34] Of course, it was more complicated than that. For one thing, E. T.'s death occurred just as Rollo was embarking on a new career. In the year that followed, he would receive his doctorate, publish an important book, be declared free of tuberculosis, and almost instantly become a force in psychology. Earl, to whom Rollo wished to prove so much, would never know.

Rollo struggled quite consciously with E. T.'s legacy for the rest of his life. At the time of his father's death, Rollo dwelled upon E. T.'s irresponsibility and what he perceived as his slick shallowness. Rollo had found a more suitable father figure in Tillich, one whose example pervaded all aspects of his life.[35] May only slowly came to see more positive aspects of E. T.'s influence— a commitment to service and plainspoken communication, a populist concern for the well-being of common individuals, and a talent for hands-on organizational work. These aspects became powerful complements to Rollo's spiritual and intellectual strivings and helped move him quickly to prominence in a psychological profession whose therapeutic horizons had widened so greatly after World War II.

17

Embracing a New Profession

The publication of *The Meaning of Anxiety* would have marked an auspicious beginning for May in any professional climate, but in 1950 the world of psychotherapy was fraught with internecine battles and public misconceptions, its philosophical and scientific commitments very much open to question. Despite the explosion of interest in Freud and other theorists in the early twentieth century, the professional practice of psychotherapy emerged fitfully from a highly charged professional and political battleground. The skirmishes within the New York psychoanalytic community of the early 1940s comprised just one front of a wider war of shifting alliances among multiple combatants. The issues were a mix of substance and turf. Concepts and techniques of psychoanalysis and various other applied psychological theories had by the 1930s begun to challenge the enshrined medical practice of psychiatry, and included school and marriage counseling, social work, the ministry, and clinical psychology. Each of these fields faced internal debates about how much and which psychotherapeutic ideas might influence training and practice. In any case, there was far more talk about psychotherapy than actual training of therapists of all kinds and practice. The Depression had made psychoanalysis and the budding fields of psychotherapeutic counseling a luxury few could afford. May's own odyssey in the 1930s illustrated both the compelling nature of therapeutic ideas and the fledgling place of psychotherapy as a professional endeavor in American society.

That all began to change drastically during World War II, when the government employed psychologists in the war effort for projects that ranged from analysis of enemy cultures and increasingly sophisticated testing of draftees to the development of "psychological warfare" techniques. The profession responded eagerly to the call, from both patriotic zeal and, not incidentally, a sense that the war validated new and significant roles, as well as increased funding in academia, government, and the culture at large. Most of all, the war raised an even more dramatic issue—treating the alarming numbers of soldiers suffering from combat stress. Psychiatrists and psychologists were called upon to improvise strategies for mentally refitting traumatized soldiers for further combat. The usefulness of "talk" became readily apparent, as did the shortage of knowledgeable professionals.[1]

As a result of the war experience, the government projected the need for vast numbers of psychiatrists and psychologically trained therapists and counselors to deal with returning soldiers. World War II had produced fourteen million veterans, and in Veterans Administration hospitals alone there were close to forty-four thousand neuropsychiatric patients. The VA hoped to hire 4,700 clinical psychologists and vocational counselors for diagnostic and readjustment services and for psychotherapy. Even before the end of the war, the American Psychological Association and the smaller American Association of Applied Psychology pressed the government for funds to train new counselors and therapists. The shortage of professionals remained a problem not only for veterans but also for a civilian population that had begun to see psychotherapy as an attractive treatment for emotional distress, marital conflict, and more generalized dissatisfactions, or as an adjunct to such traditional sources of solace as religion and friendship. Furthermore, though social workers and school counselors had come more and more under the influence of therapeutic methods, demand outstripped supply in these spheres as well.[2]

It was at the beginning of this "takeoff" stage that Rollo May set up his counseling practice. By 1948 he was healthy enough and had made enough progress on his dissertation to resume analytic training at the William Alanson White Institute. He took seminars from Erich Fromm, Frieda Fromm-Reichmann, and Clara Thompson and resumed "training analysis" with Fromm. A requirement in an analyst's education, training analysis sought to bring firsthand and useful insight into the future therapist's own psyche, as well as intimate familiarity with the experience of being a patient. May had, of course, known Fromm since the early 1940s, first in courses and in the private seminar on psychology and religion and then as a supervisor for his work at Inwood House. They had kept in touch during May's tuberculosis treatment.

Yet his analysis was destined to be relatively unproductive. It was cut short by Fromm's acceptance of a position at the medical school of the National Autonomous University in Mexico City in 1950. Fromm's move alone may have created anger and issues of abandonment that worked themselves out only years later. We know precious little about the actual analytic sessions, in part because of a lack of useful contemporaneous notes, and also because neither man chose to say much about their relationship in later years. However, hints from both sides indicate that the pairing brought out the narcissist in both parties. Fromm and his acolytes all but accused May of stealing Fromm's ideas, while May countered in private that his analyst had not written anything truly new since *Escape from Freedom*. The contrast of cultural styles (German Jewish émigré and midwestern American), a rivalry of libidos, and no clear deference to authority on May's part—and, indeed, May sharing Tillich's doubts about Fromm—all cultivated a somewhat frosty situation. Yet on the surface they remained on cordial if formal terms at least for some years.[3]

The abrupt end of May's analysis with Fromm did not slow down his rapid entry into the world of the White Institute. He finished his training analysis with Frieda Fromm-Reichmann and Clara Thompson in 1951 and 1952. And, with the publication of *The Meaning of Anxiety*, May's demonstrable achievement and professional visibility made him an asset to the institute. Thompson was particularly taken with him and wrote a stunning blurb for the book: "I have never seen the concept of normal anxiety so clearly presented. . . . He has added much clarification to some of the most obscurely formulated problems of psychology."[4] In May 1951, the institute invited him to join as a faculty member, in particular to train ministers in psychoanalytic theory. By the end of 1951, Thompson asked him to create a full ministerial curriculum while he completed his own training in the secular world of analysis.[5]

That May found his institutional niche at the White Institute through his connection to the church and Union Theological Seminary may seem odd at first for someone who had lost his religious faith. Yet liberal Protestantism had, over the twentieth century, become a community of values and institutions as much as a religious faith. In fact, it had some reason to claim its vision as the basis for public ethical and moral culture in general, often stated without the framework of faith. Training pastoral counselors and in other ways participating in the social missions of churches did not depend on avowals of faith so much as generalized senses of Christian love and charity as well as commitment to latter-day versions of the social gospel. The YMCA had pioneered this shaping of public culture, and May's participation in it came naturally.

Liberal Protestantism did not prevent him from participating vigorously in the professional world of New York's psychologists as they battled for the right to practice. Nearly a third of the nation's psychologists lived in the state, and Manhattan was the profession's most important locus. May joined the New York State Psychological Association in 1949, as the burgeoning field grappled with problems of self-definition and organization as well as the medical establishment's fierce resistance to granting psychologists the right to practice therapy. According to the NYSPA, which represented about 30 percent of psychologists, ten other groups of psychologists existed, each with memberships of twenty to six hundred. One burning issue was how to license or certify practitioners of counseling or psychotherapy, not only psychologists but also school and general counselors. Although the NYSPA had a certification board, it was still refining its standards. Most members were in favor of state licensing, but, as the *Bulletin of the New York State Psychological Association* noted, "Psychologists themselves were far from agreed as to the provisions to be included." The association thus formed a joint committee to make recommendations and, after some revision by the membership, came up with a bill that sought to turn them into law.[6]

May leaped into the fray, spending much time in 1950 lobbying in Albany for the bill. He and other members of the NYSPA team argued that it would rightfully establish psychology as an independent profession, while licensing would help prevent charlatanism or quackery. These efforts led to two stunning events. The association convinced legislators in both houses in Albany to pass a law unanimously in March 1951 that established a licensing procedure through the State Commissioners of Mental Hygiene and Health.[7] However, on April 10, 1951, Governor Thomas Dewey vetoed the bill. Lobbyists from the Medical Society of the State of New York, the American Psychiatric Association, and other doctors' organizations, as well as "a flood of opposing telegrams from physicians throughout the state," had convinced Dewey that the legislation blurred the lines between psychologist and psychiatrist and inadvertently made it easier for inadequately trained practitioners to prey on the public.[8]

The defeat underscored the power of organized medicine as well as the disorganization of the nascent psychological profession. Four days after the veto, the Joint Council of New York State Psychologists on Legislation met to formulate a new legislative campaign to counter Dewey's objections. The council also held a conference in early May aimed at mitigating tensions within the psychology profession's more specialized organizations. The invitation list itself illustrated the problem: the Association for Analytic Psychologists, Association of Psychologists for the New York City Public Schools, Group for Applied Freudian Psychology, Individual Psychological Association of New York (Adlerian), Metropolitan New York Association for

Psychoanalysis, New York Association of Clinical Psychologists in Private Practice, New York Society of Clinical Psychologists, and Postgraduate Center for Psychotherapy. May, who represented the Association for Analytic Psychology, was a strong advocate of unity.

The conference tackled many issues, including reorganizing the state association, developing accreditation standards for training institutions and certification standards for each specialization, continuing work on a code of ethics, and creating meaningful but flexible standards for membership. The new plan proposed four or five divisions reflecting various strands of the profession. Each would have at least one representative on the board of directors, with additional board members assigned according to the size of divisional memberships.

Meanwhile, preparations for legislative battles continued. The council's main opponent remained the medical establishment and especially psychiatrists, whose national organization had in November 1951 recommended support for "certification" but opposed "licensing" of psychologists. Psychiatrists argued that it was "impossible to define and delimit the practice of psychology for purposes of licensure in a way not likely to be interpreted as permitting psychologists to assume responsibilities for which they are not qualified, such as the diagnosis and treatment of ill persons."

The psychologists tried to work with psychiatrists to create legislation acceptable to both groups, but sticking points remained. Doctors made several demands: that psychiatrists hold a place on any board licensing psychologists, that patients considering treatment from a psychologist first undergo a physical exam to rule out organic causes, and that any psychologist applying for a license prove that he or she had "well-established lines of communication" with a doctor. The spirit and substance of such proposals were unacceptable to psychologists.[9]

Moreover, trust levels were low. In early 1953, a group of doctors convinced some legislators to introduce a bill that would have defined medicine as the "diagnosis and treatment of all physical and mental conditions," thus leaving only an advisory or scholarly role for psychologists in the treatment of mental illness. May, who had by this time ascended to the chairmanship of the Joint Council, organized a protest meeting for March 3 at the Hotel New Yorker. Nine hundred psychologists attended. Rollo voiced the consensus that psychologists "could not permit [the bill] to pass without surrendering belief in psychology as an independent science and profession; it would have made psychology, at least in its private practice aspects, entirely subordinate to medicine." The meeting formally condemned the legislation as "an unwarranted restriction on the legitimate activities of competent psychologists, injurious to the public welfare." In a letter to the entire NYSPA membership, May noted that "the proposed bill came as a shock not only to the Joint Council, but even to some representatives of medicine and psychiatry" who had been working in good faith toward a compromise. The *New York Herald-Tribune* endorsed the psychologists' protest on March 7, and the Joint Council began a lobbying campaign that successfully killed the legislation in committee.[10]

These events renewed efforts among more conciliatory medical doctors and psychologists toward mutual understanding, and May once again played a significant role by cochairing a research project and conference, "Psychotherapy and Counseling," sponsored by the New York Academy of Science. May and the prominent public intellectual Lawrence K. Frank recruited experts in various fields to consider the particular relationships of disciplines and professions to the broader world of psychotherapy. These "commissions" reported on medicine, psychology, social work, vocational counseling, and the ministry. They sought to articulate the best modes of inter-professional contact through explicit structures, as well as to encourage a more informal spirit of collegiality and common goals. The conference, whose proceedings were published in November 1955, produced no major conclusions or solutions but at least began to foster a cooperative vision of the psychotherapeutic and counseling professions.[11]

The psychology commission, whose members included May, Nevitt Sanford, Peter Blos, Harry Bone, Arthur Combs, and George Klein, emphasized that the American Psychological Association's code of ethics required clinicians to consult doctors concerning possible organic origins of symptoms. Indeed, they assured the conference that "what *is* done follows rather closely what *should be* done." They also noted that the profession was in its infancy and that its direction, approaches, theoretical underpinnings, and general view of human nature should encourage lively and open debate.[12] In all, while few minds were changed as to the status and independence of one field or another, each set of clinicians had been given the opportunity to humanize the caricatures by which others knew them.

May's professional home was hardly immune to such debates. Despite the fact that the White Institute was founded specifically to provide psychoanalytic training by and for non-medical practitioners, a number of its doctors carried on a battle that paralleled the struggles in Albany. In 1953, they began to agitate for limiting analytic training for all but medical doctors. At a 1954 meeting, Janet Mackenzie Rioch, an MD, sought a vote on the matter among the institute's fellows, despite the absence of the group's most visible psychologists—Erich Fromm, Frieda Fromm-Reichmann, and Ernest Schachtel, as well as May. Harry Bone protested to Clara Thompson, characterizing the move as premature and unwise. Rioch protested that she only wanted to raise the question, and then only to protect the status of the institute.[13]

The question hung fire for more than a year, but in early 1956 the institute's medical doctors circulated a "Resolution Addressed to the Council of Fellows" that forthrightly called for an end to analytic training of psychologists. They complained that the institute was "held in low regard by a major portion of the psychoanalytic community" for training non-medical analysts, and that these other analysts would "not associate with us so long as we continue a training activity which they feel is deleterious." It wasn't a question, they continued, as to "whether [other psychoanalysts] are right or wrong in their convictions—the matter is one about which reasonable men may differ—but simply that their convictions exist and have consequences which damage our influence, deprive us of the revitalizing effects of scientific discussion, injure our professional standing as physicians, and which now the high probability of the formation of a certifying board of psychoanalysis threaten to make it impossible for us to be considered psychoanalysts." In a conclusion that enraged the institute's psychologists, the doctors assured all that they would defend White's analytic heresies on "the principle of freedom of scientific inquiry" and accept the consequences. However, "in trying to console ourselves for the penalties we suffer through the training of psychologists we have searched for a principle which would sustain us," they noted. "We have come to this conclusion: *There is no principle involved.*"[14]

The psychologists soon fired back. A "Fact-Finding Committee of the Harry Stack Sullivan Society" within the institute, comprising both medical doctors and psychologists, analyzed the resolution and publicly asserted not only that its facts were wrong but that it reflected the doctrine that "*expediency and self-interest come before convictions.*" May, Harry Bone, Ernest Schachtel, and a number of the other psychologists at White circulated a more damning letter. They contrasted the "interest in experimentation," "openness to new ideas," and "courageous commitment to the importance of principles" that defined the institute's founders to the doctors' "involvement in prestige, conformity, and the following of narrow policies in theory and practice as prescribed by an authoritarian and orthodox organization." They deplored the tactics—"pressuring the signers into precipitate action . . . through misinformation and misrepresentation"—and the cause. Nor did they think that victory would gain the respect the doctors craved: "Those who are yielded to under pressure because of lack of independence do not admire their victims."[15] The fact-finding committee warned that the "*manifest* issue of training psychologists obscures a host of other problems: educational, scientific, administrative." Earl G. Witenberg, a doctor who had signed the original petition but eventually saw beyond the controversy to become one of the institute's most effective leaders, prefaced his own ideas for organizational reforms with some in-house humor: "The diagnosis that I feel can safely be made of the irrational forces let loose in these issues is one of unresolved dependency feelings commonly called incestuous problems."[16]

Even as May battled with the medical profession on two fronts, he rose to the presidency of the New York State Psychological Association on the strength of his tireless defense and eloquent vision of clinical psychology and its role in society. He also expanded his professional and public presence through lectures and publications. May accepted speaking engagements nationwide and everywhere gained a host of admirers. The success of *The Meaning of Anxiety* and May's talents as a writer also secured him a highly visible role as a reviewer of psychology books for the Sunday *New York Times*. Most of his *Times* reviews concerned books from the mainstream of psychotherapy, and he offered insightful commentary and plainspoken elucidation of psychological issues and history. He lambasted L. Ron Hubbard's *Dianetics: The Modern Science of Mental Health*, the Bible of the then-nascent Scientology movement, noting the derivative nature of concepts like becoming "clear" and the "engram" and the "bizarre length to which these hypotheses are carried." He scoffed at Hubbard's claim that his approach could "eliminate any psychosomatic illness from which you suffer (e.g., 'cleared' persons never get colds)" and "help you 'achieve at least one-third more than present capacity for work and happiness,'" as well as "raise your I.Q. substantially." May wondered "whether the author is not writing with his tongue in his cheek." He concluded that books like *Dianetics* harmed "troubled persons" with "grandiose promises."[17]

Amidst all this activity, May also found time to publish his fourth book, *Man's Search for Himself*. It originated in a four-lecture series called "Personal Integrity in an Age of Anxiety," delivered at the centennial celebrations of

Mills College in Oakland, California, in late 1952. Writing for a new, secular audience, he sought and described solutions for living in the postwar world of nuclear menace, loss of faith, and threats to individuality. He yearned to reach a wider public than he had with *The Meaning of Anxiety*. It was not simply a question of fame and fortune, but rather one of calling. In the latest iteration of a mission inspired by the YMCA and the poetry of Sam Foss, he wished to bring to everyday Americans the wisdom he had found in the difficult texts of Nietzsche, Freud, and Kierkegaard.[18]

In this endeavor he had the support of O. Hobart Mowrer, with whom he enjoyed a friendly and mutual mentorship. May submitted an early draft of *Man's Search for Himself* to W. W. Norton, which offered him a contract. Mowrer suggested May also submit the manuscript to Harold Strauss, editor in chief at Alfred Knopf, and wrote to the editor in support. While Strauss evinced "considerable admiration" for May's work and recognized his importance in the field, he rejected the book on interesting grounds. "As a man of some sensibility I feel that only artists can deal successfully with moral values," he wrote in his report to the editorial board. "The most famous statements of moral philosophers, theologians, social scientists and what not, and especially of those writers from the Renaissance to the 19th Century who were moralistically inclined, seem compelling to me only to the extent that they are art." Strauss felt that May was guilty of the very act of which he accused others: "intellectualizing the truth . . . dealing abstractly with experience." Two other in-house reviewers expressed similar views about May's style. They felt that May had too much the touch of a psychologically informed moralist and not enough that of an artist. Strauss also felt the book would not sell well.[19]

On this last count, Strauss was wrong. Published by Norton in January 1953, *Man's Search for Himself* was a bestseller within a month of its release. It presented a vivid and serious inquiry into what May termed "the loneliness and anxiety of modern man." The book featured the mix of anecdote, broad theory, and exhortation that over a decade before had lent power to *The Springs of Creative Living*. What changed were the religious, philosophical, and professional bases of his vision. The former minister who had once recommended Christ as the "therapist for humanity" had become a new and important voice in psychology. He sought meaning in personal exploration and courage stripped of theological content and reliance on higher powers, placing the search for authentic life within a broad spiritual and philosophical framework. *Man's Search for Himself* envisioned a human condition that valued religious and ethical tradition but sought their application to new and frightening circumstances. Common themes of contemporary sociopolitical analysis emerged in the book: conformity, human isolation, loss of an inner sense of self, the separation of reason and emotion, the oppressive burdens of bureaucracy and mass culture, and the dangers of totalitarianism. May cited Fromm's work on authoritarian societies and Riesman's kindred sociological study *The Lonely Crowd* (1950), which (in May's words) described the transformation of a dominant American personality from "inner-directed" to "outer-directed" and resulted in the rise of a palpable sense of "*passivity* and *apathy*."[20]

Man's Search for Himself was a striking contribution because of its rich mix of cultural and historical context and because of what May saw as the key psychological problem of the age: "*Emptiness*." He "mean[t] not only that many people do not know what they want; they often do not have any clear idea of what they feel." They "feel swayed this way and that, with painful feelings of powerlessness, because they feel vacuous, empty." Even sex had become for many "an empty, mechanical and vacuous experience." He feared those forces that were turning individuals into ciphers akin to T. S. Eliot's "hollow men." May saw this as a characteristic of the population in general.[21]

The aching resonance of "emptiness" epitomized May's own approach. He valued the sociopolitical analyses of Fromm and Riesman but sought a more intimate rendering of a pent-up urge for individuality and escape from "emptiness and boredom." *Man's Search for Himself* achieved its ends through anecdote, references from literature and media, and pointed juxtaposition of abstraction and affecting personal detail. May told the story of the Bronx bus driver who became a local hero by driving his empty bus to Florida rather than on his usual route, just to declare his exasperation with routine. He noted a *Life* magazine article called "The Wife Problem," which demonstrated how much pressure corporations put on the wives of executives to lose themselves in the cause of their husbands' careers. Popular music, May's patients' dreams, and great modern and classical writers—Aeschylus, Auden, Camus, Dostoevsky, Faulkner, Fitzgerald, Kafka, Kierkegaard, Wordsworth, and many others—all helped define the problem of emptiness. He even tried out a Kafkaesque fantasy of his own, "The Man Who Was Put in a Cage," in which a king imprisoned a man (but in a comfortable cage) just to see what would happen to him. At first the man protested, but eventually he came willingly to lose his freedom and value the security of his fate. "He had accepted the cage," May wrote. "He had no anger, no hate, no rationalizations. But he was now insane." Most poignantly when one considers he might have had E. T. consciously or unconsciously in mind, he recounted the tragedy of Willy Loman in Arthur Miller's *Death of a Salesman* (1949). Willy's obsession with being "well liked" led, as one of his sons noted as they buried the salesman, to the modern fate: "He never knew who he was."[22]

May's vision for an escape from emptiness involved a courageous revaluing of the self that would lead to a truer sense of human solidarity, freedom, and love. In such sections as "Rediscovering Selfhood," "The Goals of Integration," "Freedom and Inner Strength," "The Creative Conscience," "Courage, the Virtue of Maturity," and "Man, the Transcender of Time," May appropriated ideas from psychology, religion, and philosophy in their varieties as well as their convergences. The great traditions, along with alienated prophets of modernity, sketched individualized paths to self-knowledge and love. Rejecting both a return to tradition and an extreme existentialism that ignored the past entirely, May sought authenticity and ethical action in the resonance of tradition within freedom. "Some persons will be frightened by the freedom in such an ethics of inwardness," he noted, "and made anxious by the responsibility which this places on each man's decisions."[23]

May strove to reestablish that sense of wholeness once formed through external rules and obligations in order to nurture oneself but also to foster the love of others and to feel at one with humanity. His vision assumed an essential order expressed in ritual and mythological systems internalized over millennia of human existence. "Here is the seeming paradox," he argued, "which no doubt everyone knows to be true in his own experience, that *the more profoundly he can confront and experience the accumulated wealth in historical tradition, the more uniquely he can at the same time know and be himself.*" Such an argument also presupposed a self, a consciousness beyond Descartes's rational "I think, therefore, I am." Rather, he expressed kinship with Spinoza and his idea of human beings as *sub specie aeternitatis*, or, in May's words, that "a person acts 'under the form of eternity' to the extent that his actions arise from his own essential character."[24]

In linking the finite self, with all its limits as well as its possibilities, to the eternal self without a formal theology—and in fact, only through a courageous search for meaning amid doubt—May's work most of all reflected a debt to Paul Tillich. Tillich's *The Courage to Be*, published about the same time as *Man's Search for Himself* and sometimes jointly reviewed with it, worked through similar themes in more formal ways. However, the differences were striking. Tillich stressed the need for finite human beings to experience the God beyond God, the God who was not the "God of theism" or of the churches but rather the very "ground of being" beyond even the imagination of theology (except Tillich's own). May was satisfied with an individual reaching some authentic sense of his or her own unique "being," one that only in an indirect if powerful manner seemed at one with Eternity.[25]

Furthermore, in one dramatic moment, Tillich argued that this search for personal "being" and the "ground of being" could only be carried out within a Christianity that had returned to its radical Lutheran roots. Only a church that "raises itself in its message and its devotion to the God above the God of theism without sacrificing its concrete symbols [could] mediate a courage which takes doubt and meaninglessness into itself." In short, it was "the Church under the Cross which alone can do this, the Church which preaches the Crucified who cried to God who remained his God after the God of confidence had left him in the darkness of doubt and meaninglessness." Or, as Tillich concluded, "*The courage to be is rooted in the God who appears when God has disappeared in the anxiety of doubt.*" These stirring final passages were a powerful antidote to the confusion and the sense of powerlessness endemic to modernity. Yet they might also be read as a defiant last-ditch defense of the church's singular authority in mediating the connection to the "God beyond God" and the very "ground of being," a defense made ironically necessary by the historical, psychological, and cultural arguments in the body of the work. Indeed, within a decade Tillich was exploring Zen and in other ways moving well beyond traditional Christianity.[26]

Rollo May had made that transformation earlier, and no such declaration of fealty to any church or theological stance appeared in *Man's Search for Himself*. The "courage to be" in May's work became the courage fully to be oneself, to face the truth of death and of the finite details of one's life, and to allow the potential for love and embrace of others. "Being" itself did not hinge on a particular creed or theology but was confirmed collectively for May by the wisdom of the world's literature—all of which pointed to an ineffable but real order of things beyond human definition. Yet, for May, human action and courage were the main issues and the practical battleground of "being," especially the courage to face truth in spite of fear and doubt. This argument gave a basic Freudian paradigm a new, more philosophical and ethical twist. Quoting a letter from Schopenhauer to Goethe, May noted the philosopher's identification with Oedipus, who pursues the truth of his fate to the end: "The philosopher [must] interrogate himself without mercy. This philosophical courage, however, does not arise from reflection, cannot be wrung from resolutions, but is an inborn trend of the mind." May agreed with Schopenhauer on the origins of this urge in an "inborn capacity for self-awareness." However, he emphasized that its utilization did not come naturally: "Such probity is an ethical attitude, involving courage and other aspects of one's relation to one's self; it not only *can* be developed to an extent but *must* be developed if a person is to fulfill himself as a human being." [27]

May's reworking of courage and "being" marked a move away from Christianity per se (and from Tillich) toward an enriched sense of ideas that had dominated his thinking in the past. For instance, he had once found Matthew Arnold's "Dover Beach" a supreme statement on love's place in a disintegrating world:

> Ah, love, let us be true
> To one another! For the world, which seems
> To lie before us like a land of dreams,
> So various, so beautiful, so new,
> Hath really neither joy, nor love, nor light,
> Nor certitude, nor peace, nor help for pain;
> And we are here as on a darkling plain.

Such sentiment now seemed to him inadequate and even destructive. "When 'love' is engaged in for the purpose of vanquishing loneliness," he asserted, "it accomplishes its purpose only at the price of increased emptiness for both persons." Rather, love must be rooted in "a delight in the presence of the other person and an affirming of his value and development as much as one's own." Only then might one create "one's own joy and happiness in the relation with him." Such mature love depended on a hard-won sense of "being" on the part of each individual, which enabled the possibility of the ecstasy of love, "that moment of self-realization when one temporarily overleaps the barrier between one identity and another. It is a giving of one's self and a finding of one's self at once." [28]

May eventually came full circle on the question of the human condition in modernity. Having begun with an emphasis on the eerie modern absence of shared values, myths, and beliefs, by the end he concluded that in some sense, the struggle for full humanity had pervaded every age and that perhaps contemporary society allowed the brave a greater latitude for finding their individualized sense of being than in times past. In a curiously triumphant penultimate moment, he declared: "*Does not the uncertainty of our time teach us the most important lesson of all—that the ultimate criteria are the honesty, integrity, courage and love of a given moment of relatedness?"* It was as if he had turned "Dover Beach" inside out. Instead of lovers clinging to each other against the chill of modernity's "darkling plain," the individual's embrace of "being" and "relatedness" in a "given moment" might vanquish fear. "If we do not have that, we are not building for the future anyway; if we do have it, we can trust the future to itself."[29]

Man's Search for Himself received mostly enthusiastic reviews in the popular press. The *Herald-Tribune*, noting some of its thematic affinity to Tillich's *The Courage to Be*, lauded it as "in the best sense popular, uncluttered with jargon of the trade," and "touched with humor and imagination, infused with wide culture." The all-important Sunday *New York Times* review recognized that "much of this diagnosis has been made before, but seldom, if ever with such persuasive clarity." Viewing it as a "companion volume" to Tillich, A. Powell Davies, minister of All Souls Unitarian Church in Washington, DC. wondered whether "creative modern thinking" was "moving at an unexpected moment into spiritual unity." Davies ended on an extraordinarily positive note, calling the "Preface to Love" chapter "sorely needed" and "sheer wisdom." Others were less sanguine. The *Columbus (OH) Dispatch* found the book disappointing because it offered no clear way out of the modern predicament. "He has failed to point out any real values and goals," the reviewer noted, "and has engaged in so much double-talk that it becomes difficult to decipher just where he does stand." The reviewer concluded that, having read *Man's Search for Himself*, the "average man" not only would have moved "no closer to finding himself" but "might be a little farther away."[30]

The reaction of religious journals divided along denominational and theological lines. An in-house review by Seward Hiltner in the bulletin of the *Pastoral Psychology* Book Club (May was on the editorial boards of both the book club and *Pastoral Psychology* itself) called it "certainly one of the best, most readable, and most far-reaching books that have ever been written to help a reader to help himself." Comparing it to Fromm's work, Hiltner found that "theologically speaking, May's work [was] more satisfying because the position taken is always implicitly and explicitly Christian. Its historical references will seem much more accurate to the theologically-trained reader than similar sections in books by Fromm and other psychological and psychiatric writers." *America*, a Catholic magazine, disagreed. In a joint review of *Man's Search for Himself* and *The Courage to Be*, Father Gerald Van Ackeren found the books "stimulating" yet suffering "from inadequacies which make their analyses and solutions basically unacceptable to a Catholic." He agreed with May's assessment that modern anxiety and emptiness originated in "a lack of any compelling set of values." Yet he found that "with no concept of the supernatural or original sin," May wrongly attributed the malaise to "parental suppression of personal self-asserting and freedom." "Having, apparently, no notion of a transcendent and personal God to whom man is ordered," Van Ackeren argued, "Dr. May lacks the only ultimate orientation for human life." Indeed, the reviewer noted the influence of Tillich in May's thought before decrying the vapidity of the theologian's own book. "In his insistence on the absolute primacy of freedom," Van Ackeren concluded, "Professor Tillich seems to forget one of the basic lessons of the Gospel: it is *truth* that makes men free."[31]

Perhaps the most probing "religious" review came from David Roberts, a professor at Union Theological Seminary and an important advocate of the relevance of psychotherapy to modern Christianity. In 1950, Roberts had published *Psychotherapy and a Christian View of Man*, a key text for more than a decade in the world of liberal Christianity. Like May, he was a protégé and close friend of Tillich, had participated in the wartime religion and psychology seminars, was deeply drawn to Kierkegaard, and published in the early issues of Simon Doniger's pathbreaking journal *Pastoral Psychology*. He knew Rollo as a colleague and friend.

Roberts lauded *Man's Search for Himself* for its presentation of the issues, especially its mix of literature, theology, philosophy, psychoanalysis, and clinical anecdote. "His style is eminently readable without being watered-down," Roberts noted, "and he conveys some difficult and profound thoughts without becoming either technical or condescending." He especially appreciated May's discussion of dependence, the nature of freedom, and the "development of a creative conscience and effective religious living," as well as the chapter on "love" and "eternity." At the same time, he wished that May had made his own theological opinions more explicit: "Some may feel that his discussions of guilt and of the content of faith are bound to be incomplete until he comes to terms more directly with doctrinal questions," he wrote. More important, he felt that while *Man's Search for Himself* emphasized freedom from "all forms of slavery (including religious)," May's next book should consider the place of "*sound* forms of dependence upon 'community' and divine grace."[32]

The compelling clarity of *Man's Search for Himself* reflected a new confidence and maturity that May had gained as he rebuilt his life from the shambles of disease and marital discord. Not coincidentally, it was also written at a moment of renewed romantic passion. Between 1945 and 1950, the slow rebuilding of body and soul allowed for little in the way of casual affairs or loving reengagement in his marriage. This hiatus ended, however, as early as 1951, as he entered into a delightfully intense affair. Unfortunately, Rollo had fallen in love with the wife of David Roberts. For both, it involved—in May's own words from *Man's Search for Himself*— the "courage and love of a given moment of relatedness," though it was fraught with less sure senses of "integrity" and "honesty." Rollo met Elinor Roberts within the social whirl of Union, probably at one of the Tillichs' parties. Ellie possessed a petite and flinty beauty enhanced by intellectual and emotional acuity. The daughter of a designer and a musician, she had found her most profound expression in art since childhood. She came to New York to study at the Art Students League. She and Roberts married in 1945 and had three daughters in quick succession. As a rising voice in Protestant theology and dean of students at Union Seminary, David Roberts traveled frequently and spent long hours at the office. This alone might have caused Ellie enormous strain as she raised their children. However, he was also prone to crippling bouts of depression. Indeed, his interest in psychoanalysis and Kierkegaard stemmed from his own struggle to hold back a creeping darkness within. For Ellie, marriage had become motherhood and the love and care of an admirable but wounded soul, her own needs buried by his.[33]

Rollo presented a compelling contrast, one whose sense of romantic adventure spoke directly to Ellie. Her own passion as a creative artist was like a magnet to him. They made love, listened to music, recited poetry, talked about literature and art, and carved out trysts carefully attuned to the schedules of patients and babysitters. Not since his romance with Isabella Hunner in Greece had he allowed himself such surrender. Both Rollo and Ellie were too committed to their families to seek divorces, yet neither could deny their need for each other.

It remains unclear just how much David Roberts knew about their relationship, but his depression deepened in the early 1950s. By 1954, he checked himself in for treatment at Austen Riggs Center, the famous residential psychiatric treatment facility in Stockbridge, Massachusetts. Roberts convinced his doctors he was stable enough to return to New York for Christmas. Soon after the new year, David Roberts committed suicide. He was forty-four years old.[34]

As was the custom of the time, family, friends, and the Union Seminary kept the circumstances of Roberts's death private. The *New York Times* obituary reported the cause as "a heart ailment, after a long illness." In a moving piece that became the preface to Roberts's posthumously published collection of sermons, *The Grandeur and Misery of Man*, Tillich hinted at the more tragic reality. Roberts keenly felt "powers in soul and society against which the good will even of the very best of us is without power," his mentor noted, and "knew the nature of these powers in many individuals, including himself." Tillich reported that just a few days before he killed himself, Roberts vowed, "If I ever should become healthy again I will be able to say what the demonic is."[35]

Few of their friends knew of Rollo and Ellie's affair. Tillich was an exception. He recommended that they keep their distance at first. Both clearly felt in some way responsible for his death. Slowly they transformed the wreck of a love affair and tragic death into an abiding friendship. Two years after Roberts's death, Ellie could write to Rollo with great appreciation but also exhaustion:

> I sometimes wonder how much feeling I'm capable of after these last years. . . . I also know that in spite of the beating my feelings have taken, they turn in your direction positively and warmly . . . the ecstatic moment does not abide, but depth of affection does and profound understanding and concern does. . . . Paul says, "You must love life." Sometimes these days I feel as close to despair that this seems impossible. Yet yesterday I saw the sun rise and knew that it was beautiful.[36]

And in February 1957: "I love him and I miss him and I understand what [Tillich] means about the relief of feeling that one is no longer needed. How often, in the past few years, I've wished for this blessed kind of relief!" A bit later in the same letter, she mentioned being moved by watching the film *Brief Encounter* on television without having to say it reminded her of their affair. She did recall that Rollo once told her that the lovers in that movie shouldn't have separated, but Ellie thought that it was not that simple. "What a mysterious process it is, falling in love, and what an almost unbearable essence of joy and pain."[37]

She wrote as she was sorting through her late husband's papers, "an endless process, and often exhausting because in so much of it is joy and grief so inextricably woven that I want to remember and forget both at once."

Coming across a paper, "Counseling and Understanding the Alcoholic," that one of David's students had dedicated to his mentor, Ellie noted that she was about to climb into bed with a Scotch on the rocks, ruefully remarking that "drinking alone is bad but sleeping alone is worse."[38]

Who can say how the inevitable but hushed guilt over the suicide played on Rollo's conscience and consciousness? In his final years and after a series of strokes, he suddenly moved from present to past, turning from those with him to an imagined Ellie, imploring aloud to her, "I wasn't the only one to blame."[39]

18

Existential Calling

Rollo's affair with Ellie Roberts and its somber aftermath—as well as a tacit détente in his marriage—remained dramas hidden behind a meteoric rise in public profile and professional influence. Indeed, the very geography of his everyday life confirmed that Rollo had arrived. He had lived mostly on the Upper West Side of Manhattan since late 1933 and continued to do so, but in circumstances that had become more comfortable and secure. The Mays now rented an apartment at the corner of Riverside Drive and 114th Street, a block's walk to Columbia University and six blocks to Columbia's Teachers College and Union Theological Seminary. Rollo's office was an eleven-block walk from home. Perched atop the regal Master Building at 103rd Street and Riverside, its windows commanded a magnificent view of Riverside Park, the Hudson River, and New Jersey beyond. Home and office were a short taxi ride to the William Alanson White Institute on East 94th Street.

As the Mays were establishing themselves in Manhattan, they also built a summer home in Holderness, New Hampshire. They had visited Holderness in 1946 and immediately fell in love with the landscape—rolling hills south of the White Mountains that eased into Squam Lake and its larger neighbor, Lake Winnipesaukee. Holderness's beauty had long attracted summer folk from Boston and New York. For Rollo, it also meant membership in an exclusive intellectual community. In 1921, the psychologist Lawrence K. Frank had purchased a summer place in the Holderness area, and over the decades that followed Frank invited an extraordinary array of intellectuals to this retreat—Margaret Mead, Gregory Bateson, Robert and Helen Lynd, Northrup Frye, and Erik and Joan Erikson, among others—to chart ways to study and improve the lot of the modern family.

Frank had become, according to Rollo's friend Harold Taylor, the "patriarch of the valley," alerting those he admired when one or another property became available in the area. Taylor, who in 1949 became president of Sarah Lawrence College, first met Frank in 1945 and by 1948 had purchased a lovely home in the area. Rollo met Frank while both worked on the New York Academy of Science report in 1955, and in September of that year the Mays purchased land in Holderness. They tore down the ramshackle remains of a farmhouse and built a comfortable summer home. Soon after, May constructed a simple writing cabin near the main house. The two structures mirrored the rhythms of sociability and solitude that the community had perfected. As Taylor put it, "We have an unwritten law that we don't call on each other unless invited." Rollo's study had no phone, and no one was to intrude, especially during morning hours devoted to writing. Over late afternoon cocktails, informal dinners, and evening gatherings, socializing and serious talk were a part of Holderness's allure. Still, it was the peace and isolation for thinking and writing that Rollo came to treasure.[1]

May's increasingly busy schedule accentuated the importance of Holderness as a spiritual redoubt. His responsibilities in New York included a full roster of patients, organizational duties at the White Institute and the New York State Psychological Society, memberships on various boards and committees, and teaching at the New School. He became a training analyst at the White Institute in June 1957, moving into ranks largely reserved for doctors. In addition, Bernard Kalinkowitz asked May, along with colleagues from the White Institute and a number of Freudian analysts, to plan a postdoctoral program in psychotherapy and psychoanalysis at New York University School of Medicine. May became part of its founding faculty.[2]

Rollo's growing fame also attracted speaking invitations nationwide. The varieties of settings and topics reflected his natural embrace of the role of public intellectual as well as his insatiable appetite for work. For example, in October 1954, he participated with Werner Heisenberg, Niels Bohr, and others in a roundtable, "Science and Human Responsibility," at Washington University in St. Louis. In January 1955, he gave a lecture, "Personal Integrity in a Conforming World," at New York's Bank Street School, and a week later traveled to Rochester to give the NYSPS presidential address, "Changing Scientific Conceptions of Man." In February, he delivered a series of three lectures at Oberlin: "Psychology and the Spiritual Problems of Modern Man," "Religion in the Age of Conformity," and "The Creative Conscience." In March, he gave the Eduard Lindeman Lectures at the New School and traveled to Cornell to deliver the talk "Crucial Issues in Contemporary Psychoanalysis." After a summer's break in New Hampshire, he accepted an invitation to speak and delivered an address, "The Idea of God as Affected by Modern Knowledge," in Lancaster, Pennsylvania. The year 1956 and beyond promised the same busy schedule, just new cities and topics. His agenda of talks and radio broadcasts in New York City alone moved at an exhausting pace.

And there were writing deadlines. "For the past two months my publishers have been literally standing outside my office door—in the persons of their messengers" he complained to a colleague at the White Institute, "waiting to pull from me this galley proof or that final draft of a preface. And as soon as this 600-page volume gets out of the way, the places in the hall will be taken by messengers from the Handbook of Psychiatry, etc., etc. This along with my lectures around the country, and my consulting . . . keep my schedule as tight as you can imagine what."

He had already cut his patient hours by a third despite great demand for his services among a clientele that ranged from anxious businessmen to creatively blocked artists, writers, actors, and musicians. Haunted by visceral memories of his collapse from tuberculosis and intermittent problems with tachycardia, he reduced his administrative roles at the White Institute. As he wrote to Lloyd Merrill, "I've decided I've got to take my overloaded schedule in hand or my health will go to hell again."[3]

May's cutbacks spoke to overload but also to singular devotion to the page proofs of the "600-page volume" he faced in February 1958. Published later that year as *Existence: A New Dimension in Psychiatry and Psychology*, the book allowed May and his co-editors, Ernest Angel and Henri Ellenberger, to introduce key European theorists of existential and phenomenological psychotherapy to an American audience. The opportunity to participate in *Existence* had come just at the moment when May, deeply attached to the revelatory insights of Kierkegaard and Nietzsche, was seeking ways to integrate the often aphoristic and contradictory insights of these philosophers into a broader and more useful "science of man" adaptable to therapeutic settings. *Existence* became for him nothing less than a new calling.

Existentialism, already a freighted watchword by the late 1940s, evoked a kaleidoscopic reimagining of the human condition that at first focused popular imagination on the ideas of Jean-Paul Sartre, Simone de Beauvoir, and Albert Camus. Existentialist writers championed "existence over essence" and bluntly noted that humankind was "condemned to be free." Sartre's version emphasized a decidedly atheistic primacy of self-creation in every act and thought. Catholic existentialists like Gabriel Marcel and Jacques Maritain sought a primary essence in authentic Christianity around which to build the existential life. Tillich set forth yet another, more Protestant path, the achievement of faith and the courage to live beyond mundane religious

life in an indefinable "God beyond God." All, however, sought to recon-
nect the unique individual with experience, choice, and action, rather than
living within the false and dehumanizing security of alienating churches and
culture.[4]

Existentialism was Janus-faced in mood. It might focus on a grim assessment of the human condition that highlighted one's aloneness in the world,
the "absurdity" of being, and suicide, a darkness amply captured in such titles
as Sartre's *Nausea* and *No Exit* or Camus's *The Stranger* and *The Plague*. Yet
existentialism also inspired, for these authors and others, dreams of liberation, social justice, and the courage to experience real freedom—the experiential building of a meaningful life from meaninglessness rather than from
stale notions, philosophies, and theologies. Darkness certainly pervaded
David Roberts's appropriation of existential thought as he moved closer to
suicide (though he allowed for more positive and heroic directions as well).
"What good can possibly come of turning away from these irrational and
Demonic forces which are menacing folk in our own time so savagely?"
Roberts asked as he defended turning to atheistic existentialism for wisdom.
"Why should we be unwilling, or unable, to face squarely the life of man in
all its vulnerability, edginess, and estrangement?"[5] For Hazel Barnes, who in
1956 provided the first English translation of Sartre's 1943 existential mas-
terwork, *Being and Nothingness*, the encounter with existentialism inspired a
sense of rebirth in many ways similar to a religious conversion. As she noted
simply, the philosophy "spoke to [her] condition."[6]

For May as well as Barnes, that humans were "condemned to be free" meant
that they must have the courage to choose a meaningful freedom. That was
the promise of the existential attitude, the promise of becoming an authentic
human being—feeling fully the joys and tragedies of life. This was certainly
the spirit in which May undertook, with Ernest Angel and Henri Ellenberger,
the writing and editing of *Existence*. May spent five years helping to secure,
edit, and contextualize essays by the existential psychotherapist Ludwig
Binswanger and phenomenologists Eugene Minkowski and Erwin Strauss,
among others. Much drudgework, occasional disagreements among the
editors, and testy correspondence with authors and translators sometimes
ensued. Yet for Rollo the process became most of all a deep immersion in
aspects of modern European thought previously unknown to him, especially
the world of phenomenology defined by Husserl and Heidegger and their
students. His preface and two introductory chapters glowed with the spirit of
discovery, which he summed up by simply quoting Keats's "On First Looking

into Chapman's Homer": "Then felt I like some watcher of the skies / When a new planet swims into his ken."[7]

Still, one might ask why he should have gazed in awe at existential psychology as this "new planet." After all, he had been acting in a recognizably existential manner even before the movement had a name. May's proto-existential style surfaced visibly in the 1920s, when he formulated a self-image as rebel against authority in the cause of truth and individuality while at Michigan State College. In Greece, as he furiously scribbled his original vision of life on Mount Hortiati the central theme was recognition of human beings as unique, not simply pawns of church-building missionary work or illustrations of simplistic constructs of science. At Union Theological Seminary and during his stint as a counselor in the 1930s at Michigan State, he cleaved to Nietzsche, Dostoevsky, Ibsen, and other prophetic protectors of a humanity threatened by established orders and herd thinking.

May studied these writers and others with Tillich, whose approach to Christianity had pointed May toward Kierkegaard's recently translated work and, in a different but complementary key, the holistic neurological theories of Kurt Goldstein. Tillich also exposed him, secondhand, to the key ideas of Martin Heidegger, the central German figure in twentieth-century existential thought. Most profoundly, his bout with tuberculosis tested these concerns and cemented his affinity to existential notions of anxiety, action, and affirmation of self in the face of death. In short, some of the central questions of existentialism, whether expressed in liberal Christian or psychological guise, had concerned May his entire adult life.

The "new planet" offered by Binswanger, Minkowski, and other existential psychologists and phenomenologists was not the philosophy per se but its integration into psychotherapeutic practice. They addressed a question May asked at the very opening of *Existence*: "Can we be sure ... that we are seeing the patient as he really is, knowing him in his own reality; or are we seeing merely a projection of our own theories *about* him?"[8] Again, the question was not a new one for May. He had displayed this specific concern for understanding "the patient as he really is" as early as his first publications on counseling in the mid-1930s, when he defined the best counseling as something of a spiritual mystery, the counselor a kind of priest, and success dependent upon an empathy that allowed the counselor to enter the mind and body of the counselee. In *The Art of Counseling*, he celebrated "empathy" as a state in which the counselor's "ego or psychic state ... had temporarily become merged with that of the counselee," one that he compared to "mental telepathy." The "cleansing experience" and "psychological nakedness" that accompanied such "empathy" were the true catalysts of healing.[9]

A rocky marriage and a lonely bout with tuberculosis certainly dampened Rollo's earlier expectations for soulful unity. Furthermore, his psychoanalytic training reframed such telepathic mergers as transference and counter-transference, a patient's or therapist's eroticized illusions and fantasies about the other. Still, May never gave up hope that genuine encounter with the patient as a living, acting, and unique person could actually emerge in therapy beyond the distortions of fantasy and also with an authenticity unaccounted for by transference theory. He continued to seek as whole and unmediated an engagement as possible—the very goal of existentialism's quest for self and its vision of kinship and difference concerning the "other."

By the late 1940s, May had begun to construct in his writings and practice a philosophically based approach to therapy and life that combined elements of American individualism, liberal Christian notions of an authentic inner life, and the tragic visions of human struggle forged from mostly German, Scandinavian, and Russian sources. Indeed, it was this still fragmented road to existential thinking that caused May at first to express only tentative connection and indeed some resistance to the postwar vogue for a philosophy explicitly termed existentialism. *The Meaning of Anxiety* made approving but only passing reference to Tillich's recent and pathbreaking articles on existential philosophy. As for Sartre, May basically parroted the views of his mentor and other critics, "not wish[ing] existentialism in this discussion, to be identified with the present-day popular conception as presented, for example, in the philosophical writings of Sartre."[10] *Man's Search for Himself* reiterated this view, especially the atheistic implications of the French philosopher's doctrine of "existence before essence," which seemed to place each individual in a world without any notion of pre-existing structures or relationships. Sartre, May argued, had helped to create "a sophisticated fad, a rallying point for the young Parisian dilettantes."[11]

That *Existence* was a logical extension of May's quest, however, belies the fact of its odd and almost accidental birth. The book was originally the brainchild of Ernst (later Ernest) Angel, an émigré Austrian Jewish intellectual whose very life typified the existential dexterity of interwar European intellectual and artistic life. Born in Vienna in 1894, Angel enlisted in the Austrian army at the beginning of World War I and after the war actively supported the short-lived Austrian revolution. He moved to Berlin to begin a peripatetic romp through the arts world of the Weimar republic—as a poet and in theater, publishing, and film. He eventually founded his own production company and directed several successful movies. He moved back to Vienna after Hitler came to power in Germany but, despite the dangers, often traveled to Berlin to see his "Aryan" wife. He was arrested in November 1938 during Kristallnacht and for five weeks was imprisoned in the Sachsenhausen concentration camp. By 1940 he was in New York.

In 1953, he proffered the idea of a book on existential psychology to Arthur Rosenthal, an upstart publisher who had just launched Basic Books. Rosenthal eagerly signed the project. Angel and Rosenthal approached May, whose affinity for the project had become clear in *The Meaning of Anxiety*. As he recalled years later of that moment, "It met my own needs and my own heart." May and Angel then recruited Henri Frédéric Ellenberger, a Swiss psychiatrist who had recently arrived in the United States to work at the Menninger Clinic. The path of Henri Ellenberger to *Existence* was more ordinary only in comparison to that of Angel. He was born in Rhodesia (now Zimbabwe) in 1905, to Swiss Protestant missionary parents, and studied psychiatric medicine in Strasbourg. He practiced in France until 1941, when he returned to Switzerland rather than live under German occupation. Ellenberger found a job in a Swiss sanatorium and, more important, became part of the Jung circle in Zurich. In 1950, he sought psychoanalytic training with Pastor Oskar Pfister, an early friend of Freud and Jung. In 1953, Ellenberger came to America to accept a prestigious teaching position at the Menninger Clinic.[12]

May thus joined two supremely talented men whose highly creative, mobile lives both before and after the Nazi period personified the existential ethic of personal action and choice. The trio embraced their project with passion but were virtual strangers with radically different pasts surveying relatively uncharted territory. Nonetheless, a working arrangement emerged. May brought a number of crucial elements to the book, the most important of which were his visibility to lay and professional audiences, his relentless work ethic and organizational skills, and, perhaps most significantly, his ability to translate complicated and often opaque ideas into clear and compelling English.

Translation was at the heart of the project. Angel, with Ellenberger's help, chose authors and selections and prepared basic translations, and May attempted to shape them into more felicitous English. This was not always an easy task. In the preface of *Existence*, May recounted a meeting with Tillich at which he showed the theologian preliminary renderings of key terms from what May called "the genius and demonic character of the German language." Tillich bridled at these efforts, exclaiming, "Ach, it is impossible!" but adding, "But you must do it anyway." May, who administered the overall project, had particular problems obtaining a satisfactory English rendering of one of the key chapters of the book, Binswanger's "The Case of Ellen West." So difficult was the task (in part because, as one of the translators noted, Binswanger wrote in a style of German prose that mimicked Heidegger) that the article went through several hands before Binswanger approved it for publication.[13]

In fact, May's two introductory essays, written with authority and clarity and informed by the enthusiasm of discovery, were the most comprehensible and revelatory to American readers. "The Origins and Significance of the Existential Movement in Psychology" began with the problem of perceiving the patient as he or she actually existed, and how Binswanger's approach to analysis sought an underlying, holistic philosophy of human existence upon which various theories of therapy might be based. However, May focused on defining a broad existential philosophical and cultural imperative more than a particular philosophy. "Existentialism, in short," he declared, "is the endeavor to understand man by cutting below the cleavage between subject and object which has bedeviled Western thought and science since shortly after the Renaissance." Here, he followed Tillich's spiritual-historical rendering in *The Courage to Be*, embracing his mentor's conception of an "existentialist revolt" before anyone named it as a movement. May's list of rebels included Van Gogh, Cézanne, Dostoevsky, Baudelaire, Kafka, and Rilke, as well as Kierkegaard, Nietzsche, and Freud. They all sought to depict, understand, or simply preserve an underlying reality that embraced instinctual, irrational, and spiritual realms of consciousness. And they provided an essential prelude especially to later, explicitly existential visions.[14]

May's second chapter, "Contributions of Existential Psychotherapy," supplied a more detailed exposition of Heidegger's concept of *Dasein*, or "being," and his elaboration of that "being" as it existed in various "worlds." "Being" and its "worlds" provided primary conceptions of human consciousness that held the total reality of a person's existence in tension. May argued that perceiving the patient in this holistic manner compelled the therapist to view the patient as more than the sum total of instinctual drives, illusions of transference, or behavioral mechanisms. Indeed, the existential approach forced clinicians to face themselves as they experienced the sometimes "very anxiety-arousing" but humanizing "encounter" with the patient. Distancing oneself from that encounter not only risked the therapist's "isolation" from the patient but also engendered a "radical distortion of reality." At this point, May quoted Sartre: "In either case the *man* disappears; we can no longer find 'the one' to whom this or that experience has happened.'"[15]

May knew that defining "the man" or "being" itself was crucial no matter how fraught with semantic difficulty. He began his own interpretation with the German term *Dasein* and its central place in existentialism and existential psychotherapy. "Composed of *sein* (being) plus *da* (there)," he explained, "*Dasein* indicates that man is the being who *is there* and implies also that he *has* a 'there' in the sense that he can know he is there and can take a stand with reference to that fact." He immediately reformulated this literal translation to more straightforward English: "Man is the being who can be conscious of, and therefore responsible for, his existence." Human beings must "choose" to be or do something authentic to their own nature and thereby "become" their true self.[16]

However, consciousness always was haunted by a struggle with "nonbeing," the awareness of death's inevitability and other, less ultimate limits to choice and action. Being and the threat of nonbeing defined the human condition and bred an ontological (that is, essential or primal) anxiety and guilt with which human beings struggled as part of their very nature. They experienced anxiety when contemplating choices to authentically fulfill their "becoming" and guilt when they proved unwilling or unable to authentically "become" themselves. May carefully distinguished between primal guilt and anxiety that might spur one to creative "becoming" and neurotic varieties that were symptomatic of failure to grow authentically or face the reality of "nonbeing." It was the job of therapy to reveal to patients the nature and danger of such neurotic guilt or anxiety so that they might make choices true to themselves.[17]

Just as important to May was Heidegger's reimagining of the worlds in which *Dasein* functioned. Freudian and behaviorist notions focused on either intrapsychic forces or stimulus-response mechanisms that in fact reduced individual volition and "being" to mechanistic and predictable outcomes. By contrast, Heidegger's notion of "being-in-the-world" placed human consciousness within simultaneous and oscillating environments. Thus a human being existed most broadly in the *Umwelt* (the "world around"), the natural and biological environment. Next came the *Mitwelt* (the "with-world") of fellow human beings within which one built a social existence. The *Eigenwelt* ("own-world") referred to perhaps the most mysterious realm of consciousness, one's relationship to self.[18]

May conceded that in practice more traditional schools of psychoanalysis had moved toward considering interpersonal and social environments, but he stressed that even the existentialists were just beginning to recognize the complexity and mystery of the *Eigenwelt*. By creating an ontology that allowed for a more complex and subjective view of the totality and simultaneity of human consciousness present in all these worlds, he hoped the existentially informed therapist could better see the patient in his or her own terms and come closer to helping that person achieve a richer and more authentic life. More specifically, he underlined existential understandings of time and history that reshaped the theoretical conceptions of traditional therapies. Freud and others rightly emphasized the power of early experience in shaping present consciousness, for instance, but existentialists argued that it was a two-way street. Therapeutic reorientation in the present, May noted, could not only counter the past's damaging power but also bring to consciousness more positive and supportive recollections of the past. Past and present influenced each other, expanded and contracted the subjective experience of time, and could set in motion directions for previously closed futures. This was perhaps the most profound focus of existentialism—how one might "become" oneself, transcending the "present" with a courageous embrace of one's potential being.

May made it clear that the existential approach did not dictate a new set of techniques in therapy but rather a new understanding of the realities and goals inherent in the therapeutic situation no matter the approach—Freudian, Jungian, Adlerian, or any other. Turning to the work of existential psychotherapist Medard Boss, whose technique was highly Freudian, May noted that the existential contribution consisted of reformulating the meaning of such concepts as transference, repression, and resistance through existential understandings of the human being. For example, May's concept of transference evolved from "a displacement of detachable feelings from one object to another" (say, the parent to the therapist) to a symptom of a person whose emotions "in certain areas never developed beyond the limited and restricted forms of experience characteristic of the infant. Hence in later years he perceives wife or therapist through the same restricted, distorted 'spectacles' as he perceived father or mother." Similarly, repression and resistance became not so much distortions of intrapsychic drives as symptoms of, in Heidegger's sense, abnormally constricted visions of worlds that might be widened through therapy.[19]

May related these and other reshapings of the therapeutic process to his overriding concern for "seeing the patient as he really is, knowing him in his own reality." *Presence* became the keyword, the presence of the therapist as "not merely a shadowy reflector but an alive human being" whose concerns during the treatment focused on the patient hour as completely as possible. To be sure, one need not master Heidegger to be an attentive therapist. May noted that his own colleague Frieda Fromm-Reichmann would quip, "The patient needs an experience, not an explanation." In particular, he highlighted Carl Rogers as a therapist not directly influenced by existential thought but who shared its basic commitment to therapy as "a process of becoming." He let Rogers speak for himself in an extensive quotation that began with a sentiment close to May's heart: "I let myself go into the immediacy of the relationship where it is my total organism which takes over and is sensitive to the relationship, not simply my consciousness." Though, as May pointed out, there were marked differences between Rogers's approach and those of existential analysts, on the points of "presence" and "becoming" they surely agreed.[20] As in Rogers's "client-centered" model of therapy, the existential approach emphasized the reality of the therapeutic relationship beyond distortions of transference, one that in its potential richness might model future senses of life for the client. "The aim of therapy," May concluded, "is that the patient *experience his existence as real*" and that he or she become "aware of his potentialities" and be "able to act on the basis of them."[21]

Initial responses to *Existence*, privately expressed to Rollo in the months before publication by those sympathetic to the endeavor, boded well for its reception. May's request for a read of his chapters by émigré analyst Edith Weigert, who herself was interested in the links between psychoanalysis, religion, and philosophy, elicited unqualified praise—"I congratulate you! You have achieved a tremendous scholarly work"—and predicted that the psychoanalytic movement, despite its biological basis, would move toward "an understanding of existential aspects." Carl Rogers praised May's summary of existentialism as "the very best I have found anywhere." Surprised at the similarities between his own work and that of the existentialists, Rogers found himself "gobbling up the pages" and thought *Existence* would be "one of the most important psychological books in this decade." Erich Fromm congratulated May just before publication, encouraged him to present at the forthcoming International Congress of Psychotherapy, and praised him as the one to "clarify involved and complicated matters for puzzled listeners, and serve as a mediator between the continents." Finally, famed Harvard psychologist

Gordon W. Allport praised the book in a pre-publication blurb for Basic Books, noting that "the significance" of *Existence* "runs deep."[22]

The publication of *Existence* in June 1958, however, initially elicited little response from mass media newspaper and magazine book reviewers, and official reviews in psychiatric and psychological journals came only after the usual lag of months or even years. The professional reviews, usually written by major figures in the fields of psychoanalysis, psychiatry, and psychology, were mixed. They often highlighted the clarity and importance of May's introductory chapters and expressed, by comparison, disappointment in the detailed and dense articles that were the putative heart of the volume. Carl Rogers, for example, unsurprisingly called May's chapters "exceptional," "clear and penetrating," and emanating from "profound scholarship and wisdom," while noting for the rest, "The act does not live up to its billing." He reserved particular scorn for Binswanger's fatalism as expressed in the Ellen West case. Henry Lowenfeld's review in the *Psychoanalytic Quarterly* praised May's introductory chapters as "helpful" but also accused them of "repeat[ing] popular prejudices" against psychoanalysis. More substantively, Lowenfeld worried that existential psychology tried to stretch the usefulness of therapy to areas traditionally served by religion and philosophy. In short: "It is naïve to expect psychotherapy to offer a cure of the disintegrating forces in a society."[23]

Surprisingly, advertising, word-of-mouth, and perhaps the loyalty of May's readers created a groundswell of interest for what in many ways was a difficult read except for May's chapters. *Existence* even reached the notice of *Time,* which in late December 1958 devoted a long article, "Psychiatry and Being," to the book, May, and the nerve existentialism had touched in professional and lay imaginations. It reported that the book had sold twelve thousand copies since publication in June and credited it and William Barrett's *Irrational Man: A Study in Existential Philosophy*, also published in 1958, with "sharply increas[ing] U.S. interest in existentialism and especially its use in psychotherapy." The *Time* piece began with a report of the late 1958 quarterly meeting of the Connecticut Society for Psychiatry and Neurology. According to *Time,* the meeting normally drew about sixty attendees, but this time the audience for May's keynote address not only filled the 220 seats at New Haven's Fitkin Amphitheater but also sat cross-legged on the floor around the speaker's podium. More listeners filled the aisles, stood crowded in the back of the auditorium, and spilled out into an anteroom and stairway.[24]

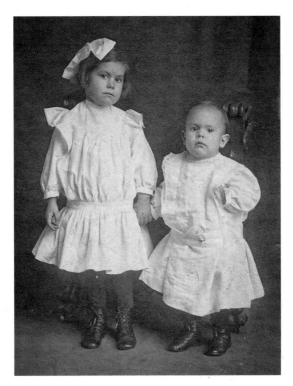

Ruth and Rollo May, ca. 1911. Rollo May Papers,
University of California, Santa Barbara.

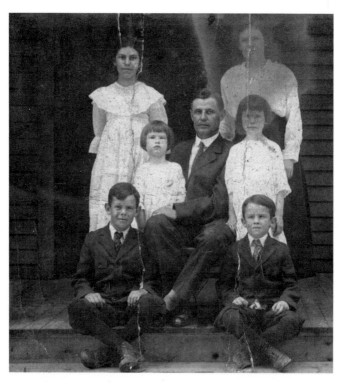

May Family, ca. 1918. *Top row, left to right*, Ruth and Matie;
middle row, Yona, E.T., Dorothea; *bottom row*, Rollo and Don.
Rollo May Papers, University of California, Santa Barbara.

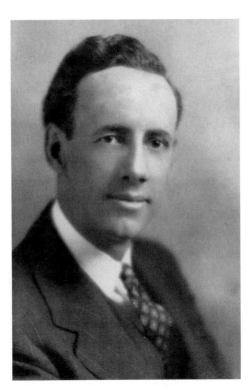

Bennett "Buck" Weaver, 1930s. © 1940
MLive Media Group. All rights reserved.
Used with permission.

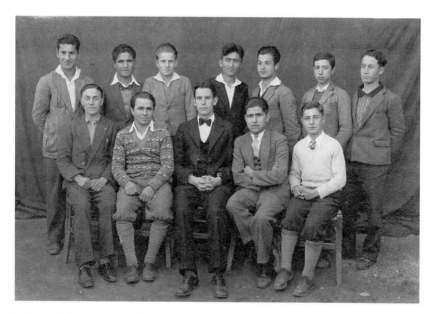

May with class at Anatolia College, 1931. Rollo May Papers, University of California, Santa Barbara.

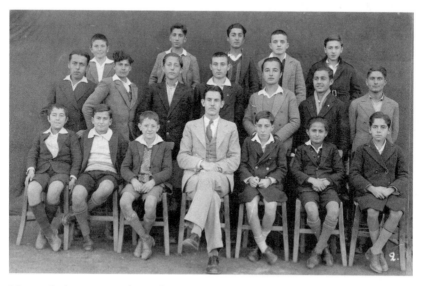

May with class at Anatolia College, 1932. Rollo May Papers, University of California, Santa Barbara.

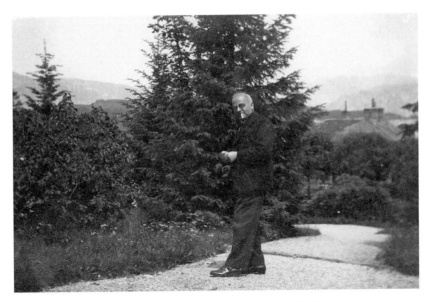

Dr. Alfred Adler at Semmering, snapshot by May, 1932. Rollo May Papers, University of California, Santa Barbara.

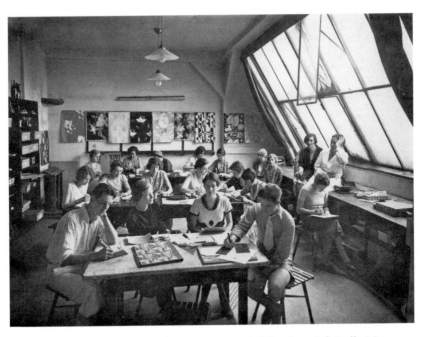

Art class in Joseph Binder's atelier, Vienna, 1932. May, *front left*. Rollo May Papers, University of California, Santa Barbara.

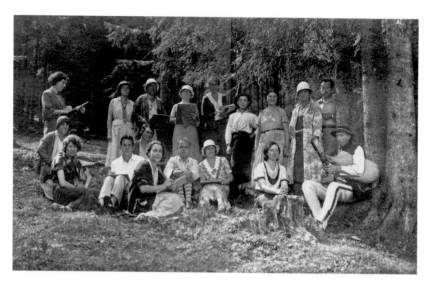

Art class, *en plein air*, May, *front row, second from left*, 1932. Rollo May Papers, University of California, Santa Barbara.

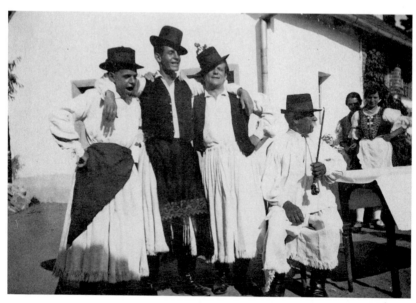

May dancing with art class in Veselí, Czechoslovakia (Czech Republic), 1932. Rollo May Papers, University of California, Santa Barbara.

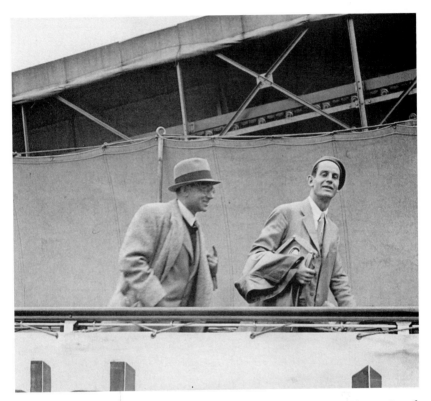

May and Binder boarding the SS *Europa*, 1933. Rollo May Papers, University of California, Santa Barbara.

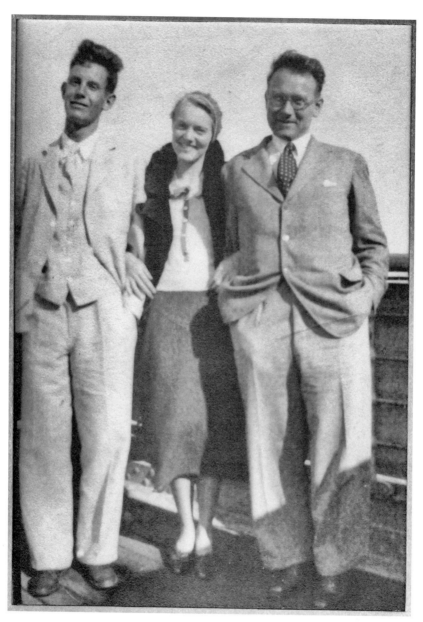

May, unidentified woman, and Binder on board the SS *Europa*, 1933. Rollo May Papers, University of California, Santa Barbara.

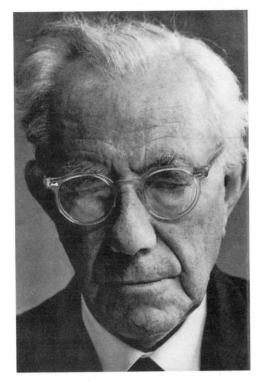

Paul Tillich, ca. 1960. Photographer unknown.

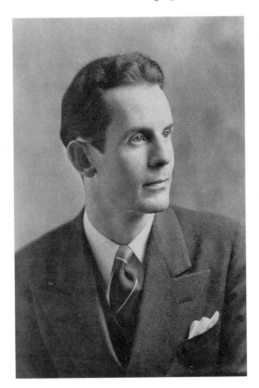

May, 1939. Rollo May Papers, University of
California, Santa Barbara.

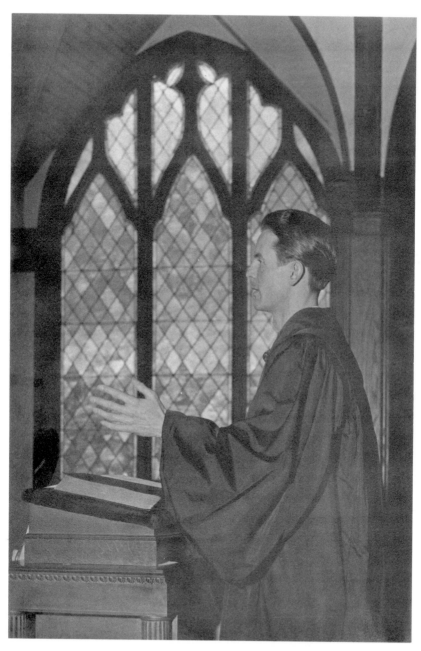

May at church in Verona, New Jersey, ca. 1938. Rollo May Papers, University of California, Santa Barbara.

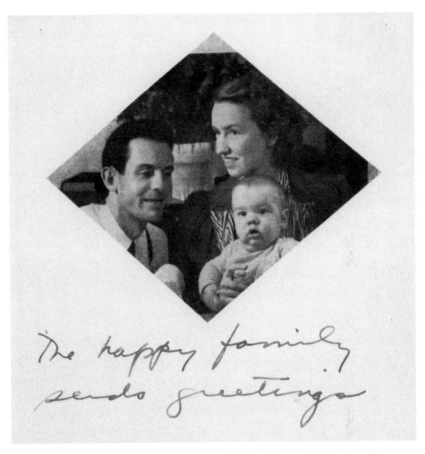

The happy family
sends greetings

Rollo, Florence, and Bob May, ca. 1941. Rollo May Papers, University of California, Santa Barbara.

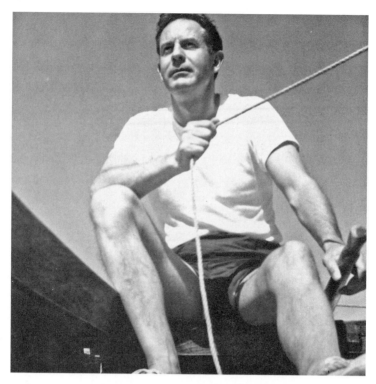

May sailing, 1950s. Rollo May Papers, University of California, Santa Barbara.

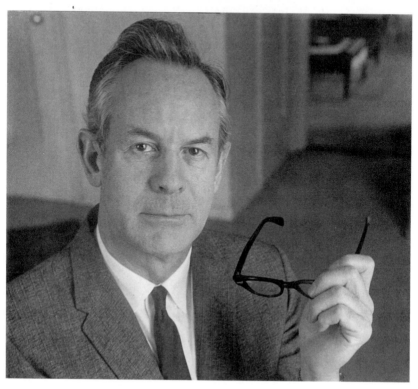

May, early 1960s. Rollo May Papers, University of California, Santa Barbara.

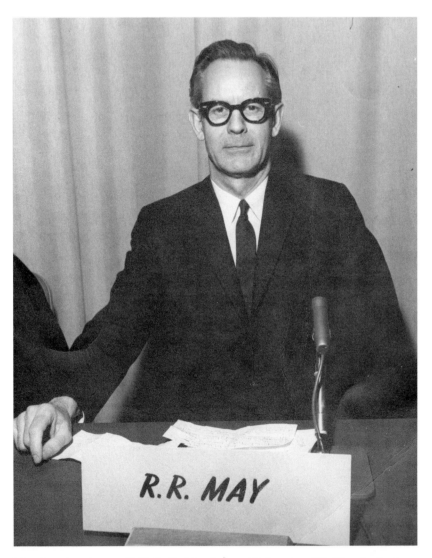

May, Los Angeles, ca. 1961. Rollo May Papers, University of California, Santa Barbara.

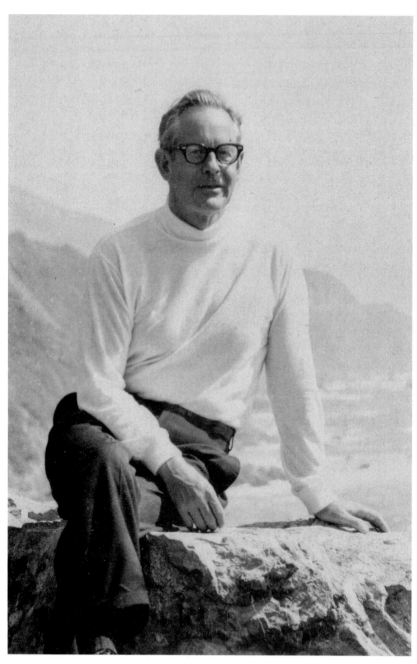

May at Esalen, 1960s. Rollo May Papers, University of California, Santa Barbara.

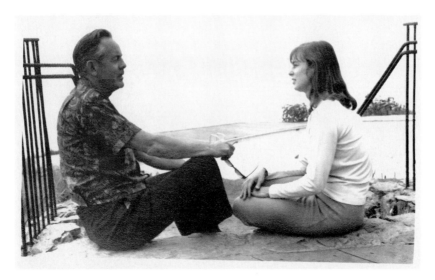

May and unidentified woman, Esalen, late 1960s–early 1970s. Rollo May Papers, University of California, Santa Barbara.

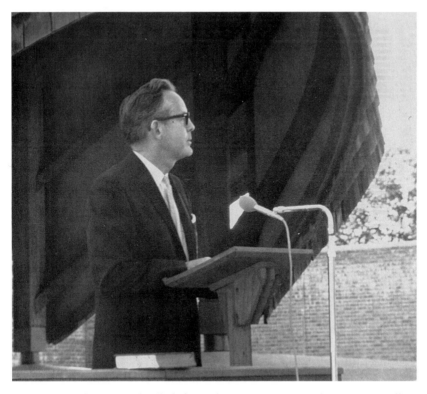

May giving eulogy at Paul Tillich funeral, New Harmony, Indiana, 1966. Rollo May Papers, University of California, Santa Barbara.

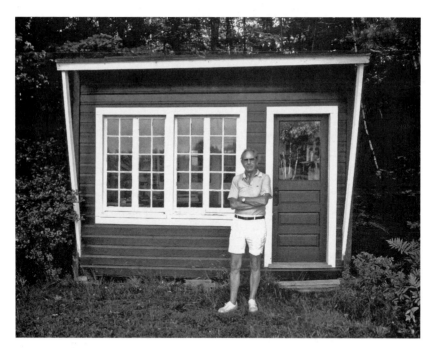

May beside his writing cabin, Holderness, New Hampshire, 1988. Photo by Robert H. Abzug.

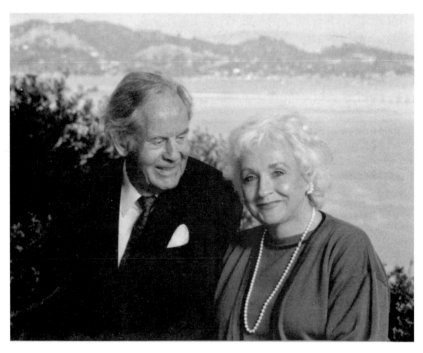

Rollo and Georgia May, on the deck of their Tiburon home, 1989. Rollo May Papers, University of California, Santa Barbara.

May's talk, "Contributions of Existential Psychoanalysis," outlined the ways in which an existential "approach" might augment common practice in American versions of Freudian and kindred methods of therapy. He used as an example the Freudian approach to Oedipal feelings of guilt and anxiety over a child's attraction to the parent of the opposite sex. The orthodox psychoanalytic cure involved understanding the lasting effect of such infantile urges through re-experiencing them in therapy, thereby neutralizing their crippling effects. While not taking exception to this appropriation of the Oedipal drama, he called also for an existential understanding of the Oedipal myth. After all, May argued, the play's great moment of realization occurs when Oedipus discovers that he has killed his father and married his mother: "The drama is the tragedy of seeing truth . . . the tragedy of self-knowledge, self-consciousness." In this and other ways, he argued, the existential lens brought a philosophical, often tragic, understanding of human nature to a more mechanistic theory.[25]

May's "skeptical" audience of professionals, *Time* reported, remained largely unconvinced that he was bringing anything new to the table. Some felt they had already incorporated the lessons of existentialism in their practice, while others rejected May's framework as more philosophy than science or medicine. May responded simply, "The trend toward existential analysis in the U.S. is only a strong undercurrent among the serious-minded."[26]

In fact, May underestimated the influence of *Existence* and kindred critiques of mainstream therapy that were developing in a variety of quarters. It not only introduced existential psychotherapy to an American audience but also galvanized a number of psychotherapists who, each in his or her own way, had sought to move beyond either Freudianism or behaviorism. Not only Carl Rogers but also Abraham Maslow, Gordon Allport, and numerous others were creating what Maslow would soon term a "third force" in psychology. They saw their work as moving beyond Freudian emphasis on pathology and biological terminology and behaviorism's deterministic straitjacket toward a conception of psychotherapy that widened the dimensions of life's possibilities. May actually shared some biographical and intellectual ground with members of this group. Maslow was deeply influenced by Kurt Goldstein's idea of the organism's ability to self-actualize and made it a key element of his "hierarchy of needs." Carl Rogers had been a divinity student at Union Theological Seminary, though unlike Rollo he dropped out to pursue a career in counseling and research psychology. Gordon Allport, never intent on a career in the ministry, studied philosophy as well as psychology and in later years sought a theory of personality that engaged larger philosophical and spiritual questions.[27]

Not surprisingly, then, the publication of *Existence* inspired a sense of intellectual camaraderie and a surprisingly American commentary. After reading a pre-publication copy, Carl Rogers focused on the contrast between May's contribution and those of the Europeans:

> I would like to say that I think that your chapters are by far the most exciting and deepest of any in the book. Alongside your description of the movement toward existentialist psychotherapy the actual writers do not show up so very well. I was interested in their contributions but they have not nearly the depth nor significance of your own chapters. . . . I think you did an excellent job of bringing together this material but it makes me wish now that you would put out a book length manuscript of your own views of therapy.[28]

Like Rogers, Maslow expressed to May just how "very much affected and influenced" he was by the book. He had not previously read any of the authors, nor Kierkegaard and Nietzsche—though he had tried and failed to understand Heidegger. Yet Maslow noted that his own "writings are in truth exist-phenom and so, in basic ways are those of Rogers, Fromm, Goldstein . . . and a lot of others in US. . . . If I knowing nothing of the European writings, come in essence to the same conclusions independently, then we are both responding to something objective in the historical situation." *Existence*, Maslow exclaimed, would have "the same stunning effect on other Americans that it had on me. You have written in American terms and so it can come through."[29]

Maslow's comments were vividly prophetic in at least one very important instance. Irvin Yalom, then a young psychiatric resident at Johns Hopkins, remembered picking up *Existence* at a moment when he "felt confused and dissatisfied with the current theoretical models." Yalom had thought "the biological and the psychoanalytic models left out of their formulations too much of the human essence." Reading May's chapters marked a turning point in life: "I devoured every page and felt that a bright, entirely new vista opened before me." Rollo had managed not only to translate the European existentialists into American English but also to pass along to others the sense of discovering a "new planet" that had set his mind afire just a few years before.[30]

The excitement and new circle of friends generated by *Existence* expanded in 1959 and the years beyond, bringing May into contact with independent initiatives and leaders who were quickly moving toward the creation of psychology's third force. Maslow's letter to May had underlined to May how little he knew about the work of his American contemporaries and their compatible strains of dissatisfaction with psychotherapy, and he responded with both a mea culpa and a plan. He admitted that he had "the bad habit of not reading enough in the persons I agree with" and having "a one-tracked [*sic*] mind" when working on a major project. He vowed from then on to "make clear the close relationship" between existential psychotherapy (*Daseinanalyse*) and the ideas of a growing number of American psychologists. "I would love to consider getting together with you and Carl and a very small group of others," he declared, "when we could really go into these matters and take steps we need." They soon took a giant step by planning a symposium on existential psychology for the annual meeting of the American Psychological Association in September 1959.[31]

Even before that panel had begun to prepare its papers, May was gathering a working group of like-minded psychologists to explore and promote the connections between existentialism and psychotherapy. The "organizing committee" included May, Thomas Hora, Henry Elkin, and Antonia Wenkart.[32] In February they mailed out a mimeographed call for participation in a two-day conference in April at New York's Plaza Hotel. At the conference itself the organizers as well as Edith Weigert, Ludwig Lefebre, Hanna Colm, and Clemens Benda presented papers. May's keynote address, "Toward the Ontological Basis of Psychoanalysis," set the tone for the entire meeting by reiterating the call for a therapy guided by a holistic understanding of what it means to be human.[33]

All considered the conference a success and set a date of May 9 to convene what had by now become a "council" consisting of May and Adrian van Kaam of Duquesne University, as well as Benda, Hora, Wenkart, Colm, Lefebre, and Weigert. May began by reporting on a recent trip to California during which he found widespread interest among psychologists in existential approaches. Wenkart shared her impressions from the recent Philadelphia meetings of the American Psychoanalytic Association, where she sensed a great deal of doubt about the effectiveness of traditional analysis. The small gathering then got down to business. They gave the group an official name, the American Association of Existential Psychology and Psychiatry, and decided to publish a newsletter edited by May and Wenkart. The first issue, which featured either full text or summaries of the papers given at the April conference, appeared in September, mimeographed and stapled, as *Existential Inquiries*.[34]

The next council meeting, on September 26, 1959, exuded the spirit of a revolution afoot. Van Kaam, Hora, and Wenkart all reported a contagion of interest, each from their own quadrant of the academic and therapeutic worlds. Most striking was May's report that the reception of the symposium organized with Rogers and Maslow at the September meetings of the American Psychological Association indicated to him that a "change [was] emerging towards existentialism as a reaction against Freud's positivistic dogma." The APA panel itself had been a lively exchange that largely highlighted the need for a therapy that enhanced a vision of life's possibilities and weighed existentialism's contribution to that endeavor. Entirely new was a paper by Herman Feifel, "Death—Relevant Variable in Psychology," whose work had already begun a broad inquiry into the psychology of death that inspired extensive work that paralleled and intersected with the concerns of existential psychology. The panel evoked so much interest that Random House invited May to edit and publish the papers as *Existential Psychology*, with Joseph Lyons adding a bibliography.[35]

The enthusiasm bred by such advances continued as the council discussed the next organized conference and the launch of *Existential Inquiries*. All agreed to printing four hundred more copies in addition to the "500 to 1,000" originally discussed, to be sent with a mission statement and subscription coupon to "persons distinguished in the field" or distributed to workshops and classes.[36] The second annual conference, originally planned for November 1959 but actually held on February 27–28, 1960, confirmed the widening collaboration of those interested in existential psychotherapy. In addition to papers by May and other members of the council, it featured major addresses by Tillich, Maslow, Leslie Farber, and Viktor Frankl. Scores of those who attended the conference also came to the business meeting that followed. Confirmation of success came when Van Dusen reported that the second issue of *Existential Inquiries* already had 361 subscribers, the rate of new subscribers was increasing, and the modest dues were more than paying for printing and mailing expenses.[37]

The rapid growth of the AAEPP was a significant but certainly not the only sign of interest in applying existential ideas to therapy. Organizations all over the country began to appear with similar or adjacent agendas. The week after the AAEPP conference at the Plaza, the Western Psychological Association featured a major symposium, "Existential Processes in Psychotherapy," at its meeting in San Diego. In December 1959, the new Chicago Ontoanalytic Society under the leadership of Jordan Scher hosted a "Conference on Existential Psychotherapy" at the American College of Surgeons in Chicago and another in May 1960 in Atlantic City, New Jersey, for which two members of the AEPP "council" (Benda and Wenkart) served on the sponsoring committee and gave papers.[38]

May also received a form letter in April from Anthony Sutich, a Palo Alto psychotherapist and protégé of Maslow, announcing a new publication, the *Journal of Humanistic Psychology,* for which he would serve as executive editor. Brandeis University had agreed to sponsor the journal but would not commit any funding, and Sutich indicated that, besides seeking "foundation grants and private donations," he, Maslow, and others planned to launch an umbrella organization, the American Association for Humanistic Psychology. Sutich hoped that May would support such an effort.[39]

Maslow had been working toward such a journal and formal organization for a number of years, adding each year to what became a circular list of potential allies in a movement toward a psychotherapy aimed at growth rather than, as they saw it, simple cure. Sutich's letter alluded to the difficulties of finding just the right name for the journal, one open-ended enough to invite a variety of contributions and an expansive audience, yet not so broad as to give the impression of a platform with limitless borders. Coming up with the name of the journal and association might well have been an impulsive gesture amidst growing frustration. It was a choice with which some would be uncomfortable for its lack of joining humanism with science. Yet it also was one that encouraged a culture-changing marriage of psychotherapy with personal and spiritual experimentation quite conducive to an emerging social mood. Rollo would soon engage that movement with hope but also deep reservations.[40]

For the moment, however, May's concerns centered on his work with the AAEPP, and it was already clear that success was bringing growing pains of its own. Calls for incorporation, more committees, more council members, and a more routinized organization began to appear. And then there was concern, as with Maslow's group, over its journal's name. The meeting voted to poll the membership about the title, and as it turned out, the issue under preparation would be the last under its original name. From 1961 on, the official publication of the AAEPP became the *Review of Existential Psychology and Psychiatry,* with Adrian van Kaam as editor and the journal relocated to Duquesne University. Rollo and Henry Elkin became associate editors.[41]

Rollo relinquished the editorship to van Kaam with some relief. He was more suited to the charismatic founding of organizations than to their maintenance, and the AAEPP was now on solid ground. In addition, he had recently been suffering bouts of tachycardia and all too frequent viral infections plausibly linked by his doctors to his exhausting schedule. They were symptoms he had experienced and written about before, of a life in further search of self. May's championing of existentialism over the years since David Roberts's death had not left his inner life untouched. In dialogue with his diary and evident in his writings and actions, May was experiencing an existential crisis of his own.

19

Freedom in the Face of Fate

As the impact of *Existence* spread across therapeutic worlds in America and Europe, May found himself more and more in demand. In interviews, on panels, and in invited lectures, he reiterated the basics of existential psychotherapy. However, in an important address to the 1958 International Congress on Psychotherapy in Barcelona, May tackled themes that in some ways hinted at more personal questions unleashed by his discovery of the "new planet" of existential psychotherapy. He reiterated its central goal for the patient: "an encounter with one's own existence," rather than merely "treatment" aimed at "adjustment." The therapeutic relationship ought to prepare the patient, May declared, to enter "a new personal world . . . in which he becomes able to take a decisive orientation to his own existence." Such was the confidence of his presentation that the listener might have mistakenly guessed May had already arrived in that new world. Yet as he continued to struggle with untamed demons, existentialism provided no sure answers but rather a profoundly transformative framework for confronting the unfinished business of his own identity and existence.[1]

One important development in this regard, easy to ignore but central to May's emerging sense of self, was a new and strikingly explicit embrace of an American identity, one broadcast in the title of his Barcelona lecture, "Existential Analysis and the American Scene." Like many American intellectuals of his era, May could not help but frame his vision of the world mostly within the European intellectual tradition. Throughout *Existence* and in other lectures and articles, despite fleeting references, May's orientation had been almost entirely European. Only as *Existence* began to have its magnetic effect on American contemporaries did May come to see that existential attitudes, whatever their given name, might also have roots and indeed flowerings in America.

The shift involved many layers of intellectual and emotional commitment and no small amount of paradox. May's personal road to both psychology and existentialism was paved virtually entirely by contact with Europeans—Alfred Adler, Paul Tillich, Karen Horney, Erich Fromm, Frieda

Fromm-Reichmann—and by the influence of Kierkegaard and Nietzsche. Furthermore, he entered the field of psychotherapy through theology and counseling, rather than through the dominant American world of experimental psychology. May's path was certainly also informed by a reflexive rebellion against his small-town midwestern roots, his useful perception of E. T. May as a tinhorn salesman for God, and the adoption of a new father— Paul Tillich—who spoke in elegant abstraction with a sweet and seductive German accent.[2]

Yet in the year after the publication of *Existence*, as the profession and public recognized him as the major American spokesperson for existential psychotherapy, a subtle but significant change occurred in May's understanding of himself as an American. His Barcelona talk was the watershed event. It was almost as if once he and his fellow editors had brought European *Daseinanalyse* to America, May felt it necessary to make America a bit more understandable, in a positive sense, to Europeans. At Barcelona, surrounded by flesh-and-blood therapists with little or no insight into and many prejudices concerning American culture, May became more conscious than ever of being an American. His thinking about America and existentialism began as part of his work on *Existence*, and one sees the roots of the Barcelona paper in a paragraph and a long footnote in that work. Going forward, he found it important to expand upon the differences between Europe and America in much broader and more pointed terms.[3]

May's presentation posed a paradox not just for his international audience but also for his own sense of self. "Existential analysis [had] many profound and important affinities with underlying traits in the American character," he noted, and yet American psychologists and psychiatrists had been "decidedly ambivalent" about the existential approach to therapy. How could "in some ways a very existential people" be so "suspicious of existentialism"? He began by comparing the American emphasis on "knowing by doing," in the everyday sense, with Kierkegaard's nostrum "Truth exists for the individual only as he himself produces it in action." May focused particularly on William James's "passionate emphasis on immediacy of experience" and thus his "amazing kinship with the existential thinkers."[4]

Indeed, May identified with James. He described the philosopher/psychologist as a man who possessed "a great humaneness and through his own vast breadth as a man was able to bring art and religion into his thought without sacrificing any of his scientific integrity." May credited him "almost single handed" with rescuing "American psychology at the turn of the century from becoming lost in armchair philosophizing on one hand or the minutiae of the physiopsychologic laboratory on the other." He was, according to May, "our most typical American thinker."[5]

No sooner did he call him "our most typical American thinker," however, than May noted that American psychologists "dismissed [him] with mild contempt between the two world wars," preferring instead behavioristic and positivistic approaches. Yet James represented "the underlying attitudes in America which are just below the conscious surface," and his reputation awaited a "rebirth of interest" that blossomed in universities after the war. Thus, though existential thinking in psychology had been "latent and suppressed," renewed study of James augured well for the future.

May explained both the American propensity for and ambivalence toward existential attitudes by focusing on the importance of the "frontier" in American life. He noted that many Americans were literally only one or two generations removed from frontier life. The needs of the frontier—action, courage in the face of the unknown, making decisions toward shaping one's destiny—were existential tendencies balanced by a "suspicion of theorizing, abstract speculation, or intellectualizing for its own sake." Nor did the modern quest for advancement, for spatial and economic mobility, come from "merely a crass materialism or solely a hunger for economic gain." May paraphrased Tillich in characterizing it rather as "a spiritual attitude . . . to risk one's self, to take one's destiny into one's own hands." It was rather an "optimistic existentialism," a belief "that everybody can change his life."[6]

In short, the promise of the frontier and its partial reality left Americans feeling in control of their lives, for better and for worse, and deeply in need of a practical means of controlling themselves and society. Technique and ritual played more than their usual role in consciousness. The American imperative—"to do"—was certainly an existential imperative as well, but May was less certain that his fellow citizens could afford the comfort of thinking of how "to be." Nor, May emphasized, could Americans easily embrace a "sense of tragedy in human existence." They were too busy doing and too often avoiding the costly process of thinking about being. At the same time, May did note changing attitudes in the shock of postwar realities. He admitted that a vast revival of interest in religion had become a hallmark of the era, though he doubted its ultimate value because of "its conformist character." More comforting was the burst of interest among academics and the public in the question of existence. In this interest lay the possibility that American psychotherapy might move from resistance to acceptance of the need to ask philosophical questions about the human condition. In many ways such comments were unremarkable variations on themes of American character that had emerged earlier in the decade, whether in May's own *Man's Search for Himself* or the popular historical and social scientific work of David Riesman, David Potter, and William H. Whyte.[7]

As surprising was May's willingness to criticize various European approaches to psychology and psychiatry, first of all to "propose modestly to accuse many of our existential colleagues, particularly in Europe, of being unexistential in dealing with 'the unconscious.'" Some therapists, he admitted, used the term "unconscious" as a noun to denote a realm " 'causing' this or that symptom or behavior." He argued that they misunderstood the concept. Freud, he noted, meant the term to enlarge the definition of personality beyond "the narrow rationalism and voluntarism of Victorian man." May preferred to speak of "unconscious experience," radically expanding in very Jamesian fashion the very notion of experience itself, while admitting that developing a "phenomenology of unconscious experience" would be a challenge in its own right.[8]

May's final bone to pick with his existential European colleagues was their emphasis on the theoretical rather than therapeutic dimensions of psychiatry or psychoanalysis. He made no apologies for what he admitted was an American bias toward applied science, "our concern with helping anyone who suffers, quixotic though that may seem at times." In addition, he doubted one could develop an existential psychology without dealing with real people in crisis. "We can find people revealed only in critical situations; no person will go through the agonies of baring the deepest aspects of his psychological and spiritual sufferings except as he has some hope of gaining help in finding his way out of his agony."[9] This last assertion, of course, brought May's calling full circle in ways his audience could not know. His consulting office had become poet Sam Foss's "house by the side of the road," where he could be of aid to "the men who press with the ardor of hope, the men who are faint with the strife," moving them toward an encounter with self that might bring them closer to authentic lives.

May's public grappling with American identity, certainly part of his own maturation and an element of the postwar prominence given to American culture and science, proceeded even as he pursued his artistic urges both in psychological writings and in private. Among the most fruitful areas of academic exploration centered on the question of human creativity. He was hardly the only psychologist interested in the creative process in the 1950s.

Indeed, as the eminent psychologist Henry A. Murray noted at the time, the very word "creativity" had sparked in the 1950s a "multiplicity of scientific investigations" and "well-attended conferences and symposia on the subject." Murray viewed this phenomenon as "a little vital turning point, initiated as always by a statistically insignificant minority, which, if our species is vouchsafed a future, will be apperceived in retrospect as a movement of historic import." Murray's observation lent weight to the notion that the existential question within psychology in fact was part of a broader postwar recognition that even experimental psychologists had become curious about subjective realms that they had previously deemed irrelevant.[10]

For May, of course, the question of creativity had longstanding and deeply personal roots. His fascination with the creative impulse harked back to his time in Greece, his own attempts at producing art, and his embrace of the artist as the new arbiter of truth. Christian concepts of the creative life had appeared in both *The Art of Counseling* and *The Springs of Creative Living*. *The Meaning of Anxiety* linked the creative impulse to Kierkegaard's more existential notions of creative consciousness, notions that emphasized the necessity of anxiety, guilt, and confrontation of self. He had expanded and romanticized this vision of creativity in *Man's Search for Himself*, rehearsing the emergence of the individual in three stages ("innocence," "rebellion," and "ordinary consciousness of self") and defining an additional stage, highest of all, as that of "creative consciousness of self," or, in "classic psychological term[s]," "ecstasy." Here he referred to the literal origin of the word, "to stand outside one's self," a kind of sublime objectivity seemingly beyond the narrowing subjectivity of everyday perception. Though he linked such ecstasy to the production of creative works, his main point was to allow for an understanding of those "special moment[s]" of transport that individuals experience "in listening to music, or in some new experience of love or friendship which temporarily takes them out of the usual walled-in routine of their lives."[11]

The editing and writing of *Existence* left May little time to pursue the question of creativity in a formal way again until 1958, when he participated in "Symposia on Creativity," a series of panels at Michigan State University that featured such luminaries as Henry Murray, Carl Rogers, Abraham Maslow, Erich Fromm, and Margaret Mead. May's contribution, published a year later as "The Nature of Creativity," revealed how emphatically he had come to associate the creative act with existential encounter. He also had become much more attuned to the process of creation as experienced by his patients who were artists and writers and began to focus the question of creativity more narrowly than the broad categories of "possibility" and "ecstasy." While May cared very much about creativity for "everyman," more and more he emphasized the special characteristics of what he called "actual creativity" or "true art," as opposed to relatively "superficial" forms of creativity or aestheticism that lent a "frosting" to life. "True art," he asserted, involved "bringing something new into birth." It was hardly a new topic of interest within psychology or the long history of Western civilization. As May pointed out, the participants in Plato's *Symposium* discussed the relationship between love and beauty in ways quite similar to his own discussion of creativity and encounter.[12]

May's major point was to return to an appreciation of creativity as a positive force for culture, the result of an original encounter with perceived reality in the face of popular conceptions and psychological theories that interpreted art and artist's lives as the products of neurotic disorders—as "regression in the service of the ego." Most of his patients began therapy worried that treatment might rob them of their creative edge. He recounted the time in Vienna when Alfred Adler had invited the traveling artist group to his house. Adler introduced the artists to his general theory and then to his "compensatory theory of creativity," that human beings create to "compensate for their own inadequacies." Without denying that many artists displayed neurotic disorders, May noted that such a theory dealt with the possible shape of creations but not the essential creative force.[13]

May was not alone in emphasizing the non-neurotic essence of the creative act. However, more than most of the other contributors, he spoke in direct and sometimes personal ways about particular artists and artwork and their contributions or failings. He even gave what amounted to personal critiques of the 1957 Picasso retrospective at the Museum of Modern Art and an exhibit of Mondrian's early paintings. He emphasized not only the artist's role in the intense encounter that produced great work but also that of the subject and the environment. He thus concluded "The Nature of Creativity" with an apt summary:

> Genuine artists are so bound up with their age that they cannot communicate separated from it. . . . For the consciousness which obtains in creativity is not the superficial level of objectified intellectualization, but an encounter with the world on a level that undercuts the subject-object split.

"Creativity," to rephrase our definition, "is the encounter of the intensively conscious human being with his or her world."[14]

Such an approach to art and creativity inexorably led May to another topic that was of growing concern both to intellectuals and to May's own integration of therapy with the wider topics of human communication and meaning-making: the centrality of symbol and myth in the lives of individuals and cultures. In 1958 *Daedalus*, the journal of the American Academy of Arts and Sciences, published a special issue, "Symbolism in Religion and Literature," featuring essays by some of the most respected members of the 1950s intellectual establishment: Paul Tillich, Kenneth Burke, Talcott Parsons, I. A. Richards, Alfred North Whitehead, and Werner Heisenberg. George Braziller offered to publish an expanded edition in book form and asked May to edit the volume and write an introductory essay.[15]

Editing *Symbolism in Religion and Literature* gave May the opportunity to interact with some of the great critics, philosophers, and scientists of the age, further widening the reach of his work and strengthening his growing reputation as a public intellectual. His own essay, "The Significance of Symbols," used therapeutic evidence to demonstrate the crucial importance of symbols to human consciousness and by extension to the health of human society. May called symbols the very building blocks of "self." He drew on various disciplines to argue that the sources of a person's symbolic identity included "those from archaic and archetypal depths within himself, symbols arising from the personal events of his psychological and biological experience, and the general symbols and values which obtain in his culture." Following Jung and others, as well as his own observations in therapy, he observed that contemporary society and individuals "suffered from the deterioration and breakdown of the central symbols in modern Western culture" and that the "emergence" and appeal of psychoanalysis was in part due to this deterioration. Its interpretation of dreams and re-symbolization of individual consciousness was a partial solution to a cultural crisis.[16]

In fact, May argued that orthodox psychoanalysis offered only a partial answer to the paucity of symbols by treating them as condensed signposts to the past. He summed up a more constructive vision in a manner that combined analytic, existential, and socio-psychological aspects and became the template for much of his future work:

Symbols and myths are means of discovery. They are a progressive revealing of structure in our relation to nature and our own existence, a revealing of new ethical forms. . . . By drawing out inner reality they enable the person to experience greater reality in the outside world as well.[17]

May's grappling with the question of creativity had already rekindled in him an urge toward artistic creation. Having found satisfaction over the years as an amateur painter and having succeeded in producing three books and embarking on a fourth, in 1952 May wrote what he called a "parable," a fantasy about the loss of freedom in a grand psychological experiment. He called it "The Man Who Was Put in a Cage" and published it in a professional journal. Not a stylistic masterpiece, the story nonetheless had a powerful theme—the use of psychological science to deprive a human being of true freedom—and May addressed it specifically to the psychology community. He told the tale of a king who, on a whim bred of boredom, asked himself, "I wonder what would happen if a man were kept in a cage, like the animals at the zoo." He hired a psychologist to administer the experiment, one who initially balked at the project as "unthinkable" but changed his mind after the king noted that others in history, from the Romans to Hitler, had more or less done the same thing. He would do it, the king argued, whether the psychologist agreed or not and added that he had already secured a large grant from the "Greater Social Research Foundation" for the experiment. His curiosity and appetite whetted, the psychologist relented.[18]

May then led both the psychologist and the caged man through various stages of protest, resignation, and finally seeming contentment—though when the caged man talked to the psychologist "his eyes were distant and vague," and he "never used the word 'I' any more." "He had no anger, no hate, no rationalizations," the psychologist observed. "But he was now insane." The psychologist was left with a deep sense of emptiness and remorse. He had done his job well, but now realized that he had been seduced by the king, the foundation grant, and the dream of professional prestige to do something he should never have done. He mused that he might have been better off farming or painting or writing "something that would make future men happier and more free." The alternatives seemed unrealistic, however, and he dropped off into an uneasy sleep.[19]

Some hours later he had "a startling dream." A crowd had gathered around the man in the cage, who was now shouting: "When the king puts me or any man in a cage, the freedom of each one of you is taken away also. The king must go!" The crowd repeated the chant, broke the bars of the cage, and "wielded them for weapons as they charged the palace." "The psychologist awoke, filled by the dream with a great feeling of hope and joy" but soon heard an inner voice, the voice of his "orthodox" training analyst, announcing that the dream was simply "wish fulfillment." "The hell it is!" the psychologist responded as he got up from the bed: "Maybe some dreams are to be acted on."[20]

"The Man Who Was Put in a Cage" encapsulated May's worries about the detached, scientistic tendencies in both academic psychology and orthodox psychoanalysis, concerns shared by others in the profession like Rogers and Maslow. These psychologists and others would soon find common cause with May in the promotion of existential and, later, humanistic versions of psychotherapy. The piece also reflected a growing popular concern with the conformist seductions of affluence. And the final rebellious heroics of the psychologist echoed the romantic editorials condemning conformity that May wrote for *The Student* at Michigan State.

May's parable also externalized a personal fantasy, that of writing fiction in the cause of making everyday folks "happier and more free." Rollo had dabbled in poetry, mostly about ideal women and courtship, and short fiction that suffered from wooden heroes and an overly romantic style, and these specimens had mostly remained in his files as tentative writing experiments. However, positive reactions to "The Man Who Was Put in a Cage" from friends and colleagues sympathetic to its main theme encouraged him to pursue many an intellectual's ultimate fantasy—writing a novel. Even as he busied himself with the politics of the profession, lectures and patients, and, of course, *Existence*, May managed to produce, by September 1956, a 250-page draft of "The Conquest of Apatheia," a dystopian novel along the lines of Huxley's *Brave New World*. The population of a future society has been perfected in its contentment by technological and psychological manipulation but then besieged by a literal plague of crippling apathy (apatheia) much like that which afflicted the man in the cage.[21]

Having developed a cordial relationship with editor Harold Strauss at Knopf, May sent the novel to him for consideration. Strauss found the idea "fascinating" but the execution problematic. It was, according to his internal report, "loaded with 'gimmicks' and bare of people," lacking a "plot even of a melodramatic sort, and virtually no characterization." He sent it back to May with a frank rejection letter but also asked him to keep working on it. A new draft submitted in May 1957 met the same fate, including Strauss's continued encouragement.[22]

May found time to work on a revised version of the novel even amid activities surrounding *Existence*, supervisions at the White Institute, seeing patients, and the usual round of speaking engagements. He consulted with a new friend, the writer Lillian Smith, who helped him bolster the characters and plot. He gave the manuscript a new title, "The Heart Is a Muscle," and sent it again to Strauss on December 28, 1959. This time he thought it was in "pretty good shape" with "new and rich characterizations, and the strengthened plot." Strauss found it not very "plotty" but still "good reading," and "quite <u>possibly</u> worth publishing." He sent it on to three others on the editorial board, but they were less sanguine. One totally panned it; the other agreed and added, "I just don't feel that this man has the ability as a novelist to pull such a book off successfully." Strauss rejected it again in March 1960.[23]

May revised it once more, submitting it to Knopf on February 10, 1964 under the title "The Glass God," and this time the process was short but not sweet. The publisher sent it back to him on February 25. The internal report suggested the publisher "leave once and for all." The reader's report echoed prior perusals: "Mr. May just isn't a novelist." Rollo did further revisions but by 1965 had given up the project entirely.[24]

Rollo might have simply taken no for an answer, as he did when Joseph Binder declared him no artist, and he eventually did. However, as he imagined the novel to be something singularly his and its success a measure of his authentic self, the stakes seemed immeasurably higher. Almost a year after he confidently declared the goals of existential psychotherapy at Barcelona, he struggled with his fiction and questioned in his diary whether he himself was "denying [his] own Being.... Denying it for security, for conformism, for purpose of covering up own strength." He expressed this concern not about one issue but many, almost all, key aspects of life. Even as he championed the courageous search for new knowledge and understanding of self, a gnawing feeling of enslavement to the real and imagined expectations of others and to chronic feelings of inadequacy haunted his dreams and waking hours.[25]

Such struggle, of course, was nothing new. May had quite consciously mixed painful self-scrutiny and creative intellectual and artistic exploration from his days in Greece through his career as a therapist and writer. After a relatively dormant period while recovering from tuberculosis and finishing his dissertation, the publication of *The Meaning of Anxiety* and his passionate affair with Ellie Roberts rekindled his thirst for the creative, experiential life as well as all the old conflicts over women, marriage, and "meaning." May continued to cycle between a remarkably productive professional life and feelings of anxiety, self-doubt, envy, and fear that he could never act from his deepest impulses and convictions. Indeed, they worked together as a something of an analysis in process, one that allowed both a certain amount of self-knowledge and a constant working out of problems as they arose. May's self-doubt and chronic feelings of inferiority in this period had their roots, of course, in his pushing creative forms as well as in intrapsychic dramas of childhood. In addition, insecurity and resentment had longstanding origins in his upbringing as part of a maddening familial world. Nonetheless, the boy who envied his Marine City high school chums for their Ivy League educations now hobnobbed with the eastern elite in New York and Holderness.

Most striking in this regard was his friendship with William Sloane Coffin, Jr.—Bill Coffin—whose uncle had been president of Union Theological Seminary during Rollo's student days. Coffin had done an adventuresome but ultimately disillusioning stint in army intelligence during World War II and in the CIA during the early years of the Cold War. In 1958, he had just become chaplain of Yale University at age thirty-four, only two years after graduating Yale Divinity School. May and Coffin's first meeting couldn't have been more conducive to May's ego, the newly minted Yale minister having sought him out in Holderness while visiting the outgoing chaplain, Sidney Lovett. Coffin told May that *The Meaning of Anxiety* had a great impact on him, and that first meeting blossomed into a long friendship. Yet Coffin's élite background put May on the defensive and raised fears of rejection bred of his own marginal upbringing. Nothing he had accomplished seemed capable of erasing such feelings. After an evening with the Coffins in Holderness, he admitted a need to prove he was "worth something" to Coffin and his "silver spoon" crowd. May felt "left out." "I still envy that, think I should be in on it? . . . I don't accept self as am, but should be an aristocrat?"[26]

This need to be "an aristocrat" spread to his professional life and heightened the stakes of competitiveness, exacerbating a fear that others eagerly lay in wait to cut him down. Reading a review by Philip Rieff of an edition of Freud's papers depressed him because of Freud's "great popularity" among those May construed as his "'enemies.' . . . I have such an ambition, rivalry with Freud?" He was quite aware of the "self-defeat in rivalry with these big shots," how it diminished his "simple, direct contribution." And, true to the vocabulary of existentialism, he wondered: "Can it be my aim, simply to *fulfill my own being?*"[27] Praise might alleviate the mood for a time, as when a review of *Existence* with glowing praise for his chapters arrived. "Shows how foolish all along has been my feeling of anxiety: I would be attacked, etc. Why afraid of that?" However, such relief rarely lasted long.[28]

It was as if imagined enemies sat on both shoulders, whispering insults in his ear and ready to pounce. This was especially the case as he moved deeper into the world of the New York intellectuals of the postwar era. Confident, outspoken, often Jewish and politically radical, some openly homosexual, they trampled on midwestern Protestant inhibition and self-presentation. On one occasion, his new acquaintances W. H. Auden and Paul Goodman (who had just published a massive novel, *The Empire City*) became the objects of fear. "Goodman will attack me, scorn . . . ," he wrote in his journal, "they don't like me . . . Auden, etc. I stuffy." And he imagined their reaction to his attempts at fiction: "Love to pour contempt on novel. I shouldn't be out of my corner. Stay in my field. . . . What does May think he is, doing everything, now in the paper re a novel!"[29]

Overshadowing it all was a keen sense of mortality that had not haunted him so strongly since his bout with tuberculosis. Reading an article that claimed the average age of death for professors was sixty-five and having just turned fifty a few months before, Rollo figured he had only fifteen years more to fulfill his real self. "Depression on dying," he wrote in July 1959, "not doing what my heart really wants to do . . . holding in . . . vegetating, holding back strength."[30] A year later, upon the premature death of Yona, his beloved younger sister, he recorded: "Strong feeling: how life is snuffed out, life is absurd, if just that; makes not [sic] sense unless one makes something of life which he has . . . putting aside all the cowardices."[31]

20

Kairos and Void

On February 18, 1961, Union Theological Seminary held a three-hour symposium, "Theology of the Secular," to celebrate Paul Tillich's contributions to Protestant thought and to explore the nature of an anxious moment in American culture. It seemed particularly appropriate given Tillich's 1926 appraisal of the "religious situation" in Weimar Germany, when the postwar collapse of European cultures inspired fear of anarchy but also hope for new beginnings. Tillich saw that age as a possible *kairos*, which, borrowing from Kierkegaard, he defined as a moment when "eternity touches time." He rejected traditional sources of sacred inspiration as exhausted, finding instead the explosion of artistic, social, political, and sexual experimentation rampant in 1920s Germany as holding special sacred promise.[1]

Of course, dreams of a *kairos* crumbled with the Nazi takeover. However, might not a similar moment of possibility be in the making in early 1960s America? *Kairos* was on all the panelists' lips, as was the possibility of "the void." The panelists shared the common view of the 1950s as a stultifying age of materialism, conformity, Cold War–inspired fear, and even apocalyptic dread. However, they also saw the revived civil rights movement, a nascent anti-nuclear movement, and the "discovery" of poverty as a political issue in seemingly self-satisfied America as hopeful signs. An incipient conflict of generations and a lack of common social purpose contributed to this striking mixture of pessimism and more optimistic expectancy. The election in 1960 of the young, charismatic, and Catholic John F. Kennedy to the presidency, a man who spoke the rhetoric of challenge and change, lent a piquant immediacy to the times.[2]

Hope and fear lived side by side, and May bluntly posed a question to Tillich: Might the present age become a moment of *kairos* for the United States, or would we sink into a dark void—"Kairos or Void?" Tillich saw both possibilities but reluctantly chose the latter as more likely—"much more of the void"—and compared the spiritual hunger of the age to the "disrupted reality" of Saint Augustine's time. May's position was more nuanced. The spiritual malaise of his patients, their sense of isolation and despair, certainly spoke to the presence of "the void." At the same time, May saw the beginnings of renewal not only in the appearance of civil rights and anti-nuclear political activity, but also among contemporary artists and especially the abstract expressionists, who were forging new secular symbols of meaning in "vitality and struggle." He envisioned the historical moment to be one "not only of Void but [also] when *Kairos* is emerging," and declared himself "much more on the hopeful side." Though he could not have known it at the time, May's declaration might have also served as a description of the next decade of his life.

The "Theology of the Secular" symposium was hardly noticed at the time and has been virtually forgotten since, yet it marked an early attempt to gauge the spiritual significance of what would be a major turning point in American society. "*Kairos* or Void" was just one among many understandings of the decades ahead, most of which veered toward one end or another of an apocalyptic/millennial seesaw. Anxiety and ecstasy became the very essences of what later would be called "the Sixties." The dreary, punishing drumbeat of war, riots, and assassinations shared headlines with sexual liberation, radical politics, and new religious experience in a counterculture of drugs, sex, and music whose influences spread throughout the mainstream. Breathless anthems of change and a countervailing dread of anarchy and death tangled in individual consciousness and society. In some sense it was Weimar, American-style, polarizing the nation into political and cultural blocs that attempted to grapple with a dissolution of everyday expectation and bred an anxiety born of broken illusions and seemingly imprisoning rules—what Kierkegaard called "the dizziness of freedom.

In 1961, although the unraveling had only just begun, signs of the ascendency of psychotherapy as a powerful explanatory device were already evident, and May's earnest existential message was tailor-made for the moment. In March, *Time* magazine featured him in a long article, "The Anatomy of Angst," that contrasted May's *Weltzschmerz* with what it dubbed Freud's "*Sexschmerz*." *Esquire* highlighted him as the leader of existential psychotherapy in "Who's in Among the Analysts: Or How to Tell One from the Other *Before* You Settle for the Couch."[3] Yet fame had its downside. It brought too many patient requests, too many lecture invitations, and not enough time for either family or institutional responsibilities. May found it more difficult than ever to be involved in the day-to-day life of the White Institute or the new postdoctoral program at New York University. Still, he did make time for special requests, as when in 1960 Robert Akeret, a recent graduate of

Columbia Teachers College's counseling program, asked May to lead a group of counselors in an informal seminar on existentialism. He and May formed a close bond.[4]

May's embrace of Akeret's group of young therapists was in part a reaction to the young man's energy and boldness, but it also indicated May's alertness to youth culture and his search for signs of an American *kairos*. While he maintained ties with White, NYU, and the AAEEP, he kept pushing against self-satisfaction and toward both a greater degree of precision and an enhanced field of action. He found at least some wisdom in phenomenology, a philosophical root of existentialism that shared its rejection of ideal types and simple positivism as guides to human reality. Phenomenology's founder, the great German philosopher Edmund Husserl, summarized this holistic and experiential frame of consciousness as an individual's *Lebenswelt* (life-world). Like existentialism, phenomenology inspired different approaches for different practitioners as it crossed paths with philosophy, natural science, and psychology. May had his first deep taste of phenomenological approaches in editing *Existence*, especially its pieces by Henri Ellenberger and Erwin Straus. May felt an immediate connection to Straus's emphasis on the richness of sensory and dimensional aspects of consciousness in the creation of the patient's world and the need for the therapist to understand the patient's subjective universe. He also appreciated Straus's attempts as a psychiatric researcher to describe scientifically those worlds, to pin down in some usable, if radical, empirical language the highly subjective interaction of person and surroundings that lay at the center of existential thought.[5]

Yet even as May pursued this quest for scientific specificity, he felt increasingly drawn to a group of mostly American psychologists who had greeted *Existence* with enthusiasm—Maslow, Rogers, Clark Moustakas, Anthony Sutich, and others—and who had begun to explore new approaches to psychotherapy in the American grain. It was as if his rediscovery of William James turned him toward Americans who in some sense saw themselves in the Jamesian revolt against strict empiricism. Like May, they embraced basic existential notions and rejected the pathological medical model of therapy. Even more than May, they emphasized the "growth" potential of the human psyche as it moved through stages of self-understanding and action. In meetings dating from 1957 and 1958, loosely under the leadership of Maslow, Moustakas, and Sutich, these psychologists had planned to publish a journal that emphasized what they saw as positive goals suitable for therapy, including the centrality of "self-actualization" and creativity, as well as more existentially philosophical explorations of being and meaning. May joined the group in 1960 on Sutich's official invitation. In the spring of 1961, they successfully launched the *Journal of Humanistic Psychology*. By the following year, they had established the Association for Humanistic Psychology (AHP) with James Bugental as president. While not immediately accepting new organizational responsibilities, May would soon make the AHP an important focus of his energies.[6]

Humanistic psychology encouraged an ethic of self-scrutiny, honesty, and humanity, especially in the realms of intimacy and relationships natural to the therapeutic setting. In an atmosphere where the boundaries of public discussion of sex, love, and gender relations had already begun to dissolve social norms, it was both symptom and co-creator of a new age. Not that it was all pretty, least of all on the marriage front. An ethic of "honesty" in relationships often produced not just a kind of clarity but also agonizing hurt. Decades-old relationships were questioned for the first time, and the divorce rate began an inexorable climb.[7]

May was not immune from the revolution. He and Florence had lived a frosty, turbulent détente in the mid- to late 1950s; while she raised a family and took care of the domestic scene, he breathlessly built a career. After his affair with Ellie Roberts ended and his professional life following *Existence* accelerated, Rollo's capacity for finding love with other women seemed temporarily diminished and overwhelmed by work. Perhaps there were other sexual encounters, but none important enough to mention in his journal. Struggles with a sense of meaning and mission, as well as a nagging insecurity, dominated his inner life. He had advocated the authentic life for others and, at least in the struggle, lived it himself. Still, he found it difficult to believe he had progressed very far.

He was reaching a breaking point, desperate for the intimate support he had come to assume Florence was incapable of giving him even as he came to understand the hollowness of public adulation. As he said years later, he was in "a bind about my marriage."[8] Then he encountered Magda Denes, a dazzlingly bright and driven twenty-six-year-old Hungarian Jewish refugee who, sixteen years earlier, had barely escaped the Nazis. She received a BA at City College of New York, an MA in psychology from Boston University, and a PhD from Yeshiva University in 1961. Magda was small and vivacious, her energy reflected in what May called her "tiger eyes." She was also uncompromisingly possessive and emotionally needy. They met at one of May's lectures, probably in late 1960 or early 1961. During the question-and-answer period, when an audience member criticized May, Magda leaped to his defense. At the reception after the lecture, he sat next to her as they ate. "Now, I looked into her eyes and she had this tiger expression," he recalled. "They were green. They seemed to go on forever behind her head. I was very shaken. I was captivated. She was also a very beautiful woman, but it was these eyes that I couldn't forget." She was like no other woman Rollo had known. He was smitten with her fervor and intelligence.[9]

When Rollo escorted Magda home that first night, she invited him in but resisted his advances, warmly joking that he was an "old married man." Months later, however, she called him and asked if they could get together. He took Magda out to dinner at the Roosevelt Hotel, where she revealed to him her family history, her fears and defenses, and her vulnerability. He again took her to her apartment and this time kissed her good night. Their second encounter led to occasional lunches and drinks. In the late spring of 1961, he left Florence and the kids in Holderness and returned for a few days to New York, having brought back some apple blossoms from New Hampshire. "Magda and I went out to dinner and I gave her the blossoms," he remembered. "We came back [to her apartment] and sat on the edge of her bed. I stroked her leg. Then we made love." They made love again the next night, and then Florence and the kids came home. "I fell in love with her passionately," May revealed years later. "It was with a passion I'd never known before."[10]

The affair continued over months. Rollo made excuses about staying late at the office or having committee meetings, but Florence figured it all out sometime around New Year's Day 1962, when Magda dropped by their apartment, "frantic and hysterical." Florence, in a fury of hurt and anger, revealed her own passionate affair with a tour guide on a solo trip to Europe a few years earlier. The Mays argued and cried. Rollo was crushed and, soon enough, moved out. No doubt not coincidentally, he began to experience life in something of a delirium. Magda pushed him to see a psychiatrist to check for any physical maladies (she worried about epilepsy), but the doctor found nothing. He gave a lecture at Yale but could remember only stumbling through it in a haze. "All I know," he recalled later, "is that I was almost incapable of taking care of myself."[11]

By March, Rollo and Florence were each seeing an analyst, and though May's rational self thought it a good idea, he also blamed his ever-worsening physical and mental state on Florence being in therapy. Soon enough, he was in the hospital with a hemorrhaging lung. After a week of not hearing a word from his wife, he wrote to her from the hospital, begging for a visit or some sign of caring: "Florence, are you trying to destroy me . . . ? [T]ho I'm full of sleeping pills, I lie awake asking why you haven't written since a week ago yesterday."[12] Instead of a hospital visit, at the suggestion of her analyst, Florence unleashed her rage in a letter to Alberta Szalita, Rollo's analyst and distinguished colleague at the White Institute. Szalita shared the letter (with or without Florence's permission), and it provoked a long rebuttal from Rollo that was at once heartfelt plea, condescending critique, mea culpa, and angry defense. He began by thanking Florence for finally unburdening herself of feelings that she never was able to communicate to him before. "I appreciated you very much as a completely real person," he declared, "in your anger and fury in your letter." After noting patronizingly that she was finally getting the help she needed, Rollo added: "I also felt in the letter that it took a very sensitive, gifted person to write such a burst of rage with so much color and so many nuances of perception and feeling! I hope that means ultimately your positive feelings may come out for me with the same reality and imagination." Not that he thought that all she said about him to Szalita was fair, especially "imputing to me all those wicked, bluebeard powers to destroy women."[13]

The heart of Florence's letter, of course, addressed May's affair with Magda, but for Rollo it was important to place his most recent romance in the long history of "affairs" in their marriage. The messages were mixed. He worried that her analyst must think him "a moral monster," since apparently Florence had described her own affairs as "denials" of her "humanity, a result of [his] 'pushing.'" Rollo noted that when at one point Florence had made a similar accusation to him directly, he had too cavalierly dismissed this as a reversion to the moralism of her own family and compared her attitude to that of her sisters, who had created marriages "based on structuralized hatred and resentment." Now he saw it differently but still paternalistically: "You have become radically different from them, and you must give yourself credit for this."

He expressed a vision of their marriage laced with keen and sometimes self-critical perceptions, and yet also a reluctance to relinquish an omniscient tone that sought to control the situation. May noted that when patients came to him about affairs that seemed to be destroying their marriages, most often the affair was a "symptom" rather than a "cause" of the problems. Applied to themselves, he stated simply: "The sad thing is that we have both given each other a 'starvation diet' emotionally in our marriage." He knew he hadn't provided "the support and kind of love [she] wished," which he had rationalized as protecting her from being too dependent. Now he saw that he had tried to "hold [her] off" for his own neurotic reasons.

What of affairs? May recalled his version of the history of the marriage and philosophically argued that in some cases extramarital relationships fostered "growth in love" and "development" when they didn't threaten the marriage. However, the tone quickly changed when he began to write specifically about *her* forays. He noted with approval Florence's affair with Harry Bone while he was recuperating at Saranac but also revealed how painful it was for that relationship to continue while he was convalescing in Manhattan. "I haven't entirely forgiven you for that part of it," he wrote; "I think you don't simply imagine in such situations what this does to me." Nor did he think the affair Florence had with her tour guide in Europe, one in which she said she "had felt more 'love' . . . than in 23 years of married life," helped either of them come closer to solving their problems.

Woven into the letter and especially the discussion of affairs was an unsurprising, reflexive defensiveness from an assumed position of higher wisdom. May, while referring to none of his own transgressions (they were a given), dissected and judged the quality of Florence's flights from the marriage. More striking were his admissions of hurt, insecurity, and weakness, a veritable avalanche of self-deprecation sometimes stronger than in his diary. To be sure, some of it bordered on self-pity, but more of it seemed a genuine facing of facts:

[You] haven't been able to give me what I needed—a conviction that *the* woman believed in me, that you prized me as a man (it comes as a surprise to you these days that I have never believed profoundly and really in my image of myself as a man, never believed you were genuinely and over a period of time proud of me and whatever strength I could use—which I did use.) I know I have needed to keep you out, not to accept what tentative outreaches of love you made, though you didn't express or make nearly as much as you think, and did expect me to read your mind. . . . Now I've got to work on my side of this problem and you on yours—clearing away the neurotic demands, and seeing if we can give each other the genuine kind of love we each do so much need. When you told with such enthusiasm (and "triumph"—or am I reading my mother's rejection into that?) how you could give yourself with such abandon to another man, I naturally took it as a real blow below the belt—and one I haven't yet adjusted to.

May understood how an affair could feel fresh and unfettered compared to sex within a decades-old marriage filled with resentment, but he
also couldn't help but feel that she was accusing him of being a failure as a
husband. He reminded her that he had "begged" her, "crying and broken-
hearted," to acknowledge that he been "something more (not more than
[the tour guide]—the hell with him—for I have enough sense to know what
was good there and also how limited it was)," but she would not credit May
with anything positive. This was all the more maddening, he explained, because he was ill. For two months, even before entering the hospital, he had
been "exceedingly depressed" with no faith that his "work, or capacities as
a father or husband or man, were worth anything at all." But he felt himself coming out of this funk and could "only hope" that months of turmoil
also could "be a period of the birth of some happiness and meaning and
love" between them. They would have to overcome "rage and anger and
resentment," but, he was sure, something had to be worth preserving given
that the marriage had produced "three wonderful children." He closed by
hoping for the best for both of them and "even more that it turn[ed] out
well" for her.

Amidst this turmoil, perhaps the worst moments he had experienced since
being diagnosed with tuberculosis, Rollo also faced the "abandonment" of
his analyst. Szalita went on her annual vacation in late March. May decided
to go to Majorca for two weeks to think and rest and calm down. He felt he
couldn't stay in New York with Florence unwilling to communicate with
him and Magda badgering him with her own needs. Magda even insisted
on taking the taxi ride with him to the airport, the whole way demanding he
marry her. "I knew I would go to hell in a hurry," May later reflected, "if I ever
married this woman."[14]

In Majorca, Rollo found that a French psychiatrist with whom he had had
a brief affair in 1961 was there, and they linked up for ten days. She showed
him the sights and clearly hoped to rekindle their romance. Trapped in his
mind already by Florence's coldness, Magda's neediness, and Szalita's imagined neglect, May found himself incapable of feeling. "We never made love,"
he recalled; "I never even kissed her." When she left, however, he felt so alone
and distraught that he considered literally leaping off a cliff. Only running
away from the precipice saved him. He was, as he remembered it, "skat[ing]
on the edge of psychosis." May wrote to his wife, and she didn't answer.
Desperately lonely and confused, he telegraphed Florence asking her to come
over to be with him. She replied by telegram: "UNHAPPY YOUR ILLNESS HOPE

MUCH BETTER NOW MYSELF NOT WELL ENOUGH FOR SUDDEN TRIP PLEASE REST RECOVER LOVE FLORENCE."[15]

The one constant voice of support for both Florence and Rollo was Hannah Tillich, whose views on marriage and affairs mirrored her tortured, sexually flexible, and doggedly committed history with Paul. When Rollo wrote to her from Majorca, she immediately answered sympathetically and with the hope that the climate and natural beauty might ease his pain. She noted that she had talked on the phone to Florence, who seemed "in a hard struggle now," but admired both of them for trying to put their "house in order." In a letter soon after, Hannah also indicated some understanding that her views on marriage might be different but that Florence had "been very generous and very understanding about many things in our life and your and her life." Hannah added some words of wisdom: "The only way is to understand better and to know, 'nothing is threatening but your own fears.'"[16]

Rollo's marriage, split wide open by a new level of revelation and conflict, receded into an unstable stasis. Though somewhat patched together on a day-to-day basis, it slowly fragmented with new affairs and new degrees of self-understanding on both their parts. The players changed somewhat. Magda married a fellow postdoctoral student in 1963, though she and Rollo continued to see each other. He also relied on Ellie Roberts as a dear friend and occasional lover. Here and there came transient affairs. He and Florence sometimes made love but more often kept their emotional distance. They adopted a public profile of marital stability. Only the Tillichs and a few of the Mays' closest friends understood just how troubled the marriage had become.

The explosive turn in May's marriage perhaps inspired him to pursue his professional life ever more single-mindedly. The umbrella of his work, which had been with the existentialists, shifted toward the more inclusive Association for Humanistic Psychology and its vital, revolutionary sense of mission. The great turning point was its Old Saybrook Conference, held in Connecticut in November 1964. May had agreed to give one of the seven principal lectures and in other ways to help shape the meetings. He came to Old Saybrook in the company of Norma Rosenquist, then secretary of the AHP in San Francisco, who had flown cross-country to take part in the conference. May remembered the drive from Manhattan to Old Saybrook as something of a pilgrimage. They stopped at several sturdy New England churches as they traversed coastal Connecticut. He described them later as "built by these old puritans who were sons of bitches in their daily life, but had a sense of beauty underneath." They called at one whose minister had been May's classmate at Union. It was a fitting prelude to the underlying agenda of the conference.[17]

The meeting itself inspired in most attendees the spirit of revolution. They were an estimable bunch, all in one way or another having crossed swords with the psychological establishment in the cause of placing the profession's empirical agenda within a broad human or spiritual dimension. Not surprisingly, most were concerned with personality theory or thera-peutic applications of learning theory and cognitive studies and had already made significant contributions to their fields: Gordon Allport and Henry Murray from Harvard; George Kelly of Ohio State; Gardner Murphy of the Menninger Foundation; Edward Shoben of Columbia University's Teachers College; and the core movers and shakers of the movement: Carl Rogers, Abe Maslow, Clark Moustakas, Sidney Jourard, Charlotte Bühler, and James Bugental. They were joined in their quest by two renowned scholars and public intellectuals, Columbia's Jacques Barzun, a cultural historian and critic, and René DuBos, a famous microbiologist and humanist at the Rockefeller Institute for Medical Health (later Rockefeller University).[18]

May remembered them as a group of men that he "respected and ven-erated" and, "in some strange professional way," loved. It was the love of members of a sports team or combat unit, men who would protect their comrades at all cost. "Nobody shoots a buddy of mine" was the parallel he drew. Members of humanistic psychology's early cohort certainly had their differences and expressed them. They were, however, bound by a cause far greater and a vision more resonant than what seemed at the time to be petty disagreements. That did not prevent May's usual trepidations, however; he vowed two weeks before the conference that he would make a "good talk, think well, whether they (Murphy, Allport, Rogers, etc.) like it or not." He was ready for combat.[19]

He needn't have worried. After dinner on the first night, May recalled raising the big question: "Where is there a psychology that gives a suit-able basis for psychotherapy?" Gordon Allport, struck by May's directness, answered bluntly: "It doesn't exist." These founders and their successors would seek just such a philosophical, scientific, and spiritual basis for the search for meaning that, for many at least, traditional religion no longer seemed capable of supporting. Each of the main speakers tried to define the terms of that search. Henry Murray's Friday night keynote, "A Preliminary Sub-Symposium," set a standard for idiosyncratic visions of humanistic psychology. Murray considered the various traditions and concluded that those present must remain open to each other's views and to those of behaviorism and orthodox psychoanalysis. He took particular umbrage at the blustering hostility he sensed in the proclamation that the new movement was a "third force," battling the first and second forces of behavioral/academic psychology and strict Freudianism. Murray urged the audience to build on the past and on each other to create a humane and useful psychology—useful to everyday human beings and their dilemmas. He called for an enlightened awakening rather than a revolution.[20]

In the formal comments at least, few of the other speakers—among them Maslow, Rogers, Shoben, Kelly, and DuBos—gave Murray cause for worry. While some talked of a "third force," all saw the task as building upon the advances of prior schools by providing an understanding of the living human being imagining and acting in the real world. In short, they hoped to create a vision of human consciousness and meaning that would undergird the science of psychology. Each had his angle on the problem, from Maslow's concern with a progressive order of qualitative human experience to Rogers' call for a science whose terms could approximate an individual's experience rather than a theory that defined and thereby reduced lived reality. May's presentation, "Intentionality, the Heart of Human Will," perfectly exemplified the humanistic deepening to which all aspired. May began by differentiating between the conscious, voluntary act commonly associated with the word "intention" and intentionality, which he defined as "a state of being [that] involves to a greater or lesser degree the *totality* of the person's orientation to the world at that time." He posited that "consciousness" always looked outward to the world with intent, and "intentionality gives meaningful contents to consciousness." Indeed, "consciousness not only cannot be separated from its objective world, but it is indeed *constitutive* of its world." The challenge of therapy, among other things, was for the therapist to understand and bring to consciousness the world created by his patient's consciousness, if only to help him or her modify it in light of observable realities.[21]

The Old Saybrook Conference was in retrospect a grand beginning despite some losses in the older generation of psychologists. Henry Murray concluded that humanistic psychology as a movement would not deeply affect "mainstream psychology" and that he had little to offer a group with such a diffuse agenda. Allport and Kelly were in the twilight of their careers and died three years later. Furthermore, though the conference fostered the spirit of united struggle, differences in approach and personality lingered and sometimes flared into public argument. May noted the ironies of this band of insurgents as they sought a new psychology but sometimes found it hard to get along. May recalled that he greatly respected Carl Rogers, that "all the characteristics of liking and loving another person were there, but I never liked him." And, though May always thought Maslow's "hierarchy of needs" a bit simplistic, "peak experiences" harder to achieve and less long-lasting, and in any case simply a prelude to the tougher work of finding meaning in a tragic world—despite it all, he loved Abe Maslow as a person.[22]

Nor were May's feelings simply retrospective, reflecting later ambivalences about humanistic psychology. They were those of a man whose own philosophy "took in" tragedy, anger, and limits as well as "growth." One memory of Saybrook highlighted an issue that had already been broached between May and Rogers and would continue to be a source of vexation. May remembered being in the men's room at the Old Saybrook Inn as he and Henry Murray relieved themselves at adjacent urinals. They had just listened to tapes of Rogers treating schizophrenics in the calm, nonjudgmental manner that was at the core of Rogerian therapy. At the time of the presentation, May commented that it sounded like good therapy but that at some point Rogers should have expressed some anger, if only so that the patients would feel free to get angry at him. Rogers, true to form, took in the criticism with perfect Rogerian lack of affect. Murray and May exchanged impressions as they peed: "Murray said, 'Did you see Rogers' feet going up and down? What was wrong with him?' [May] said, 'He's trying to get angry.' [Murray] said yes, he probably was, and it did not succeed." May concluded that Rogers "was practicing anger, but he never got any place with it."[23]

Still, the sense of mutual endeavor remained. On the final day, after a glorious dinner at Wesleyan University hosted by its president, Victor Butterfield, the participants all drank a lot and the camaraderie returned. "Each one of us had a point of view that was different than the other," Rollo recalled. "Each one of us believed in human beings as humans, people that were going to live and die, whose birth was magical and whose death was final." They all felt—atheist, agnostic, and believer alike—a religious fellowship that came, according to May, from "putting everything you've got on the line. . . . We went away from there with the conviction that we had met colleagues, friends whom we loved." They didn't know where it would all lead, but they did know it was "for keeps."[24]

"For keeps"—it was a remembered feeling that spoke to the escalating intensity of the times. At the unsettling heart of the matter was violence—the attacks perpetrated on civil rights workers; the assassination of John F. Kennedy; a war of attrition in Vietnam; and domestic disorder unleashed by fear, anger, and the unpeeling of corruption and injustice lying just below the surface of American society. A crumbling vision of everyday life presented a potent mixture of "void" and, as May had predicted, also nascent *kairos*. Prophetic voices emerged, May's among them. His course on existentialism at the New School, always well attended, now attracted overflow audiences. In 1965 WBAI in New York broadcast the entire series.[25] Fame opened doors in the early 1960s art scene where had had once been simply a consumer of concerts, shows, and recitals. Founders of the new Society for the Arts, Religion, and Contemporary Culture (ARC) appointed him as a charter fellow in 1963, an honor bestowed as well on poet W. H. Auden, architect Phillip Johnson, and Alfred Barr, director of the Museum of Modern Art.[26] He involved the American Association of Existential Psychology and Psychiatry in the arts by organizing "Imagination and Existence," a conference held in late January 1966 at the Barbizon-Plaza Hotel. May, the artist Ben Shahn, and research psychologist Morris Parloff led the proceedings, which closed with a panel discussion titled "Imagination and Existence," with discussants Shahn, Saul Bellow, Jacques Barzun, and Stephen Spender.[27]

It was also in this period that May forged a friendship with Joseph Campbell, then a professor at Sarah Lawrence, whose 1949 book *The Hero with a Thousand Faces* had become a classic in the study of myth. Campbell was a friend and colleague of Harold Taylor and on ARC's board of directors. The Mays shared evenings with Campbell and his wife, Jean Erdman, at avant-garde theater and dance performances. Campbell's upper-middle-class Irish American brio and his wife's extraordinary career as a dancer contrasted markedly with May's more awkward, small-town reticence and Florence's homebound world. An undeniable attraction of opposites developed. "There was some kind of real love between us," May recalled. "He would hug me and kiss me on the neck. I think he's a very handsome man. . . . I'd say he loves me and god knows what."[28] However, it was a tempestuous friendship, one that built upon visceral attraction and a simmering competitiveness further entangled by radically different political and social attitudes. May noted Campbell's anti-Semitism as well as his elitism, not to mention his outspoken anti-feminist tirades. In the end, however, they kept in touch despite duels over politics and, later, over the question of myth that so deeply intrigued both of them.[29]

Most notable were May's and Campbell's contrasting positions on Vietnam, especially after the Johnson administration escalated American troop levels and bombing missions in April 1964. At first protests were scattered and promulgated mostly by longstanding pacifist and radical groups. However, every month brought new voices, larger demonstrations, and increasing antiwar sentiment on college campuses. Campbell found the sudden appearance of antiwar activity at Sarah Lawrence a frightening turn, destructive of what he considered the university's true values. May had the opposite reaction, renewing a social gospel and socialist activism born at Oberlin and Union but mostly dormant since the early 1940s. May's commitments were shaped by his friendship with William Sloane Coffin and others at Yale, who spoke out early against the war as part of a broader critique of Cold War policy. He joined Coffin as well as Harold Taylor, John Hersey, and even Cold War "realists" like Reinhold Niebuhr in a campaign aimed at college campuses, Americans for Reappraisal of Far Eastern Policy, which planned to hold regular rallies and information sessions on Vietnam and the broader issue of relations with China.[30]

While his public and professional worlds were expanding, May faced not only a failing marriage but also Paul Tillich's advancing years. Upon retiring from Harvard in 1962, Tillich accepted an appointment at the University of Chicago's Divinity School at age seventy-six. He embraced his role at Chicago as if he were ten or twenty years younger—taught new courses, completed the last volume of his *Systematic Theology*, and gave major lectures across the country and internationally. He continued to explore the question of world religions in order to better see Christianity, even as an earlier trip to Japan and exploration of Buddhism weakened the exclusive hold Christian tradition once had on him. Yet by 1965 physical decline had set in: heart disease and an aging, frail body conspired against his still vital mind. Still, he persisted, and on October 12, 1965, delivered a lecture, "The Significance of the History of Religions for the Systematic Theologian." The audience could not have been disappointed by the lecture's final, affirming point amidst the growing turmoil of challenges to every establishment. Tillich emphasized the freedom attained both from honoring tradition and escaping enslavement to them. After questions and answers, Hannah and Paul Tillich retired to their apartment with a few friends and went to bed at about 11:30. Around 4:30 a.m., Paul Tillich suffered a massive heart attack. He was rushed to University of Chicago's Billings Hospital, where he responded to treatment but eventually died on October 22, 1965.[31]

May had last seen Tillich a month before, during a weekend visit to East Hampton just before Paul and Hannah headed back to Chicago for the school term. By then it was clear that he was in decline; both sensed the possible finality of their encounter. In this last meeting, Tillich finally as much as said May no longer needed him. Having heard May's lectures from the New School on the radio, Tillich declared: "Now Rollo [is] a Master." Hannah refused all requests from friends and even the children to visit Tillich in the hospital, a painful sign to all that death was imminent and an example of her fierce possessiveness in these final hours.[32]

Soon after Tillich's passing, Hannah asked Rollo to deliver a eulogy at the interment of his ashes in East Hampton. The death of his mentor and the honor given to him as eulogist marked in substance as well as ritual a great passage in May's own life. He returned from the ceremony to put his house in order, cleaning his office high atop the Master Building and pondering the debt he owed Tillich as well as the powerful freedom, real and in fantasy, that his death brought. On October 28, less than a week after Tillich's passing, May began to explicitly differentiate himself. Rather than grapple with questions of God, he noted in his journal, he focused on "what is distinctively human in man." His engagement would be with people, "not 'Truth' for own sake" or "God for his own sake; but these as expressions of the dignity, greatness, nobility, tragedy and baseness of man." Nor would he promise cheap happiness or, as he saw it, "Fromm's oversimplifications" or "any oversimplifications" that ignored "the tragic, the demonic, the qualities that give man depth, that save him from shallowness." He loved Tillich because "he represented exactly this depth in all realms," but now it was time for May to "come to [his] own purpose in life" by devising ways to bring that depth to the care of souls and the reimagining of society. Now was the time to envision a *kairos*.[33] Less than a month later, he addressed the subject in more personal terms:

I start a new page; a new life, a new birth of freedom? Free from needing to carry Tillich; free from needing to carry an emotional debt, or from temptation to depend upon him. . . . Free to use all I learned, free to step out with courage, daring, to learn, to work with the rigor he taught me, to love and feel with the depth I learned from encounters with him. Free to love life as he did . . . free to bring eros, philia and agape into every encounter . . . free to leave Flo, live on my own, to use my courage, my open world, my horizon. . . . I pause, meditate, dream, wonder between sloth and work . . . perhaps there is a being between sloth and work, which is *being*. . . . These things need to be lived out: now to test the courage, and the perspective and inner balance, to do so. [34]

May performed his final act of formal mourning and celebration on Pentecost Sunday, when Hannah again asked him to be the eulogist. Tillich's ashes were moved to their final resting place in New Harmony, Indiana, where the Owen family (direct descendants of the utopian socialist communitarian Robert Dale Owen) had asked Tillich whether they might construct a Peace Park in his name. May delivered a solemn, loving, and affirming address, one that characterized the broad appeal of Tillich's ideas and presence beyond the worlds of church and theology. He recalled the scene on Pentecost at a dinner marking Tillich's retirement from Harvard. At the end of the dinner, as Tillich rose to address the distinguished assemblage, a spring shower suddenly commenced. Lightning flashed and thunder boomed, often drowning out Tillich's words and lighting the gothic statuary adorning the main hall of Harvard's Busch-Reisinger Museum. "Nature itself seemed to surround Paul Tillich and confirm him with exactly the demonic and the earth-bound elements," May remembered, "from the depths of the universe which were the sources of his own deepest thoughts and feelings." He lived in "eternal essences" but also in "the mud and the rain of our day to day earth."[35]

May elaborated on the Pentecost theme of "speaking in tongues" as a metaphor for Tillich's own ability to speak to the concerns of so many different souls and groups in the culture. He seemed to have a special appeal to those in his own profession, May noted, for "*he spoke out of our broken culture, but he spoke believing.*" Tillich demanded fealty to no particular theology but rather modeled a life rooted in both faith—no matter how constructed—and grit. Therapists, trained in the sciences, found themselves "yearning for *meaning*, for help in the capacity *to care.*" They sought, in Tillich's words, a "belief-ful realism." "In these professions," May continued, "which must remain related to science and the earth-bound aspects of man or they are lost, it is difficult to sustain a 'belief-ful realism.' . . . Paul Tillich gave us the capacity *to believe*, even though honest men differ in the content of beliefs. He taught us the importance of *ultimate concern.*"[36]

Curiously, as May turned to Tillich's next contribution to therapists—"his emphasis on the meaningfulness of the demonic"—he switched tenses in referring to Tillich. "Tillich not only recognizes the *demonic* with which we must deal," May noted, "but he makes it an integral part of his philosophy. He not only stands within our anxiety, guilt, and despair; but he points out that these are an inescapable part of man's life as man; we do not need to be guilty about despair, not anxious about our guilt." It was as if May was affirming the present and future importance of his ideas. He described the ultimate effect of Tillich on clinicians as almost religious, making it clear that therapists could help but could not become gods. "I think our work with people we seek to help is then interfused with a quality of deeper understanding and mercy—and if I may use this term without hubris, a quality of grace," he suggested. "Thus, it seems to me that Tillich is the therapist for the therapists." May concluded by focusing on Tillich's love of human beings and humanity, his loving wisdom of a piece with that of Oedipus in his final days at Colonus, when the aged king said to his daughter, "and yet one word frees us of all the weight and pain of life: That word is love."[37]

21

The Dizziness of Freedom

When May wondered whether Tillich's death marked "a new page; a new life, a new birth of freedom," he meant something more than a simple change of professional direction. At fifty-six, in the prime of what most would have considered a life of intellectual and professional success as well as public influence, he still felt as if he hadn't written or acted from the profoundest center of his soul. Now was his chance, as he saw it perhaps the last chance, to contribute wisdom that spoke from that core of his being without compromise. He still carried within him the spirit of his declaration on a Colorado mountaintop in 1936, that "the world calls—I must give," and that he must be part of a great succession that included Whitman, Ibsen, Van Gogh, Adler, Rank, and Jung. Though tempered by life and psychoanalytic understanding, his heroic calling remained intact. It was perhaps one reason that while Tillich saw mostly a "void" in 1961, May could see the outlines of a new *kairos*. Perhaps not in 1961 but certainly by 1965, he saw the opportunity to take a significant role in shaping a radically new era.

May's first bold engagement with the times came in opposition to the Vietnam War. When the Committee for a Sane Nuclear Policy (SANE) proposed a March on Washington, May immediately signed on, and on November 27, 1965, marched with twenty to thirty thousand others to the White House. A small delegation of demonstrators met politely with three representatives of the Johnson administration to discuss the war, after which thousands rallied at the Washington Monument. The *New York Times* noted ironically, "Most of the crowd would not have been out of place at the Army-Navy game. There were more babies than beatniks, more family groups than folk-song quartets."[1]

It was in retrospect a curiously poignant moment for May, one that underlined his position between generations. Among others at the rally was Norman Thomas, the aging six-time Socialist Party nominee for president, whom May admired while an undergraduate at Oberlin. Thomas, thirty-five years May's senior, had attended Union Theological Seminary and became a minister before directing his sense of mission to socialist politics. Thomas's appearance symbolized the passing of an older circle of Protestant liberals and radicals who had put their stamp on the culture with a coat-and-tie civility still dominant in the first major protests against the Vietnam War. Only on the fringes of the march were signs of a growing radical antiwar movement, forged by a generation coming of age in an era of assassinations, ghetto riots, military escalation, and liability to the draft. Though the Students for a Democratic Society and various other campus-based antiwar groups had already been born, they so far had received relatively scant attention in the press.[2]

May remained staunchly committed to the antiwar movement, but his original contributions and most passionate involvement remained in the realm of psychology and culture. Once again, he found himself between generations. Those who brought existentialist and similar philosophical orientations into humanistic psychology and beyond—Carl Rogers, Abraham Maslow, May himself, and others—were elder statesmen, wisdom givers, who had not always imagined the radical applications that merged religious, psychological, and body therapies as means to enlightenment and well-being. The gateway for May, as for many in the mid-1960s, was Esalen Institute. Michael Murphy and Richard Price, two young devotees of Asian religion, had transformed a small hot springs resort at Big Sur into the epicenter of a new religio-psychological culture built upon Eastern philosophy, massage and other body work, encounter groups, and consciousness-expanding drugs, as well as goals and ideals derived from humanistic psychology. In contemporary parlance, Esalen had established itself as the capital of the "human potential movement."

Esalen's location alone—an easily missed turn west off California's Route 1 as it snakes high above the Pacific Ocean at Big Sur—could transform the soul. Verdant steep ravines and coastal forests spread toward the ocean, ending in spectacular cliffs that dwarf secluded beaches and crashing waves. Esalen sits at the edge of one cliff, its baths affording an enchanting view of the ocean beyond. Michael Murphy's grandfather bought the property, which had been known as Slate's Hot Springs, in 1910 to use for family vacations. There was no easy access until Highway 1 reached Big Sur in 1935, after which the area became a gathering place for a small number of avant-garde artists and writers living in modest cabins, most famously Henry Miller and friends. In the 1950s, it attracted such Beat generation notables as Jack Kerouac.

Mike Murphy grew up in the much less exotic coastal town of Salinas, though he spent much of each summer with family at the hot springs. As a star student at Salinas High School and devoted altar boy at the local Episcopal Church, he imagined a future as a psychologist or doctor. However, in the early 1950s, during his sophomore year at Stanford University, he went to the wrong classroom and found himself in a lecture not on psychology but on Asian religion. Murphy sat transfixed as the professor, Frederic Spiegelberg, recreated the philosophy and universe of the Vedic Hymns and the life of the Brahman, the supreme Hindu god. He stayed on for the rest of the course. Murphy became a devotee of Spiegelberg's classes and ended up particularly interested in the philosophy of the contemporary Indian mystic and activist Sri Aurobindo.[3] He longed for direct spiritual experience and in 1956 journeyed to India to join the ashram founded by Aurobindo. After returning to the Bay Area he joined a growing community interested in Buddhism and other Asian traditions. Murphy soon met Richard Price, coincidentally a Stanford classmate and also an acolyte of Spiegelberg. In 1961 the two moved from San Francisco to the Murphy property at Big Sur, mostly abandoned and in something of a shambles. By 1962, they had come up with the idea of Esalen Institute. It would bring together alternative thinkers in religion, psychology, science, and just about any other realm, those who envisioned a more comprehensive, spiritual, holistic sense of human existence and, indeed, the life of the Earth.[4]

It was telling that Paul Tillich had in a significant way unknowingly enabled Murphy's awakening and the course of events that led to Esalen's founding. Tillich and Spiegelberg had become close friends at University of Marburg in the 1920s, and Spiegelberg later credited Tillich's idea of God as the "ground of being" for placing his own startling religious experiences in a framework from which grew his interests in the East. In 1937, Tillich arranged American employment for Spiegelberg so that he could flee Germany. He taught at various institutions, including Union Theological Seminary, before securing a permanent position at Stanford. Murphy returned the favor in Tillich's last year of life, inviting him to lead a weekend workshop on the dialogue between Eastern and Western religions in February 1965. Tillich gave two lectures, each followed by workshop discussions, "Self-Actualization and Self-Transcendence" and "Symbols of Eternal Life in the East and West." At the end of a long journey and friendship, it seemed that Spiegelberg and Tillich's divergent spiritual paths finally overlapped.[5]

May's first visit to Esalen was already in the works at the time of Tillich's workshop. Murphy finalized plans for May's lectures for August 27–29, 1965. He would be the first in a series of weekend conveners on the theme of "frontiers of human development." May described the themes of his workshop as "the function of will and intentionality in human growth; the meaning of choice and freedom; the exploration of creativity in relation to the unconscious; and the dynamics of relationship in encounter, transference and empathy." The weekend went well, but it was unlike just about anything he had ever experienced, challenging his senses and intellect in ways that soon became apparent. The air of freedom and experimentation—drugs, nudity, and casual sex—in pursuit of sacred (some would say pagan) totality caught him by surprise. This first time at Esalen, he pulled back somewhat and mostly observed when it came to the world beyond the workshop. However, the allure of such freedom ate at his mind and body.[6]

One direct manifestation of Esalen-inspired change came soon after, when he wrote to a White Institute colleague, Charles C. Dahlberg, to congratulate him on winning a $150,000 grant to study LSD in therapy. This was before LSD was banned for use in scientific experiments and also when its popular reputation as a transformative psychedelic drug was spreading through American culture. Like marijuana, it was illegal for general distribution but readily available from street dealers and home producers. Research scientists had been interested in LSD for decades; psychotherapists in particular hoped it would break down clients' resistances in therapy far more quickly than talk alone. May's interest in LSD focused on "the meaning and nature of consciousness [and] unconsciousness." Did he wish only to "observe," or did he mean to inch his way toward "observation" of its effects on his own consciousness? Esalen whetted his appetite for a direct experience, but also reminded him of deeply entrenched self-imposed limits that he both felt secure within and wished to shake off.[7]

Tillich's death, social and political turmoil, and Esalen all rekindled May's interest in refining his sense of calling. One morning in October 1965 he woke up at 4:00 a.m. and "realized suddenly" his "life's purpose." "To further, work for, support, create what is distinctively human in man," he typed in his journal, and elaborated for a single-spaced page on just what that meant and did not mean. He was concerned with science, especially psychological science, only insofar as it helped expand human possibility, and certainly not to control behavior. "My interest[s] in art, religion, the spirit are part of this devotion," he added—"what gives man beauty, form, meaning in his life." He also struggled to shed what he saw as his own destructive competitiveness. He no longer hoped to be the "greatest psychologist in the country," narrowing his ambition to being "the best possible therapist, analyst, I can be;

the best healer; the best knower of the human soul." As always, self-critique followed such declarations, and the ensuing months found him scrutinizing his behavior for signs of defensiveness or competitiveness that sapped his courage to find "my form in life."[8]

Mostly such thoughts remained confined to his journal, but on at least one occasion he shared his hopes and fears with one of his oldest mentors, Herman "Hy" Reissig. Reissig had become a lifelong friend after May had interned with the minister in his first year at Union. Ten years May's senior, Reissig had just retired from an activist life in church organizations to the relative leisure of Lakeland, Florida. Rollo and Florence, their marital problems still under wraps, joined the Reissigs for Thanksgiving in 1965. May did confide details of a more general personal crisis to Reissig and his wife. He poured out his soul to them, revealing that his declaration of a "life's purpose" was a hope, not yet a reality. Too much work, too little direction, fear of death, the nagging dream for "Messianic fame" that defied all reason—"God is dead, I must take over"—why couldn't he just relax, coast, enjoy his success? Or: "My religion gone, no sanctions, no criteria: marriage unsure; and so I keep going so fast I never have to stop to be, to feel, to know who I am." The Reissigs listened attentively but in the end could only counsel that he get some rest.[9]

Rest, however, was not May's style. Rather, he ran himself ragged seeking the elusive peace he hoped a true connection to being might bring. Surprising moments of illumination did occur, as when he took Florence to hear Mahler's Symphony no. 5 at Carnegie Hall. "It spoke to me, I felt and had relationship with Being in the music. . . . pure tones, pure beauty and color," he wrote a day after. "To be at this moment, like last night, what I am, the Being that comes out of me, to live it, speak it, be honest with it, devoted to it . . . that is the opposite to anxiety about death." He rediscovered with new words an insight he had decades before, that anxiety might "jar" him into a "relationship with Being." Fear of being himself "at every moment" imprisoned him in that death anxiety: "When I afraid to speak up to a patient, (something unpleasant, will elicit angry, contemptuous retort); when I afraid to speak up in an argument, afraid to argue vs. Fromm. . . . When I afraid to love, afraid to take a chance doing something with Flo, drawing her out, planning something . . . then I afraid of death." He found, in fact, that he enjoyed the music "with" Florence, and "she enjoyed it herself." So much for his "old idea that I can't live fully because she holds me back." Perhaps, he mused, he held *her* back.[10]

The moment of Being with Mahler was short-lived. Two days later he was suffering from an anxiety attack and his old medical nemesis, tachycardia. He was preparing to give a talk, "Personal Identity in an Anonymous World," at Texas Technological College (now Texas Tech University) in Lubbock. Texas Tech was hardly a mecca for New York intellectuals in 1966, but the prospect of a public presentation elicited New York fears. He worried that "every one will be there to jump up and say, full-of-shit," ready to "slay" him. "*They all like Ruth, waiting the chance to show I am stupid, to erase me*" he observed in his journal, "(esp. the Jewish ones, and the experimentalists—the two 'sharp' types, as her intelligence was sharper than mine)." Not surprisingly, it didn't work out that way in Texas. The *Daily Toreador*, Tech's student newspaper, reported that May received a "standing ovation," despite his criticism of data-driven education at a tech school and condemnation of the government's "no exit" strategy for the "questionable" war in Vietnam. (The same issue of the *Toreador* featured a comic strip sendup of antiwar demonstrators.) May himself reflected: "They show me I worthwhile, I valued, have something to say, am read, and am loved."[11]

May's surprise at such adulation indicated to him that he still suffered from serious strains of neurotic bondage. He sought a "new birth of freedom" from the darkness that was plaguing him—envy, competitiveness, a sense of inferiority to the "big shots," self-inflicted loneliness, and, perhaps most of all, deep feelings of entrapment by his mother and Ruth that colored all of his relationships with women. None of these were unusual human frailties and were certainly common enough among clients of psychotherapists. Nor was it surprising that they crowded in on him just at the point when he sought a creative breakthrough. In fact, May's constant rehearsing of neurotic patterns in his journal had long before come to be a goad to creativity, as if by keeping such problems conscious he warded off at least some of their ill effects and provided a constant example of psychological complexity against which to write. Digging deeper into his psyche—repeating and expanding upon old tropes—seemed to free him.

The contrast between May's public demeanor—calm, earnest, with tonalities ranging from grave to bemused—and his private agonies, then, invites more complicated explanation than that he was simply a tortured soul. However genuine the torment, May's private meditations played an extremely important and positive role in the creative process. May's self-analysis dramatically externalized issues common to writers and artists as they sought to overcome inhibitions and express themselves with honesty. Unconscious or half-realized fears of castration, destruction, ridicule, or something un-imaginably worse all had the potential to stifle creativity. May's strategy was to grapple with them every day to and create a private drama of martyrdom and possible triumph over them. It certainly had the elements of a Christian drama but also those of existential struggle. The cast might be different, but the central issue was the same. May sought to defy the gods and demigods of his life, the ones to whom he gave so much power and the defiance of whom would afford him authenticity.

In fact, by most standards the mid-1960s were an extraordinarily pro-ductive era in May's professional life. He continued to see patients, conduct classes, do committee and supervisory work at the White Institute and NYU, and give lectures all over the country, mostly without outward signs of crisis or exhaustion and almost always to adoring audiences. He taught summer school at Harvard in 1964. He published a very successful collection of his essays, *Psychology and the Human Dilemma* (1967), worked on a new edition of *Existential Psychology* (1969), and created with Leopold Caligor, his col-league at the White Institute, a unique experiment in dream analysis eventu-ally published as *Dreams and Symbols: Man's Unconscious Language* (1968). This was, of course, in addition to constantly revising his lectures at the New School and producing variations on older presentations as he accepted invi-tation after invitation for public appearances.[12]

Nor did his simmering rage against Ruth and his mother, now in her early eighties, deter him from continuing to be their backbone of support. Rollo visited Matie periodically in Michigan, corresponded with her, listened pa-tiently to her complaints, sent her money, and traded news about the rest of the family. Ruth, who now fancied herself a religious prophet, was more of a problem. She had moved to San Francisco in the late 1950s and eked out a living, but she was prone to chronic delusions; for example, she reported that she was "writing a book on Yoga and Creativity" and assumed in her commanding way that Rollo would write a preface. (The book never mate-rialized.) When she related an "Acute Nervous Breakdown" in the fall of 1967, Rollo generously referred her to friends in the area for help, and Norma Rosenquist Lyman, with whom he had traveled to Old Saybrook, called her to see if she could be of aid.[13]

May's public lives, whether professional or familial, were not fronts for some more genuine self expressed in his journals. Rather, his inner dialogue represented an urge toward breaking through to new understandings and syntheses. May felt as if he were treading water in his marriage and, perhaps even more so, in fulfilling his calling. His latest books, essays, and lectures created variations on themes in his work from the late 1950s. Yet as each year in the 1960s passed, sexual, political, patriotic, and generational assumptions seemed to melt, and old answers no longer made sense. New art, new music, escalating military and political violence, disaffection, and generational struggle—all seemed of a piece. *Kairos* and void often seemed indistinguishable. Yearning had turned into open rebellion, a collective wrecking ball of hope and despair.

It was this new reality that May wished to address in a brave new book. He had shown a brief outline to the Tillichs in early 1964, while Paul was recovering from multiple ailments in a Chicago hospital. Hannah wrote to Rollo of her conversation with Paul about the plan, since he was too weak to write it himself. Both Tillichs thought May's subject, creativity in its broadest conceptual and cultural context, was too expansive, and they suggested a narrower and more academic focus: "phenomenology: a psychology of creativity."[14] By late November 1965, after Tillich's death, May had gone in the opposite direction, further generalizing its scope and calling it "Love and Will." He garnered appreciative comments on some preliminary chapter drafts from Bob Lifton and Gordon Allport, though Lifton worried about its "moralistic" tone that "if more extreme, would be 'pompous.'" May took the critique to heart, promising himself to "identify with the suffering patient" more both in therapy and in writing. He would then no longer be judging from "above" the situation but rather "stand with him in it."[15]

As May sought an involved engagement with the potential reader, self-analysis became a more significant tool than ever. He concentrated on his fear of women and the power he perceived they held over him. He felt particularly sensitive to their criticisms and in need of their encouragement. On those grounds, his own wife had become an impediment. In fact, just a few days after the Mahler concert, where he had felt a glimmer of harmony with Florence, Rollo excoriated her for calling his latest writings "hard to take" and "about sick people." She picked at his punctuation—"'n[e]w puritans' should be in quotes'"—and damned him with the faint praise "Oh, you write well." Thinking of Florence and numerous others, he asked: "Can I free myself of giving women power to undermine me . . . ? When [has] Florence ever liked anything I did?" No matter who he included in this circle of women, his meditations on the problem all led back to his tortured relationships with Matie and Ruth.[16]

It wasn't so much that May thought expunging women from his life was the answer. His imagined enslavement to Ruth and Matie almost guaranteed his need for connection to strong women even as it instilled fear. He sought women who praised and encouraged him, who took his side in battle with unwavering loyalty. They might act as muses, intellectual companions, lovers, informed admirers, or some combination of all of these roles, and the more supportive the better. Not surprisingly, during this period he received significant support for his ideas and his communicative skills not only from Magda Denes but also from Ellie Roberts; Dorothy Norman, the photographer, writer, and liberal activist; Mary Hall, who interviewed May for *Psychology Today*; Doris Cole, a professor of religion and philosophy and friend of the Tillichs; and especially from an intense relationship with his former patient Jessica Ryan, the writer, actress, and wife of actor Robert Ryan. Each in her own way was the good sister, mother, or lover as opposed to those censorious women closer and more hostile to his calling. Yet each had to keep her distance lest she become too threatening.

May's heightened sense of the importance of women in his life also helped him begin to work out the origins of his often distanced and problematic relationships with male colleagues. Though hardly accurate (except perhaps in the case of Tillich), he saw himself as always playing a secondary role to his male mentors and friends, an impression in part related to his fear that if he truly spoke his mind, "they" would destroy him. Despite May's growing fame, paranoia preceded every lecture he gave in New York. He described his anxiety before a talk at NYU in virtually the same terms as he had before his Texas trip: "They'll be ready to shout out, bull shit, what nonsense, they'll laugh in the middle, hoot me down." Fueled by envy of Paul Goodman (author of *Growing Up Absurd*), Erich Fromm, and Susan Sontag and what he saw as their ability to hit hard and say exactly what they felt, he again turned to a glancing anti-Semitism—he blamed "Jews, practiced in cutting down"— an unsurprising target given the predominance of Jews in Manhattan's psychological, intellectual, and artistic communities. Once he had verbalized these feelings, he noted again that it wasn't so much the Jews but really fear of his sister Ruth, brilliant but crazy, who liked nothing better than to "laugh at [him], cut [him] down. . . . She always cleverer."[17]

Much of his anxiety also involved class, regional, religious, and ethnic roots. He became more and more conscious of his modest midwestern Protestant upbringing—its reserve and euphemistic expression, as well its assumption that it represented the true American culture. May's outer sense of confidence masked an endemic mixture of admiration, envy, and fear of eastern elites and, increasingly, émigré and first-generation American Jewish (and in some cases Catholic) intellectuals. May bravely tried to come to grips with these feelings in his self-analysis. In fact, his efforts to overcome his inhibitions and sense of inferiority were well served by self-revelation even in its uglier moments, when he expressed his prejudices only to question and free himself of them.

These cultural dramas had practical significance that ranged beyond dreams and self-reflection. Most obvious was an inexorable pull toward California. Though May had built ties and friendships in the Bay Area and Southern California throughout the 1950s and early 1960s, most recently in the AHP and AAEP, he remained centered in New York. However, the quick succession in 1964–65 of the Old Saybrook Conference, May's first trip to Esalen, and Tillich's death began to loosen his ties to Manhattan. Compared to the tensions accompanying professional worlds in Manhattan and the growing disaster of his marriage, the Bay Area and Big Sur—far from his usual chorus of real and imagined critics—came to be both a respite and a field for risky experimentation. Still, the West and Esalen upset May in a different way. Though clearly revered as a prophet by those at Esalen, May felt old and staid compared to the youthful vigor, sensuality, and visionary optimism on display.

His feelings toward Mike Murphy were particularly complex. They spent meaningful time together on May's first trip to Esalen in August 1965. "Our conversations turn me on," Murphy wrote to May in December 1965; he was especially appreciative of the older man's advice to "be ever more assertive. It feels good." And, invoking a ritual of assertiveness more Esalen than May, Murphy proudly noted: "I even beat my chest like Tarzan every time I step out of the shower."[18] In turn, Murphy's presence at Esalen recalled for May days of simple affection at YMCA camp. He imagined Murphy as the "feminine counterpart to me, the little boy back in camp, sweet-faced, I liked to hold his hands, sexy, warm, nice to pet—I want Mike to say I like you most of all, want them to say George [Leonard] says that too; they should cuddle up . . . not sex. *But he is the spitting image of the boys I used to feel adolescent sweetness toward.*" However, when Murphy visited him in New York in April 1966, May was tired, tense, and depressed. In came Murphy—"light, free, aerial, seems not to be depressed . . . always 'on,' stimulated, things always great," and, worst of all, touting Maslow as "the best." The founder of Esalen became "a rebuke always. . . . I old and tired, 'tired writers of the east,'

they the adventurous, daring, young culture, believe in joy, soaring, richness. . . . I heavy, feet on earth, hanging." May realized that the "rebuke [is]
inside me" but feared that it could be true: "I too heavy, I let myself drag."[19]

Sparked perhaps by his inner wrestling with what Murphy and Esalen
represented, May began to meditate in general on his relationships with men.
As he confided to his journal in June 1966, the prospect of intimacy even
with his male friends and colleagues frightened him. After a "good; warm;
human" dinner at the home of Leslie Farber, an ally in the promotion of existentialism in psychiatry and psychotherapy, May wondered whether he
had prevented his "competitiveness" from "bursting out," as he thought it did
whenever he got "too close to a man." May worried that such intimacy would
compromise the "freedom, independence" he won "by being all alone . . . isolated on my mountaintop, myself only to take care of myself." Afraid of being
swallowed up by others, he preferred to stay on the "mountain peak." Indeed,
May feared that his friendship with Mike Murphy would compromise his
own self-identity. He felt "compelled to go along with Mike's plans, *his* attitude toward life" and "even guilty, anxious because I wasn't the 'joy-loving-
LSD' type he was." Rollo felt caught between his own generation and the one
whose freedoms beckoned. His guilt and attraction, intellectual instincts and
libido, feelings of moral superiority and jealousy, remained at war.[20]

Of the endless variations to these questions of power and freedom, one
that May himself rarely considered stands out: his ability to embrace those
who presented no threat. He could be a warm and loving spiritual guide from
the mountaintop. His openness to Mike Murphy came in part from the fantasy that Murphy was like one of the needy YMCA boys in summer camp.
This was also true for his favorite students. Take the case of Robert Akeret,
who was an advanced student at the White Institute. Akeret asked and May
agreed to meet a group of students at his office high atop the Master Building
in an innovative seminar. May would play tapes of therapeutic sessions with
his clients, opening them to discussion as if the trainees were his supervisors.
Satisfying moments came also with meditation, one in particular that May
associated with his forthcoming return to Esalen in August. There he sat, in
the "quiet, coolness, brightness of early morning" in Holderness; "silence
everywhere, which is the time when Being speaks eloquently, clearly, immediately." He prayed in silence to be "free" from his dreams of glory and the
"hurry, haste, pressure to win" before he died. "May I rather, be part of Being,"
he declared to his journal, "and then *give back what I have to give*—the only
thing really called for from me."[21]

May owed his practice of meditation to Esalen, and he may have begun meditating on a regular basis on his first trip to Big Sur in August 1965. It soon became a habit and a source of solace. Furthermore, Esalen's broader challenge to social norms expanded upon an alternative vision of life that had begun to influence him mightily at the Old Saybrook meetings. To move from Old Saybrook to Big Sur, however, involved a great leap—not only physically but also generationally and culturally. May's consciousness had been deeply affected by thirty years in Manhattan and an intellectual life dominated by dark neo-orthodox and existential themes emanating from Europe. His turn to existentialism, powerful as it was in his conceptualizing a therapeutic breakthrough to authenticity and growth, still relied on bleak grays for its dominant philosophical aesthetic. To be existential meant to be alone, to grapple with the shadows of one's life, and to be blessed with no certain reward except struggle. For May as for so many others, the crowds, grittiness, and concrete of New York embodied the existential mood. So too did the sensibility of Eugene Ionesco and Edward Albee onstage and abstract expressionism in the galleries. One can only imagine Esalen's effect on his sense of possibility, enveloped by its dramatic natural splendor and its search for transcendence. Some part of him felt a quest for the new, in Walt Whitman's words, "Facing west, from California's shores, / Inquiring, tireless, seeking what is yet unfound."[22]

Rollo's journey from New York to California was neither easy nor linear, nor was it ever quite complete. Yet it loosened the hold of repression and at times took him to the borders of a new and almost paranormal consciousness. In July 1966, a bout of loneliness in New Hampshire was triggered by Florence and their daughter Carolyn returning to New York. He saw reacting to this aloneness as a rational choice between self-pity and self-affirmation, but by the afternoon May began sinking into what he called a "schizophrenic panic." It was one of "utter desolation," tense and wandering, "not alive, a film between me and life, *a vague abyss*." He feared that he had moved beyond anxiety's panic to some more irretrievable state, and for the first time pondered the "pre-verbal" shock of a mother's abandonment, of "loneliness and desolation," what he must have experienced in his earliest years. "While outside this panic," he wrote, "there is no way of imagining myself in it. While in it, no way of imagining how it would be outside it." He walked into his son's room and felt the "whole world gone . . . dead forever . . . no possibility whatever of meeting them in any world." And, then, startlingly, he declared: "Like coming home from camp, I was in and of a world, meant everything to me, would never happen again." Coming home from camp meant leaving friends and friendly counselors and reentering the void of Matie and Ruth.[23]

"Then!" That is how he typed it in his journal, discovering that he had been actually "playing with his panic" for "'bitter-sweet' reasons" of his own. He was purposely keeping himself imprisoned by mother and her surrogates to prove that he remained "loyal to her, needed her, tied to her, and she to me." The very consciousness that he *chose* to stay within the "pre-verbal" stranglehold of his mother made him see that "*getting over it [was] an act of will.*" He could choose to know the world through his "own self," to break through the veil and see "the mountains, trees; affirm what I doing." More profoundly, it meant "loving myself, experiencing myself as a person I like . . . breathing becomes relaxed and pleasant . . . muscles a kind of very mild, suffused joy (ecstasy in very minor key—since that is the feeling of being one's self in transcendence of oneself)." Words were inadequate to describe the revelation. He was simply "happy," whether sitting on the patio or walking around the house in the late afternoon gentleness of air and sky. The panic had vanished.[24]

Self-doubt quickly returned, but even so, his sense of the world had explicitly become a dialogue between hope and despair. For every twinge of doubt, he began to produce contrary evidence. For every enemy who crushed his confidence, a friend declared his greatness. Dreams and fantasies of coldness and failure warred against self-affirmation. Adding it all up and finding ways of countering the "fatal habit" of seeing himself as "no good," he managed to focus on a virtue more modest than his unrealistic dreams. He might not be a Freud, a Tillich, or even a Fromm when he wrote, but only he brought to his work a certain poetry. He had been disappointed, for instance, in his eulogy to Tillich at New Harmony until a friend raved about how "the poetic stuff 'undid' her." Another praised its "tenderness." Perhaps that, he thought, was his "unique contribution."[25]

A week later, in August 1966, he was back at Esalen to lead a seminar and workshop, "Dimensions of Consciousness." The focus was on phenomenology as "the science that begins not with impersonal objects but with acts of consciousness, and endeavors to discover objective reality by the deepening and enlarging of subjective reality." The total experience was somewhat less abstract. Apparently he gave in to the "tug," and his fears of "being swallowed up in the morass" didn't materialize. Rather, he imbibed. Soon after returning home, he pondered the meaning of his having had sex with three different women ("good but not that great") and taken LSD. The lesson: he knew he was still attractive to women and that, through drug-induced insight, he could "cut loose."[26]

In the wake of this trip, he pondered a new life without Florence. "Days go O.K.," he noted at the beginning of an informal separation. "I awake lonely, empty; but not angry and tied up . . . at least future is open, can mould it."[27] In dreams he fought the usual battles with himself and others in bed and at the dinner table, not only Goodman and Sontag but also May's good friend Bob Lifton and other Yale faculty. Florence's appearances in his journal and dreams waned. In his waking notes, May moved decisively toward wrestling with his writing, his significance, and those neuroses that stood in the way of his saying what he wished to express. He and Florence still met, mostly in Dr. Spector's office, and rehearsed their complaints. However, for Rollo, their marriage seemed a thing of the past, electrified only by his attachment to their children. On January 7, 1967, May told Florence that he thought they "must" legally separate. He began to imagine seriously a world where he was finally free to meet and get along with many people, untied to a condemnatory wife, enjoying what he saw as his final chance truly to be in the world.[28]

On March 9, 1967, while in San Francisco, Rollo decisively crossed a psychological Rubicon when he decided to take a full-blown LSD "trip" supervised by Norma Rosenquist Lyman. She had been involved in psychedelic drug research for a few years in the Bay Area. He hoped to break through from everyday being to Being itself. That didn't happen, but much did. Rollo's record of the trip reflected both his own consciousness and that of the times. He rested on a couch, and others lay on pillows on the floor. As the acid took effect, he initially felt lonely but quickly moved to join Norma and her husband, John, and, taking each by the hand, drew them to himself. "I felt I had mother and father, being accepted by each," he wrote, also noting that he could accept being accepted by them. Norma, feeling a similar escape from loneliness, began to cry, but John, "in his conflicts, despair, wasn't feeling anything." Rollo and Norma tried to help but could not break through to him. Someone turned on a cacophony of loud and dissonant music, and as the acid overtook him, Rollo "couldn't stand it." It was as if the music underlined his helplessness in the face of John's passive despair. He saw Norma's husband's condition as a judgment on himself, a "return of my feeling I have to take responsibility for everything . . . mother, father, from time I born: have to take care of her, makeup for him; and, if don't, I am no good."[29]

The acid's power continued to build and swept May into its vortex. He asked Norma to switch the music to Mozart, but then changed his mind. He decided it would be "good if I could take this assault on my nerves." "Maybe music good for the others," is what he said to Norma, but he "meant: I would like to live thru it." And then the music took him to a psychedelic edge: "It pounded on me, cut me—sharp notes came like razors, against my skin, muscles, like I being beaten, big men in only loin cloths, bald-headed, brown, oriental (like Yul Brynner) beating me. . . . Every note out like lash of whip. . . . I could feel even the pleasure in the pain of the whip."

He tensed up to the point of orgasm, "like a woman being forced to have intercourse, raped, sharpness of the penis in me, terrible pain but a greatest pleasure at the same moment, liking, crying out for the pain." Pleasure and pain, repeatedly inflicted for a timeless moment by devils with horns, demons, Viking-like brutes, and then came "a white queen," who ruled all. "These brown devils walked by," he recalled, "each taking a stroke in fucking her, she lying there (half on a throne) each shoves his erect penis in, strokes and then the next comes by and does it, continual stroking for her, but many different brown, huge devilish men." He allowed the scene to "engulf" him, tear him apart "in a dungeon, in hell itself," and it was only then that he "regained" himself. "I could be strong like the devils, I could exchange blows as well, I could experience the zest ecstasy of demonic battle," he remembered, "of the pleasure of giving great blows, pleasure even of being hit while you are also giving the blows." The pleasure and pain were unimportant, "only the release of power, muscle, living out the demonic life in me. The men's world, with abandon."

As the LSD eased off and the music stopped, he remarked to Norma that he had lost all fear. "I've been in the base of hell, endured all the pain until death, or thought I would die, torture, cutting," he declared, "and I could come thru it, and what is more do It myself and like it." Norma changed the music to Gregorian chant, which May felt was a "pallid" accompaniment compared to what had just transpired in hell. Nonetheless, it brought him visions of a "joyous cosmology," with "God on the clouds throwing flowers about, casting them here and there like Ophelia." However, as the LSD wore off and he changed drugs—tokes of marijuana to ease out of the acid state—May recorded a disturbing impression. Others in the room seemed less important and even annoying distractions. "I in my own world," he remembered. "Didn't even like them particularly while under the Marijuana. Sharpens vision at price of giving up the real interpersonal world."

Of course, in his own mind, all that he had experienced, including the frightening moments under the spell of LSD, were now part of his real world. The drug's effects, after all, replicated unconscious issues albeit in their most extreme forms, and in doing so sharpened May's will on marriage and writing. A joint meeting with Florence's therapist (something that had become a Monday ritual) just after his acid trip left him depressed and ornery. "Feel I'm being trapped back into same old marriage," he complained, "caught by both of them." Only meditation brought temporary relief, and by evening the orneriness was back. He went to an ARC meeting and drank too much. Irritated with others, often feeling empty when alone, he imagined himself like a caged squirrel on a wheel, a self-sentenced Sisyphus. His dreams turned apocalyptic. In one, he was giving a speech on a raft when a wind came up, boards crumbled, and he sank in the water. He flailed to get above the water, but his heavy clothing dragged him down—and he awoke from the nightmare understanding that he feared the power of Ruth and Matie and madness, and that staying with Florence would drag him back into the morass.[30] A month later he witnessed in his dreams "cliffs falling down, burying people."

Yet the helter-skelter of contrasting images and moods, intensified by the experience and memory of LSD's surreal liberation and by periodic attacks of tachycardia, also had the effect of freeing May's imagination. His writing flourished, and his fantasies, waking and dreaming, became more colorful and complex. He allowed himself to feel more tenderness toward Florence, recognizing at times that she was her own person, though perhaps not the one he should have married. It was, however, a kind of love designed as well to assuage guilt. After an hour with her analyst in late May 1967, he vowed to give up the fantasy that Florence would commit suicide if he left her. He had to base his own sense of self on something more positive, not "the arrogant belief mother-and-Flor-can't-get-along-without-me—that I do not act actively, love actively, at all. . . . Oh, cravenness. . . . Oh guilt? re Ruth?" May felt free to love Florence for who she was but also realized that he had gained the freedom to "leave Flo anytime." Still, as Florence's analyst suggested and May half seemed to agree, in this new mood, over the summer and in the peace of New Hampshire, they could " 'try out', see how living together goes."[31]

The summer in Holderness did not go well for the marriage but was productive for Rollo in other ways. It gave him time to work out interior dramas that moved him toward literally separating from Florence and pondering in general the relationship between his most creative moments and the men and women in his life. She arrived in late June and stayed past the Fourth of July. He experienced moments of good sex and the security of bodily warmth, but mostly, more acutely than ever, he sensed the widening gulf that lay between them. She would sleep late, and when Rollo asked her why, she would answer, "What is there to get up for?" Florence also condemned his LSD experience—her response was simply, "Can't get over the shock." "I depressed when I alone around her," he confessed to his journal.[32]

May found relief only in his writing cabin. He had a conference paper to prepare for the upcoming meetings of the American Psychological Association and ideas for his new book. At work he encountered the usual highs and lows, especially in regard to the APA paper. May reported to his diary that "writing went very well . . . an hour of real ecstasy when I felt hitting something of great importance." He fantasized that it was so "brilliant, I'd even get elected pres. of APA over this." The very next morning, however, writer's block set in. He was sure that it was because he was "afraid of success" and more comfortable being in the position of "second man . . . still stay a boy among the men." Even when the writing came, he felt the pull toward distance and abstraction rather than saying what was really on his mind in full force. And then: "ALL BECAUSE I AFRAID TO BE A MAN WITH THE MEN ** WANT ALWAYS TO BE A BOY STILL, A SMILING BOY BESIDE THE MEN * THE Interpreter—carrying on . . . Christ—why don't *I* form the world I live in—I leave it to the shitty Fromm, [Paul] Goodman, *This is why they are my daimons.*" In the end, he judged the paper a mediocre effort, the victim of "'protestant perfectionism': I must always continue doing better, can't get behind in race, like mathematically grading myself. . . . (What narcissism! That I must never make a mistake—always the right one, the right act, the right answer! the right word in writing!)"[33]

At the very time May was calling Fromm and Goodman his "daimons," he was working out a more general and original definition for the "daimonic" that would appear in his next major book, now definitively titled *Love and Will.* He had been happy with the traditional concept of the demonic as a force of evil and used it in this way in prior work. However, the events of the time, this strange mixture of *kairos* and void abroad in the land, as well as the fearless exploration of his own thoughts and dreams, pushed him toward seeing an energy that might be molded toward good or evil, creativity or destruction, or even creative destruction. He came to see the heart of his LSD trip as just such a window on the daimonic's primal force.

This was especially true in the realm of sexuality and most of all in relation to men. In January 1965, for example, after a particularly vexing day of silence while sharing the same apartment with Florence, he realized (as he did on occasion) that he was perhaps mostly to blame for the mess of his marriage. He suspected he truly didn't know how to love a woman. In dreams that night, he imagined himself "screwing" a "guy, younger than I . . . as if he were a girl" and added a vague reference to a boyhood experience with his brother Don. He thought it meant that he was "castrat[ing]" himself in relation to other men. In another dream that night, he had sexual desires toward an older man (he speculated Norman O. "Nobby" Brown or Jacques Barzun), doing the elder's sexual bidding. However, he also wrote a somewhat cryptic addendum: "To admit homosexual desires, relationships. . . . To admit, and be with the men, on love relationship, homo or not, like this one with Don, not with the bullying." In various dreams in this period, he found himself in bed with friends like Bob Lifton and Alfred Barr or with the wives of competitors like B. F. Skinner. In late December 1966, he dreamt he was in a meeting with Norman Cousins: "He threw his arms around me, held me tight like a woman a long time. . . . I uncomfortable. [When] we pulled apart, I saw his face just like my father's . . . he wanted to go to men's room . . . I with him." The following week he observed, "Need to make friends with men . . . almost none now."[34]

As he advanced his writing on the daimonic, explicitly sexual dreams became more complex and threatening, heightened by triangular struggles with both perceived enemies and friends, and with bisexual feelings that only rarely had come to consciousness before. He had resisted his deeper feelings for friends—the student of myth, Joseph Campbell, and the radical psychologist R. D. Laing—"that's why I so driven with women, have to *have* them." And women became vivid threats. In one dream, Florence pointed out a snake near their stone wall. When he looked closer, he saw the snake coiled in a hole in the rock that he identified as the vagina of a friend's wife. He remembered it as a "hideous dream" and added—"snakes in the vagina. Don't get in—I still have such fright of them? Or of women having affairs, young women like M, leaving old men." To which he added: "This dream comes at same time as: I have excellent, and *new*, ideas for book—my mind working great, deeply, strongly, originally."[35]

His dreams of the daimonic sometimes replicated the frightening imagery of his LSD trip not only in its sexuality but also in its evocation of violence. He fought an unconscious war that echoed the reality of Vietnam and ghetto riots:

There is to be a big battle, with swords; I the leader of one side. Negroes in it, also very big men (the daimonic?) . . . It was to start in a.m., (like night before in War and Peace) I afraid I would be a coward—swords—would I know how to use it . . . I knew once it got started it (or rather I) would not be a coward. Though also: if we had gunpowder, etc., could ambush the other side . . . Awoke, heart fast, thinking: "Why not fight forever—I have it to give!"[36]

It also left May wondering what the battle would be about. On July 14, Bastille Day, a week after dreaming of swords and impending combat, he had dinner with his friend and colleague Leslie Farber, Farber's wife, and David Bazelon, a brilliant social critic. Discussion turned to the future of American society. Bazelon had just published *Power in America*, a vision of a destruction of a traditional class structure at the hands of technology and a "new class" of technocrats and bureaucrats. May expressed particular concern that in Bazelon's dystopia, "people would lose all old reasons for living, acting—ambition to get money—work—success goals—to succeed—prestige." He worried that all that he had accomplished and earned would mean nothing in his final years.[37]

After listening to Bazelon, in fact, he wondered whether his "whole way of life [was] wrong, empty," in that he worked hard "like a scholar still" in fear of being attacked for not proving his points. That was "the trouble with daimonic chapter—I start out with good idea—then I get anxious, guilty, run to 'scholarship' to prove 'this and that' and turn into a 'grammarian.'" The motive was "wrong"; it was an "escape from *my* living." The lesson: "I have to reform my myth of life—hard work in itself won't do it." He yearned to express himself directly, not through the obfuscating lens of scholarly arguments. "Is my 'envy' of Goodman that he represents *my* daimonic? Obsessed by him . . . why not identify with? Same of Fromm." May recognized that "part of me wants to be direct, free, living out feeling, conviction of the moment. . . . And: to take life as Old Testament enjoyment—cup runneth over."[38]

Not incidentally, as tensions and creative juices mixed and merged, May seemed more and more open to the peace and natural beauty that drew him to Holderness in the first place. He delighted in the "sheer joy" of taking a friend's young children to the lake, to just pause and "come to my own being." He "felt at home again" and could imagine the "rest of these days and years—what joy to look, to see—to be able to write what I want to; to know I can say it and people will read." Later in the year, as he walked to his office one brisk November morning, the "early blue light in morning, wind, all so clear, open, fresh, beautiful," seemed to give him courage to change: "I affirm life—whatever I can with Flo and me—or with someone else—; affirm my writing—with courage, the hell with the great book, do it as it is *me*, assert my being; and nature, beauty, friends. . . . If this could be the morning the switch is thrown!?(!)" It wasn't so simple. A few days later, in therapy with Szalita, he experienced "devils all around fighting each other. . . . I depressed, in conflict, tension—all day along. Evening crying: could strike at Flo, she so stoney."[39]

And then, almost two weeks later, palpable reality hit. On November 30, 1967, May wrote: "Flo took seven sleeping pills Monday night—three nights ago. . . . I stunned for day and a half. . . . She: cry for help—and I don't answer?" It happened on the Monday after a genial family Thanksgiving. As a result of Florence's suicide attempt, Rollo "almost decided [he] could manage the marriage." He was shaken by both the act and his thoughts as he fantasized about the freedom he would have gained had she been successful. "Terrible cruelty," he wrote, "as cruel as the demons which beat me in the LSD—the demons inside me . . . and I *am*, I use them, I as cruel." He discussed Florence's condition with her analyst and concluded that it was the prospect of happiness, dashed quickly by a minor argument on Sunday—a seesaw of hope crushed by reality—that drove her to despair. In a sense, it was a reprise of a pattern that began with their courtship, May by turns embracing and rejecting her. In her mid-twenties, Florence could blithely call his bluff to end their relationship and so ensure his return. Thirty years later, in her mid-fifties and worn down by a life devoted to their children and his career, she attempted suicide.

May did not respond as he had thirty years before. He was no longer the fledgling minister but rather a man in his late fifties contemplating the years left to him. A month and a half before Florence's suicide attempt, he pondered what it would mean to leave her. "Is it the element of acting for myself I interpret as so catastrophic, so much a revolution; acting not for mother, or duty to family, or society; but for my own wants?" He was riven with the guilt of hypocrisy, of being married but having "only this friend-brother-sister-toleration relationship." He wanted to be free of guilt, free of constraint, free in the way his daimonic models, Fromm and Goodman, were—free to leave their wives and, as he saw it, engage fully in life. Florence stood in the way of his fantasy of freedom and fulfillment. Rather than rallying her husband to her side by taking too many sleeping pills, she had unwittingly confirmed his need to remove himself from the marriage.[40]

This was made easier by the fact that May's work on the book he hoped would be an authentic commentary on the human condition was approaching completion. An intensifying and mutually supportive relationship with the actor Robert Ryan and his wife helped a lot. The Ryans were in tune with psychology's growing cultural import, and their fervent admiration for him gave May a sense that he might reach a much wider audience than before. They were warm, laughed a lot after a few drinks, and could talk about the world without reference to theoretical issues or internecine rivalries among psychologists. Furthermore, they reinforced the political side of May's consciousness, encouraging his condemnation of the Vietnam War and, more forthrightly than most in the psychology world, his focus on the relationship of psychological problems to the poverty and injustices revealing themselves every day in urban violence and the battle for civil rights. Jessica was herself a talented novelist and children's book author and had been enamored of May since their therapeutic relationship commenced a few years earlier. Now she was a dear friend, demanding of his attention but also supportive of his work's plainspoken writing intentionally beamed at the elusive intelligent lay public.

As his marriage moved toward dissolution, May was also gaining everwidening recognition in a world hungry for explanations of the increasing turbulence around them. Nothing cemented his place on the emerging cultural horizon like the singular attention he received in *Psychology Today*, a new glossy magazine with serious intentions that premiered in May 1967 and would be a mainstay of popular media through the 1970s. In its first issue, publisher Nicolas H. Charney declared that psychology, while not "a panacea for the world's ills," nonetheless offered important insight into the human condition. However, it had too often been presented to the public in "pompous and unnecessary vocabularies" and in "jargon" that prevented communication of important ideas. Charney wished to bring into public view the best current research in psychology in readable and compelling form. "It is time," he concluded, "to let the air in, and this is the major purpose of *Psychology Today*." Though it drew upon a variety of research traditions, the incoming breeze was largely humanistic. The magazine's first issue even featured a reprint of "Human Potentialities," a visionary article by Aldous Huxley, the author of *Brave New World*, who since the 1950s had been experimenting with psychedelic drugs. Esalen's Richard Price had heard a version of Huxley's article as a lecture at the University of California, San Francisco, in 1960. Huxley's clarion call to conceive of "the world in terms, not of national power, but of basic human needs and the human potentialities which may be actualized when (and only when) those needs are satisfied," affirmed all that humanistic psychology and Esalen hoped to accomplish.[41]

For May, the appearance of *Psychology Today* was fortuitous, as was the bent of one of its editors, forty-three-year-old Mary Harrington Hall. Hall, a veteran journalist and managing editor, found May's work particularly intriguing. She was also charmed by May himself, and he by her, and they formed something of an intimate bond. May was one of three psychologists Hall chose to interview for the September 1967 special issue "Focus on Man," honoring the seventy-fifth anniversary of the American Psychological Association. In addition to May, she singled out E. G. Boring, then an eighty-one-year-old Harvard historian of psychology and former editor of the *American Journal of Psychology*, as "Mr. Psychology," and B. F. Skinner, the great modern-day advocate of behavioral psychology, as "Mr. Behaviorist." Predictably, May was "Mr. Humanist." Boring represented the rich past of psychology, Skinner the present ("very much the man of today"), and May "the man of tomorrow." Boring concurred with her choices for the APA anniversary—not only his own but also the "great new psychologists [Skinner and May]. . . . One says their names and thinks, *Zeitgeist.*"[42]

Hall treated May as some mix of matinee idol and renaissance intellectual. She described him as a "striking man, and tall, with deep brown eyes that are both piercing and gentle. He is delightful company . . . yet his personality remains elusive, fugitive in the sense that a fluid watercolor is fugitive." She stressed the breadth of his training, especially in religion, philosophy, and classical antiquity. As for his professional standing, Hall wrote that "for many years, he has been one of psychology's persistent pioneers." She made May feel comfortable, and that comfort unleashed a passionate personal vision of cultural disintegration and possible renewal. Much of what had gripped him in existentialism lay at the center of the interview in telling, sometimes autobiographical terms. Asked about his "goal in psychology," he replied that he wasn't in the business of "effecting cures" (though he saw the usefulness of therapists who did) but rather of helping "the patient to rediscover himself," to "find out what it means to be human." It was a task on the outer edges of professional psychology, much more in the realm of religion and philosophy, but that was the whole point. The culture, sacred or secular, he argued, no longer delivered the myths that allowed people to imagine meaningful lives. The myth of American self-reliance, he argued, had turned into the hollow rags-to-riches drama of Horatio Alger, which in turn was destroyed by

Arthur Miller's *Death of a Salesman*. "That play, which was written in 1948," he revealed, "shook my very depths. I knew my father's world was dead."[43]

May saw the alienation bred by conformity overpowering what was left of the old values. He indicted most therapists as being part of the problem by helping, with presumably the best of intentions, individuals "fit in." There was no room for the rebel, nonconformist, or "oddball." May had been making this point, identifying personally with historic figures like Jesus, Freud, and Socrates, since his editorship of *The Student* at Michigan State. He declared in the Hall interview "that every human being must have a point at which he stands against the culture, where he says, this is me and the damned world can go to hell." He illustrated the problem with the question of homosexuality, which had become a focus of controversy among psychotherapists in the early 1960s. "In our current society," May noted, "we'd have cured Socrates of it, or Plato, or Alcibiades, and if so there probably wouldn't have been any Platonic dialogues." His main point was that he wanted his patients to be able to choose their sexuality based on knowing themselves, not on the basis of a "cultural judgment" of others that denied their humanity.[44] He warned Skinner and the behaviorists to "beware lest they help create a mechanical society" with no room for unique individuals. May chided Carl Rogers's denial of the tragic in life, reporting that when May asked him, "What about *Romeo and Juliet*?" Rogers replied, "They wouldn't have committed suicide if only they'd had a little counseling."

As for psychologists in general, he accused them of ignoring "almost completely the problem of power in race relations." The exception he pointed to was Dr. Kenneth Clark, the African American psychologist whose research helped influence the Supreme Court in its historic 1954 desegregation decision, *Brown v. Board of Education*. Race was very much on May's mind in the summer of 1967, Detroit having just exploded in a deadly race riot. May noted that Clark's most recent work, *Dark Ghetto: Dilemmas of Social Power* (1965), was one of the few books that considered the psyche of socially powerless individuals in relation to those with power.[45]

Despite the enormous boost the *Psychology Today* interview gave him, as well as the publication of an excerpt from the forthcoming *Love and Will* in the February 1968 issue, Rollo remained vulnerable to criticism from friends within the profession. Ernest Schachtel, an eminent psychologist, felt the interview in *Psychology Today* was too much a love letter and May's answers too "negative" and self-serving. Magda added that one of her patients "criticized [him] all over." He was so unhinged by Schachtel's remark and the manipulative way that Magda delivered the message that he briefly thought he was losing his mind. And so it went for the rest of the year and into 1969: the helter-skelter professional life of publishing and lecturing, large and appreciative audiences, endless grappling with critics real and imagined, the demons inside and his own daimonic energies, and unsteady progress on "the book."[46]

And, then, in early April, seemingly to fulfill a promise to himself that he would decide by the time he was sixty, Rollo declared that he wanted a divorce. He and Florence began what was by law still an adversarial process. May described the meeting: "Yesterday with Flo and lawyers. . . . An awful experience—everybody cheating everybody—no human trust at all . . . all that *was* good between Florence and me is lost, betrayed, down the drain." The haggling continued until they signed the agreement in late July. "At last it is over," he wrote. "At last freedom to be what I am, to live out what is truly me . . . only if I have the courage to live against loneliness, to accept non-being, to affirm myself . . . against all negativity, let me see now if I can affirm my existence." The quiet affirmation of the decision reflected exhaustion and sadness, a mood compounded by coming home to the news that Mary Hall had committed suicide the day before at the age of forty-five. It was an act that surprised those who thought they knew her, Rollo included, and was a sobering endnote to a day that began a new chapter in his life. [47]

22

Love and Will

In late summer of 1969, May submitted the final edits for *Love and Will* to W. W. Norton and began to make the rounds of radio, television, and other media interviews. Each new appearance inspired frightening dream dramas and waking struggles. The book was in but not yet out, and even when his advance author's copy arrived the same day as a party in Holderness, he struggled to balance joy and disappointment. Despite a congratulatory toast by Robert Ryan and hearty cheers from others, he felt empty, the paradoxical vacuity that he ascribed to a focus on accomplishment rather than Being. He returned to New York on September 13, almost exactly on the book's publication date, and soon after the Ryans threw him a lavish launch party at their new apartment in the Dakota on Central Park West. By early October he had achieved a certain peace: "Whatever happens now—in the lap of the gods. Long sleep last night; rested. Whatever I do now, part of a new life. Got divorced two weeks ago; at the same time as publication—a new life at 60."[1]

This new life for May and the publication of *Love and Will*, of course, were shaped by the most intense period of cultural and political turbulence since the Great Depression. The seams of American society were beginning to split wide open even as May was writing. Stalemate and increasing casualties in Vietnam by late 1967 brought Democratic Party challenges to Lyndon Johnson's nomination for reelection, and early in 1968 Johnson declared that he would not run for reelection and instead concentrate on seeking an honorable end to the war. The assassinations of Martin Luther King, Jr., and Robert F. Kennedy in April and June, as well as campus demonstrations at Columbia and other colleges and universities, added generational warfare and defiance of authority to the more specific antiwar and civil rights campaigns.

What ensued instead was a dizzying miasma of a cruel and costly war in Asia and an explosive home front. A mostly youth-oriented counterculture of drugs, open sexuality, and apocalyptic spiritual seeking—something like a Tillichian *kairos* mixed with darker themes of addiction, overdose, and disappointment—set itself against the void of violence both foreign and domestic. The contrasts were sometimes startling. In August, a half million people converged on Bethel, New York, for the instantly legendary Woodstock Festival. *Time* elicited from May the accurate if incomplete appraisal that the Woodstock love-in was "a symptomatic event of our time that showed the tremendous hunger, need and yearning for community on the part of youth." *Time* noted that May compared the "friendly spirit favorably with the alcoholic mischief ever present at a Shriners' convention but wonder[ed] how long the era of good feeling w[ould] last." Just months later, he had a partial answer in the equally symbolic music festival at Altamont Speedway in Northern California, where the Rolling Stones headlined a show that ended in Hell's Angels mayhem and death.[2]

Amid intimations of hope and fear and the grinding presence of Vietnam, *Love and Will* addressed an existential theme long central to May's work: the individual's quest for a meaningful life in modernity. However, what May and others had once envisioned as a struggle against implacable forces of depersonalized authority now appeared in a different light. As mostly youthful critics pummeled each myth of authority, law, and structure in American life and revealed a record of injustice, hypocrisy, and death, the entire culture lost itself in a world of crumbling assumptions, unbridled anger, and newfound if sometimes chimerical freedom.

May wrote *Love and Will* just as the seams were splitting and called upon the venerable traditions of the West to understand a crisis that was widening even as the book made its way to press. Thus it differed from many other approaches of the era in adapting existential themes of encounter and choice, of meaning and caring, to the incipient cultural anarchy of the 1960s. May made few references to politics and Vietnam, mostly to illustrate more philosophical points. Nor did he endorse drugs or rock and roll as a road to social bliss. Rather, May consulted the grand sweep of Western thought, from the Greeks to the latest sociological study, in order to decipher what had happened to love, meaningful life, and community. In that sense, *Love and Will* encompassed the cultural critiques of such other works of the late 1950s and 1960s as Norman O. Brown's *Life against Death* (1959) and *Love's Body* (1966) and Herbert Marcuse's *Eros and Civilization* (1955) and *One-Dimensional Man* (1964).

These and other books had begun to attain a kind of prophetic status among radical academics and students, laying the philosophical basis for the New Left and an emergent counterculture. By contrast, *Love and Will* spoke directly to the personal and social concerns of middle-class Americans. It demanded no loyalty, strictly speaking, to an intervening ideology, only to the general notion of twin crises of intimacy and social cohesion. For *Love and Will* to be relevant, one simply had to share in an almost universal sense that things were falling apart: events, technologies, and outdated values were in the saddle, relations between the sexes were chaotic, and too often individual response to these disturbing developments was passive, apathetic, or violent. May had little to say about the great social and political movements of the day except as they impinged upon or illustrated his central theme. This lack of a specific political theory, for some potentially a weakness, was the source of a paradoxical strength. For middle-class America, whose vision of society began with assessment of individual spiritual and psychological health, *Love and Will*'s viewpoint was congenial to the broadest of America's reading publics.

In part, this breadth of audience had to do with the fact that May was one of the few popular interpreters of the age whose life and consciousness had been formed within the culture of Protestant Middle America. Marcuse, Fromm, and Erikson were Jewish émigrés who had escaped Hitler's Germany. Maslow was the son of Jewish immigrants. Their voices and perspectives were striking because of difference as well as substance. By contrast, May spoke the native social, cultural, and emotional tongue of middle-class America. While he cast himself as a rebel against the narrowest aspects of that heritage and drank voraciously from the well of European psychoanalytic and social criticism, his visions of the world and of life deeply reflected his midwestern background. And, more than his other recent work, *Love and Will* intoned its message in the voice of a minister.

Indeed, at its heart, the book was a prophetic sermon, a modern jeremiad, preaching a vision of decline but also promising a road to renewal. It organized the contradictory impulses of the age into a message of dark hope. May revealed the contrapuntal nature of the book in a short foreword that set human consciousness in relation to nature. He invited the reader to imagine his summer retreat in New Hampshire, describing the world around him as it came alive each morning. A "hallelujah chorus" of birds—the song sparrow's chirp, the goldfinch's "obligato," the wood thrush's unbounded warble, and the beat of a woodpecker on the beech tree. Against them all, the loons on the lake "erupt with their plaintive and tormented daemonic." These sounds of nature evoked in May the "everlasting going and coming, the eternal return, the growing and mating and dying and growing again." Not so humanity, May noted, for man's possession of consciousness forced it to "transcend the eternal return." It could not simply and mindlessly repeat the cycles of daily living. "In this transitional twentieth century," he declared, "when the full results of our bankruptcy of inner values [are] brought home to us, I believe it is especially important that we seek the source of love and will."[3]

Like the chorus of birds, the main body of *Love and Will* played itself out in musical form—dark themes, complicating variations, and cautiously hopeful resolution. The central motif was an old one stated in new terms, the fate of human consciousness in an age of doubt and transition. May pointed his readers toward a paradox. Once, the culture offered love and will as the solutions to life's problems. Now the solutions had become the problem. In "our schizoid world," the old sureties were gone. Love and will, instead of being integrated into the fullness of culture and relation, had become distorted through alienation. Profound love had been translated into its lowest common denominator of sex. The power of will had been crippled by the modern age's increasing sense of individual powerlessness.

May located authentic contemporary cultural enrichment only in the realms of modern art, music, and literature, where the very alienation and agony of modernity had been translated into creations evocative of the age. Cézanne, Van Gogh, Picasso, and Auden managed to refract their creative talents to illustrate the torn state of modern consciousness and the modern realities of alienation and emptiness. However, for most, modernity had bred only a dull numbness, disorientation, apathy, and impulse toward violence. Beneath this gray surface lay a much more complicated reality. Patients in therapy often offered the most candid insight into broader dilemmas, May argued, and he used such evidence to present a new description of the problem of modernity that might lead to "a new basis for the love and will which have been its chief casualties."[4]

What did love and will, at least in May's usage, really mean? May discussed love first, arguing from cultural convention that there were really four types of human love: libido, eros, philia, and agape. Libido simply referred to the sex drive, while eros represented the pull of love toward creation or procreation. Philia was brotherly love and friendship. Agape stood for the love and care of human being for others, friends or strangers, which in Christianity mirrored God's love of humankind. May proposed that authentic human love, in its fullest sense was a "blending" of all four. The modern age had distorted, trivialized, and alienated each manifestation of love from the other.

In the first five chapters, May analyzed modern love and proposed ways of reuniting and reasserting all its aspects. He began with sex, noting that the Victorian neurosis of repressed sexuality had been replaced by an almost oppressive openness in contemporary discussion and expectation of sex. While applauding the new sexual freedom for its honesty, he argued that internal anxiety and guilt had replaced older, more externalized manifestations. Concentration on technique, performance, and frequency had severed sexuality's relation to feeling. "Sin used to mean giving in to one's sexual desires; it now means not having full sexual expression," he noted. "Our contemporary puritan holds that it is immoral *not* to express your libido." Sex without love had replaced love without sex as a personal ideal. May did not advocate turning back the clock but worried that the emphasis on pure libido helped to close "our senses and imaginations to the enrichment of pleasure and passion and the meaning of love."[5]

May illustrated the problem with case histories of four women and two men, each with some form of sexual dysfunction. The women didn't feel much during sex, and the men were impotent or reported that sex lacked any "bang." Physical pleasure and communion had little to do with their motives for sex. Two of the women used it to "hang on" to their men; another saw sex as "something nice you give a man." The fourth, a bit lustier, expressed both generosity and anger when she had sex. The two men mostly felt the need "to demonstrate their masculinity." All wandered in the sexual wilderness, diminishing the richness of the act itself by making it the instrument of neurotic (though culturally encouraged) behavior.[6]

To May, this acting out in the sexual realm pointed to other underlying motives—the "struggle to prove one's identity," a "hope to overcome [one's] own solitariness," and a "desperate endeavor to escape feelings of emptiness and the threat of apathy." He argued that these were motives and consequences of even the richest relationships. The problem was that the culture had concentrated more and more on physical signs of success—erection, orgasm, multiple orgasm—to the detriment of the human relationship symbolized by the sexual act. One might even choose to "*feel less* in order to *perform better!*" Thus came the inevitable confusion of one of May's patients, whose impotence belied his own self image as a "screwing machine." Impotence was the natural result of the alienation of sex from other forms of love.[7]

May's chapters then moved to a detailed analysis of these estrangements. "Eros in Conflict with Sex" explored the alienation of sex from love. "Love and Death" argued that in an age when "sexuality" became tied to assertions of identity and a quest for security, human beings were less likely to experience the piquant relation of sexual surrender, death, and rebirth. Indeed, he asserted that the "obsession with sex serve[d] to cover up contemporary man's fear of death." Other aspects of modern sexual life carried double meanings. For instance, in addition to its liberating gifts, contraception, by separating sex from procreation, allowed human beings to repress or ignore those aspects of sexuality of which childbirth and the creation of life itself were emblematic. In short, death, tragedy, passion—the things that once made *Eros* a "*mysterium tremendum*"—had in the modern world been written out of the sexual act.

May sought to reinvigorate the meaning of *Eros* by viewing it as part of an even more elemental force—the daimonic. He quoted Plato—"Eros is a daimon"—and defined the "daimonic" as "*any natural function which has the power to take over the whole person.*" Whether creative or destructive, angry or ecstatic, the molten force of the daimonic lay at the root of both creation and destruction. In this sense, the daimonic became something of a cultural id, the engine of what Freud called *Eros* and the wish for death. By denying the existence of so potent a drive in the human psyche, human beings risked losing their sensitivity to the relationship between creation and destruction. They became apathetic and potentially dangerous innocents. Surrender to the paradox of attraction and fear, of acceptance and rejection, of the loss of self in the other, made all aspects of love and life more profoundly human.[8]

As for will, paradoxes abounded. May saw the central crisis as the widespread inability to formulate some sense of wish or intention and then work toward that end. He had no great love of the nineteenth century's concept of "will power," as if things were as simple as choosing a goal and achieving it. Freud's theories relegated motivation to the murky world of the unconscious and, for some, destroyed the idea of independent will. For them, humanity lived by unconscious and unstoppable drives. For May, psychotherapy should have been but only rarely was an exercise that freed one to want and then to will. An individual gained such freedom, he argued, not by passively understanding that one's actions were controlled by invisible forces but by learning to shape one's larger and smaller actions with an understanding of the power the unconscious wielded. Thus "will" might be reborn by uncovering one's unconscious blocks to fulfilling those wishes and, through such insight, serve one's own more authentic wishes. Wish and will were the keys to May's vision of reconstruction. In place of the narrow margin of choice promised by Freudian psychoanalysis and in defiance of the conditioning recommended by behaviorists, May sought a therapeutic goal that resulted in a creative reimagining of goals and futures appropriate to a revivified sense of self.

May's approach to getting to that state involved the existential idea of intentionality. He defined it as "the structure which gives meaning to experience." "Intentionality is the heart of consciousness," he argued, "out of which comes the awareness of our capacity to form, to mold, to change ourselves and the day in relation to each other." Intentionality was thus the bridge between the objective world and the subjective inner self. It allowed individuals to move toward investing meaning in objects, individuals, and actions. Through this reopening of the possibility of human assertion, May revived will as a concept that comported not so much with the nineteenth-century sense of self-reliance as with a modern vision of psychological possibility. "Intentionality," he concluded, "itself consisting of the deepened awareness one's self, is our means of putting the meaning surprised by consciousness into action." That action could in turn build a better world, one where "in every act of love and will—and in the long run they are both present in each genuine act—we mold ourselves and our world simultaneously." And, finally, he declared: "This is what it means to embrace the future."[9]

Love and Will attained its power and popularity not just from its frank discussion of the cultural crisis and its modern, spiritually uplifting solution to questions of sexuality. By embracing the entirety of Western thought, it also restored a reassuring cultural memory to its readers. Its liberal references to Greek myth, biblical stories, and a wide selection of philosophers defined a kind of intellectual collage, preserving tradition in the style of modernity. Indeed, May declared on the very last page of the book, "We stand on the peak of the consciousness of previous ages, and their wisdom is available to us."

It took a while for *Love and Will* to gain public notice. There were only a few reviews when it came out in September 1969, perhaps due to its rich, densely packed kaleidoscope of ideas. Even the *New York Times*, where May's own reviews had appeared regularly, did not immediately run pieces in either its daily or Sunday edition. The first major review, by the insightful psychoanalyst Anthony Storr, upset May. Storr began with apparent praise, calling it "a tract for our times compounded from the author's wide culture and clinical experience." Nonetheless, he questioned the connection between neurosis and art and deemed "pathological" what he saw as the book's "advocacy of allowing erotic passion full throttle." Storr's final judgment mixed shrewd observation and a grudging measure of admiration: "This book is more a profession of faith than a scientific treatise, but as such it has a value."[10]

Nonetheless, May's editor at Norton reported to him that despite the slow start in the press, the book was selling thousands of copies. In early December, May witnessed proof of its success when he boarded a plane and saw *Love and Will* in a fellow passenger's hand. The biggest gift of all, however, was bestowed by the *Times* literally on Christmas Day. The opening flourish by John Leonard read:

> Rollo May's extraordinary book was ignored by this column when it first appeared three months ago, for which some of us should have our space-bar thumbs chopped off and fried for hors d'oeuvres. It is wise, rich, witty and indispensable; a meditation rather than an apocalyptic seizure; a text on consciousness as well as an approach to psychotherapy; an argument for the fashioning of a set of values appropriate to our biological, historical and individual selves, as we apprehend them in the fitful modern gleam; an escape from determinism. It should not only have been reviewed: it should have led any list of important books published in 1969.

Leonard proceeded to give an incredibly appreciative, complete, and nuanced summary of the book, taking his daily column space for two days to do so. His Christmas Day installment emphasized May's vision for repairing the world. In Leonard's rendition, "care—not sentimentality, which is the satisfaction we take in recognizing an emotion, in thinking about it; but rather the genuine experience of the object of that emotion—is the only base upon which to build our ethical skyscrapers."[11]

Thanks to Leonard's review, word of mouth from longtime fans, and newcomers who might have heard a May lecture or an interview on the radio, *Love and Will* made its way on to the bestseller lists. It won the Ralph Waldo Emerson Award of the Phi Beta Kappa Society for 1970. The following year, surely on the basis of both May's past work and the success of *Love and Will*, the Division of Clinical Psychology of the American Psychological Association honored him with its Distinguished Contributions Award for 1971. *Love and Will* quickly became required reading not only in psychology but also in philosophy and theology courses. It appealed to disaffected youth, to those of the counterculture who supposedly did not trust anyone over thirty, and to otherwise unremarkable citizens who felt confused and dismayed about inner conflicts and recent events.[12]

One might well ask what made *Love and Will*, a sometimes complicated evocation of the human condition, so compelling a read. A criticism from the eminent psychoanalyst Leo Rangell offers a clue. "It is difficult to know who is speaking in the book," Rangell noted with a faint odor of condescension; "May the psychoanalyst, May the theologian or May the existentialist." Stated another way, May spoke simultaneously in all three tongues.[13] It was precisely the inimitable combination of ministerial, philosophical, and analytical voices that struck a chord with so many. In fact, just how personal the responses to the book were was revealed in the fan letters that came pouring in from men and women of all walks of life. They attested to its therapeutic or, in some cases, religious power. Somehow, May had imbued his expository prose with the feeling of actual face-to-face therapy, a style that suggested May's own vulnerability and fellow suffering.

No wonder, then, that the book might elicit ecstatic reactions. One woman declared that reading *Love and Will* had changed her life "in a flash." Another thanked May "for opening up a whole new dimension in [her] life," indeed for turning her away from suicide. Still another claimed she had more than read *Love and Will*—she had "absorbed it, ingested it, devoured it" and "awoke in a clear, almost blinding light." She was "blinded" by "healing" tears: "I no longer feel I am a voice crying in the wilderness, for you are there to hear, to listen and to understand! You are wonderful! You are magic!" An eighteen-year-old artist from Montreal found in *Love and Will* an appreciation of her lonely quest for creative expression and identified another compelling quality of the book: she trusted him with her feelings because of the many "deeply personal" passages. "In this sense you have also trusted me," she wrote, "for you have also exposed your own feelings."[14] Still another fan passed along the thoughts she had written down in Mexico: "I have recently read a book. I wish the man who wrote it could know how much I thank him for writing it. It touched my blood. . . . He gave me a way to understand some parts of my life that were barren, cut off, hateful, so that I wasn't ashamed of them. I saw how they were connected to everything I value and love."[15] May even heard from one of the women over whom he had obsessed at Union Seminary in the 1930s, who broke a decades-long silence to express her delight in the book and reminisce about Harry Bone, Reinhold Niebuhr, and sitting together in seminar in 1935.[16]

The majority of letters came from women, but the book could evoke similarly ecstatic responses from men. William Douglas, a professor of psychology and religion at Boston University and a leader in the field of religious studies, wrote that it spoke to him "in a transforming and renewing way" and added a page-long poem:

> A Tribute to Rollo May—after having re-read LOVE AND WILL
> and really experiencing it
> in the depths of my being
> and his daimon met mine
> in the context of the BEING
> that unites our separate beings[17]

This dizzying acceleration of fortune, fame, and divorce began to spin May's world almost out of control. He continued to accept speaking engagement after speaking engagement and found time to conceive of at least two new books, in addition to teaching at William Alanson White, NYU, and the New School. Of course, he also struggled with his own world of love and will, fraught as ever with hesitation, fear, and desire by the loneliness of ending thirty years of marriage. At sixty, he wondered whether he would be attractive to women and, for that matter, whether his tachycardia would interfere with his sexual abilities. In addition, there were the women who already existed in his life. Being married to Florence had freed him to be intimate with others without much worry about demands or expectations of marriage. Now single, he feared that Ellie Roberts, Magda Denes, Jessica Ryan, or Dorothy Norman might see her chance. He wanted none of it, but, it must be added, rarely did they express such wishes. He was at times achingly lonely and sexually starved, wondering what the future held.

Then, in the fall of 1969, after delivering what he later regarded as a disappointing lecture at a conference in Hawaii, he noticed a beautiful blonde in a muumuu running after him as he attempted to escape the hall. She wanted to know his views about Camus. Weeks later, at a workshop in San Diego, she reappeared and reminded him of their prior meeting. Her energy and beauty was such that he needed no reminder. Her name was Ingrid Scholl. They talked and talked, and Rollo felt viscerally attracted to her. She was bowled over by his fame, good looks, and interest in her. In her mid-thirties, she immediately noted that she was living with the man with whom she had come to the workshop but also made it known that it was an "inconsequential" relationship. In December he called from New York to suggest they visit Furnace Creek in Death Valley National Park, where he could paint and she could enjoy the stark beauty of the desert. They met at the house of his brother Don,

now a painter and illustrator based in Los Angeles. For May it felt like an un-
deserved dream. As he wrote soon after, she was "glorious, much too beautiful for me." He worried that she would back out. [18]

Ingrid didn't disappoint. Off they drove for five hours to Death Valley. As
she took the first round of driving, Rollo buried himself in the map rather
than face his aching desire. He then took the wheel, and Ingrid "nuzzled
close, affectionately." They reached the resort, checked into their room,
showered, and Ingrid emerged from the bath "a dazzling creature" dressed
in black satin. Dinner was mired in expectancy and nervous banter, Rollo's
voice lost to laryngitis. They then they returned to the room and in the dim
light made love. They made love again in the morning, toured the ranch
and surrounding desert—its barren beauty of borax and rock formations—
returned for dinner and dancing, and made love again and again, and for two
more days toured, painted, talked, and made ecstatic love. He remembered
her saying, "I didn't know this could really happen . . . an orgasm with a man."

Physical desire and satisfaction wrecked the well-honed defenses of both
and punctuated the weekend's passion with moments of remorse. At one
point Rollo felt "resentful" for no apparent reason, while at another moment
Ingrid became so "despondent" that she ran to the phone and called her
sister. A frustrating round of lovemaking made her angry—"I hated it!"—
and left both feeling lonely. Ingrid's attempt to lead while they were dancing
bothered Rollo. Later, an argument about Nietzsche upended a time of quiet
reading and could only be resolved in bed. At her home after four days in the
desert, the sex was better than ever, driving May to write: "She discovered
me, how to make me ecstatic, how to carry me away, how to make [me] delir-
ious . . . and I fucked her with all my power—and it was wonderful." He told
her over breakfast that he didn't deserve her, and she replied, "Just like me?"
They made love once more the night before he returned to New York in early
January, and both evinced wonder at the transport that had enveloped them.
Yet Rollo began to feel deeply ambivalent, aching for Ingrid's body but worried and jealous.

In fact, once in New York he continued to pick apart his life, especially his
relationships with women. In a declaration typical of his most self-pityingly
heroic moments, he sought to "accept the loneliness" and "the cruelty which
is mine, and is part of life." A few weeks later, while at Oberlin for a lecture, he
had a dream that laid bare his deep ambivalence about women. In the dream,
he came upon his son Bob as a baby, having been beaten "unmercifully" by
Bob's (imagined) four-year-old sister, "lying in puddle of water." He knew

the dream was about Ruth. He asked himself whether he could approach a new relationship with an emotional tabula rasa instead of the fear, anger, and helplessness ingrained by the unfortunate experiences with his mother and Ruth? That meant not only trying to filter out the ways in which his visceral reactions to Ingrid repeated the past but also attempting to see Ingrid for who she was and acknowledging her own motivations and fears.[19]

Rollo needed clarity. He began by consulting with intimate friends who might help him see his recent relationships and his life in some new light. A long talk with Dorothy Norman convinced him that his stormy relationship with Jessica Ryan and the underlying tensions with both Ryans were not his problem but issues emanating from their own complicated marriage. His guilt came from his need to "play god." With her encouragement, he vowed to resist the Ryans' anger and blame and began to create a kind of home-baked Nietzschean justification for living a new, guilt-free life. May imagined for himself a liberating ethic, one in which his devotion to work overrode all else, including commitments to others, to find "'new' work, 'new' self, 'new' development." It was indeed a "'new' ethics—or ethics for the elite." The entangling emotions that affected others need not get in the way of his life's mission, or so he thought.[20]

May didn't have to wait long to test his new, "above it all" resolve about life and relationships and to experience its limits. Initial signs were reaffirming. *Love and Will* kept selling and remained for weeks on the *New York Times* bestseller list. About the same time as his conversation with Dorothy Norman, he was told that his book was one of five finalists for the National Book Award in Philosophy and Religion. A few days later, he heard that Erik Erikson's *Gandhi's Truth* had won, but, after a first wave of "bitter disappointment," May experienced a new sense of freedom, "a new surge on my consulting—a new interest . . . and zest . . . sharpness." At the National Book Award cocktail party, he even allowed himself a little "forced jollification" and accepted with equanimity the compensatory congratulations of those present for his "runaway best seller."[21]

Yet guilt-ridden doubt continued to plague him, especially over his relationship with Jessica Ryan and the accusation of both Ryans that he hadn't given Jessica enough credit for her assistance in the writing of *Love and Will*. Echoes of Robert's "dark depressed rage" and "*his semi-psychosis*" haunted Rollo. He tensed when Jessica called, assuming she was about to go on the attack and furthermore that she had the "right" to "hold a gun on me—make me think I'm a shit." Instead, she phoned to say what a great and good influence he had on "young people," including her son Tim. May could only blame himself, his masochistic need to be disliked, and his use of it as an excuse to be unfaithful and isolated from real intimacy. His short-lived vision of a Nietzschean heroic future ended, at least for a moment, in a flourish:

> *But it is my guilt*—that eats at me—not Robert's accusations
>   Christ, let me accept that part of it—and give me some light . . . some light.[22]

Rollo tested himself further on a trip to visit his mother in late April 1970, as always overseeing the welfare of Matie and Ruth even as he decried their tortuous influence. No surprises greeted him in Michigan. Matie remained the negative, critical soul of his imagination and reality, belittling his successes, criticizing Ingrid without meeting her, even suggesting to May that he "would look younger" if he cut his hair. He was caught in a bind, recognizing the roots of her darkness—"an orphan girl—no status in life (no family, no place where she belonged, where she had right to be herself)"—and yet having to live his own life imbued with her damaged soul as an inheritance. "I no good because I from her," he wrote; "I carry the taint, I have to apologize. . . . I carry her burden."[23]

One road of escape was suggested by Dorothy Norman, who encouraged May to take a chance on Ingrid "and get what you need, what supports and satisfies you." He called Ingrid regularly, but reservations continued to surface, fueled by the contentious moments of their epic trip to Death Valley and by their phone conversations. In one call, she told him that she stopped seeing her psychiatrist. He feared that without therapy she would give him up.[24] The summer of 1970 reignited old fears, especially after a frank conversation with Ellie Roberts in which she warned him that he was getting older and might lose his "vitality," that Ingrid might be attracted to others. He faced a quandary. If he made her "alert sexually, alive, aware, she might want to find other, more potent men. May recognized his jealousies were "age-old stuff," that he felt it about each woman in his life and, in terms of competition, "toward every man—young enough, etc. to be attractive." As if to confirm his trepidation, the next night he called she was out (at a woman friend's house). The night after it was the same story. And so it went through the summer and fall, highs and lows and indecision. He made several trips to see her in Los Angeles, and with each encounter his ambivalence grew. At the same time, his sense of vitality, energy, even if fueled by anger, was like an elixir. He discussed his dilemma with the Reissigs in August, and at first thought they were "vaguely against her," which May resented. He reminded himself that it was his decision to make alone.[25]

Ingrid was impossibly beautiful to Rollo, a badge of honor for a sixty-one-year-old thrust into the supposed freedom of divorce. She was also "imperious," angry, and clearly protective of her right to be with other men and women in ambiguously romantic ways. May assuaged some of his jealousy by imagining her "the one who doesn't kiss on the mouth, who saves that for me, who lets herself go sexually only with me and who feels sexually only with me." Deciding about a future with Ingrid meant measuring his own manhood as much as deciphering Ingrid's behavior. Indeed, the very same evening he rebelled against the Reissigs' lukewarm reception of Ingrid—"I have to make the decision, and stand by it—make it succeed"—his torment returned. He dreamed that he caught Ingrid having dinner with a "man, employer, tall, clean-cut," and at the end of the dinner "he kissed her, she returned it on mouth. I assumed they had been to bed." And, penciled in: "I was very jealous."[26]

By November 1970, May seriously considered ending the relationship despite plans to see Ingrid for the holidays. He consulted a psychiatrist friend in New York, who warned him that things did not bode well, but that he need not worry. May was, he noted, among the most eligible men in New York and shouldn't be pining over such a difficult and unrewarding relationship. Furthermore, he pointed out aspects of Ingrid's personality that Rollo reluctantly agreed were there, especially "her hostility and aggression" and "very little capacity to love." May himself saw "a repetition of Florence in some ways . . . covered over in mechanism by her beauty, her charm, her foreign ways." His nostalgia for the free lovemaking of Death Valley reminded him of his idealization of Isabella Hunner. He vowed to end the relationship but still planned to see her at Christmas. Yet, though doubts never ceased, the pull toward Ingrid was too great. He proposed, and they married in Holderness on July 8, 1971.[27]

23

In the Maelstrom

Even as *Love and Will* captured the imagination of hundreds of thousands of readers, May could feel events moving somewhat beyond that book's universe of assumptions. The calamitous events of 1968 highlighted an underlying challenge to the legitimacy of established authority and norms in just about every quadrant of life: racial, sexual, personal, and political. The divorce rate climbed, the pill allowed for riskless sex, book and movie censorship all but collapsed, children ran away from home in droves, and religious cults recruited those in despair. At the same time, the arts, popular culture, and the elbow room of personal freedom expanded, all within a hope for personal, spiritual, and cultural transformation. A decade before, May and Tillich had calmly discussed whether *kairos* or void would dominate the future. As it turned out, both prophecies were confirmed in a frightening and exhilarating swirl, all to the drumbeat of urban riots and casualty lists from Vietnam. Many thought William Butler Yeats's famous lines from "The Second Coming" captured the moment:

> Things fall apart; the center cannot hold;
> Mere anarchy is loosed upon the world. . . .[1]

May's sympathies were clearly on the side of protest and freedom. He had always considered himself a rebel, whether as editor of *The Student* at Michigan State or within psychology itself as an advocate of existential and humanistic psychology. Yet May's reaction to this palpable unraveling of the social order was complex. He had relied on an unspoken assumption that, despite differences of race, culture, religion, and gender, one could write collectively about men and women of all kinds, that they shared a "human condition," and that human needs and desires could be addressed without reference to social or cultural particularity. He also believed in a liberal concept of American democracy, flawed but open to change and ultimately united in basic values. Yet every day the news brought evidence that America might better be defined by the fissures within—divisions that seemed to be clustering into racial, generational, religious, cultural, sexual, and political civil wars.

However, May was firmly committed to protest within the bounds of civil discourse. He expressed his strong allegiance to the antiwar movement through writing and nonviolent protest. He attacked Vietnam policy in newspaper pieces and, no matter the ostensible subject, in virtually every one of his public lectures. In May 1972, he participated in a sit-in at the Capitol in Washington, risking arrest (police took about a hundred of the group into custody) to deliver a "Petition for Redress of Grievances" to Congress. He found himself increasingly uncomfortable with more confrontational, revolutionary, and, just as important, overly media-savvy campaigns. He bridled at the Yippies, Students for a Democratic Society (SDS), and other radical groups "performing" protest with anti-American fury and open endorsement of the North Vietnamese cause. Nuanced discussions had turned into slogans, mass demonstrations and counterdemonstrations, violence, and sometimes death. To May, the debate over the war was spinning out of control.[2]

On the civil rights front, May had actively supported desegregation and civil rights in general, albeit in a style typical of a liberal white professional. Rollo's closest personal connection to the cause came through his friendship with Lillian Smith, author of *Strange Fruit* (1944) and *Killers of the Dream* (1949), a southern white woman and intellectual who early on openly dared to champion desegregation. May also participated in fundraising events for the Student Nonviolent Coordinating Committee (SNCC). However, at that point he claimed no special insight to the core poison of racism. Like most white Americans in the North, he knew few African Americans, and aside from living adjacent to Harlem and thereby having at least glancing familiarity with black culture, he knew little about the everyday life of black America.[3]

By the late 1960s, however, May had become deeply disturbed by the escalation of racial unrest playing out on urban streets across the nation, uprisings that shocked whites with nightly news images of ghettos aflame that underlined black discontent but also courted violent suppression by police and the National Guard. Not only in cities but in prisons as well, racial suppression—mostly white on black, as in the murderous quelling of a prisoner revolt at Attica prison in 1971—shocked May and many others into thinking for the first time about the central role of violence in American society. The Reverend Martin Luther King's espousal of nonviolent action brought some comfort to the white community. However, more radical black organizations, most notably the Black Panther Party, began to espouse active armed resistance to the racial status quo. And police authorities responded in kind. The report of the commission charged by President Johnson to study the causes of urban unrest ominously summarized what African Americans had always known: "Our nation is moving toward two societies, one black, one white—separate and unequal." Few predicted a peaceful separation.[4]

Of a different order was the sexual revolution symbolized by the advent of second-wave feminism but also involving access to contraception and especially the pill, "no-fault" divorce, the rise of an increasingly significant advocacy of gay rights, and the progressive collapse of most forms of censorship in literature and the media. Feminism especially posed dilemmas for May and most men and women in its challenge to legally sanctioned inequality and defiance of the sexual hierarchies and gender customs embedded within virtually every aspect of social and personal consciousness. In short, these forces combined to grant personal freedom from the state, expected behavior, and assumed values to a degree never seen before in American society.

In principle, at least, these developments comported well with the ability of the individual to make the kinds of personal choices May and other existentialists had advocated for almost two decades. In fact, May and his colleagues had provided inspiration for one of the most formidable founders of second-wave feminism. Betty Friedan began "The Forfeited Self," a key chapter of her epochal book *The Feminine Mystique* (1963), by quoting May's essays in *Existence* and otherwise relying upon May, Maslow, Fromm, Goldstein, and other pioneers in humanistic and existential psychology in making her feminist case. May repaid the compliment in *Love and Will* when he embraced *The Feminine Mystique* and the founding of the National Organization of Women as part of a broader quest for personhood.[5]

Nonetheless, as a sixty-year-old male with strong fears and desires concerning women despite an existential commitment to authentic connection between men and women, he wondered in *Love and Will* whether the new feminism had not given up its part in true sexual intimacy through "the struggle to prove one's identity." He argued that feminism "had helped spawn the idea of egalitarianism of the sexes and the interchangeability of the sexual roles." Woman had "clung" to equality "at the price of denying not only biological differences—which are basic, to say the least—between men and women, but emotional differences from which come much of the delight of the sexual act." He worried that women were following the path of men by endorsing a sexual life freed of commitment that promised liberation but that had already led, according to May, to a numbed and often impotent masculinity.[6]

He was rudely awakened with the new militancy of the feminist cause. In fact, he played a minor role in what has become a legendary moment in the history of radical feminism. It occurred during his first appearance on *The Dick Cavett Show*, in its time considered the thinking person's version of late-night TV. Cavett, who displayed a combination of Yale sophistication and boyish midwestern charm, chatted about the issues of the day with intellectuals, artists, actors, and musicians. On March 26, 1970, his guests included May, *Playboy* magazine's Hugh Hefner, the psychedelic rock group Jefferson Airplane, and two radical feminist journalists, Susan Brownmiller and Sally Kempton.[7]

The show began with a song performed by Jefferson Airplane and an amiable chat between Hefner and Cavett about Big Bunny, the *Playboy* corporation's new private jet, and its onboard delights. May then joined the group and launched a somber but direct salvo at Hefner and *Playboy* and also at the lead singer of Jefferson Airplane, Grace Slick. "*Playboy* takes the fig leaf off the genitals and puts it over the face," he asserted. "The faces of these lovely girls have no expression. They are withdrawn, detached. And this goes along with the feeling in *Playboy* that the aim is to play it cool, not to commit yourself, don't get caught." As for America's youth counterculture: "The trouble with love in our day, as it comes out in, say, the hippies," he asserted, "is that they have spontaneity, but they don't have fidelity. They don't have commitment, responsibility." Hefner agreed that "the best kind of sex and the best kind of love includes involvement." But he also thought that there should be "a time of exploration and play" in one's twenties, and enriching that time was Playboy's mission. May painted the situation in darker shades of male fears, emptiness, and impotence, while Hefner countered by noting the findings and curative therapies of Masters and Johnson. Hearing the reference to Masters and Johnson, Grace Slick chimed in: "Wire me up and fuck me wired!"—with the appropriate bleeps from the ABC control booth.

Alongside the youngish (not yet forty-five), pipe-smoking Hefner and Slick, thirty, May, wired indeed but relatively mute, seemed distinctly from another era. His words seemed sermonic amidst the more jocular banter about love and sex. An observer of the show described him as "looking and sounding like a benign Barry Goldwater." Indeed, as the evening unfolded, he grayed into the background. May's assessment of *Playboy* gave way to an assault more in tune with the future. Susan Brownmiller, an emerging feminist journalist soon to be famous for a pathbreaking book on rape, *Against Our Will*, and her writer companion, Sally Kempton, entered the conversation circle and began a full-bore attack on Hefner. He was her "enemy," a man who had "built an empire based on oppressing women." All the men—Cavett, May, and certainly Hefner—seemed startled, and each in his own way smiled uneasily. Hefner responded by conceding the past oppression of women but countered that *Playboy* wanted to liberate them, all the while addressing Brownmiller and Kempton as "girls" and then "ladies," instead of as women. Countering Hefner's claim to fostering gender equality, Brownmiller challenged Hefner to attach "a cottontail on your rear end" but stop claiming to be a liberator of women. Slick seemed to be shocked in her own way and jumped in with her own sense of men, one in which the male became the object and woman the chooser:

> Some of them are great, some of them are crummy. Why do you have to form a theory? Some of them look at you as a sex object, fine. You fuck them. The ones who like to both go to bed with you and talk to you, you do both of those things. The ones who like to make music and talk to you and go to bed with you and write, whatever you do—draw . . . ? I don't see where the problem is, maybe because I don't see what you're talking about. Yet. I don't see the problem. Yet.

The audience applauded, and Cavett invited the Airplane to perform another song.

May saw both Slick and Hefner as going down the wrong paths, but all three (and Cavett) shared in the shock of Brownmiller's anger and directness. Though the target may have been Hefner, each man on the panel and probably in the studio audience shook under the force of her anger. Indeed, in its wake, Cavett smiled nervously, and May and Hefner shared an off-mike chortle. For her part, Grace Slick was jarred by Brownmiller into her sex-centered riff as much in defense of her own proclivities as in dismissal of feminist anger.

May's response to the increasingly radical challenge of the women's movement, its reach into every level of personal, social, economic, and political experience and expectation, was complicated. He could not help but be both excited and fearful of feminist hope and rage from his own life and philosophy. His often tortured relationship with Ruth and Matie exposed him to the plight of strong and talented women, ones whose gifts sat wasted because of society's domination by men. Despite their demands and slights, May never shirked the role of protecting and supporting both throughout their long and difficult lives, whether rescuing them at the time of E. T.'s leaving the family or bailing them out of difficult personal and economic situations. Nor did he neglect Yona, his less problematic younger sister. These familial roles had engendered in him a self-image as protector and emancipator of women, as long as he remained in charge. At the same time, he sought peace and security in marriage, rejecting more challenging women as mates in favor of Florence, who seemed more likely to bend to his will.

The influence of his mother and sister lived on in May's dreams and self-analysis, but by the 1960s and 1970s their lived realities bespoke more pathos than power. Matie lived near her youngest son, Pat, who had become a small-town doctor in Howell, Michigan. She worked full time until she lost her job in 1967 at age eighty-three. Still a bit directive, she had mellowed to the point of praising her son and delighted in hearing about the successes of his latest books. Rollo, Don, Pat, and Pat's children's families supported her through a gradual decline. She died in 1974, at the age of ninety. Ruth's last years were stormier. She moved to San Francisco in the late 1950s, involved herself in various fringe religious and health movements, but hit a dead end in September 1967—she called it an "Acute Nervous Breakdown"—while writing a book on "Yoga and Creativity." By the 1970s, Ruth had moved to Placerville, California, where she and some other friends ran a small meditation retreat purposefully located "on certain magnetic lines of Force." Rollo helped keep her afloat financially, but, plagued by delusions and physical neglect, she died in 1979 at the age of seventy-two.[8]

Just as important to his attitude toward women and gender in general were the educational and professional worlds he inhabited and the era in which he grew to adulthood and professional standing. From the 1920s through the war and a bit beyond, progressive notions of gender roles, sexuality, and marriage had begun to appear within the culture, often promoted within bounds by liberal church groups such as the Y. Although the YMCA, Oberlin, Union Theological Seminary, and the emerging profession of psychology were populated and mostly dominated by men, they were not totally closed to women. Both Oberlin and Union were coeducational. Several women psychoanalysts—Clara Thompson (whose work Betty Friedan relied upon), Frieda Fromm-Reichmann, and Alberta Szalita—directly supported his career. Even May's seemingly traditional marriage to Florence soon turned into something more open, though mostly dictated by his preferences. Most of these relationships had substance beyond sex. For example, May's relationship to Ellie Roberts proved to be one of the longest and most intimate of his life, even after Dave Roberts's suicide poisoned the sexual part of their relationship.

Furthermore, the atmosphere in all these realms engendered a broad, if mostly unspoken recognition of and respect for a variety of sexual preferences and styles. May's important emotional relationships with Buck Weaver and Charles Wager, both married but most likely closeted gays, spoke to the ease with which men in the academy might commune intimately with each other in a fluid if sometimes awkward space without explicit reference to one's sexual preference. May sometimes expressed his deep love for Weaver and Wager without ever raising either the fear of or desire for a physical relationship. Nothing in May's diaries indicated suspicion that they might be gay or that it even mattered. These mentorships and friendships continued a form of male friendship not uncommon in earlier eras, before the rigid medicalization and definition of same-sex relations as pathological and destructive of the social order.

Of course, such relationships were hardly the majority view of homosexuality, but May stepped up to resist more conservative norms. No wonder, then, that May's advice to Elver Barker in the 1940s was to seek his authentic sexual identity. No wonder, too, that May supported protestors during the Stonewall rebellion of June 1969, in which gays in New York vociferously protested an early morning police raid on a Greenwich Village gay bar and ignited an explosion of activism that openly battled the almost universal existence of sodomy laws against homosexual behavior and rights. Indeed, soon after the Stonewall incident May shocked a small group meeting held in Herman Reissig's Greenwich, Connecticut, church to discuss *Love and Will*. A member of the audience asked, "How can we stop homosexuality?" May replied: "I don't see any reason why it should be stopped. A homosexual is not the worst thing a man can be."[9]

May imagined himself, then, as a champion of gender inclusion, whether for gays or women. His adherence to existential psychotherapy's central goal of leading an individual, no matter their gender or sexual preference, to allow them to experience an authentic and full sense of self—joy, anger, creativity, self-recognition, and true visibility to others—also counted. However, not surprisingly, May's conception especially of women could not help but be informed by a lifetime of living in a world of powerful men, whose power in part found confirmation in doctrines of gender difference and hierarchy. In short, May's vision of gender equality, no matter how well intentioned, emanated from a male perspective that claimed an omniscience challenged directly in the 1970s by Susan Brownmiller and many others.

One woman deeply affected by feminist militancy was Ingrid, whose upbringing in postwar Germany predisposed her in some ways to a freer attitude toward female identity and sexuality than the American norm. Her energetic embrace of life also fit perfectly with feminist exuberance. Her marriage to Rollo was a whirlwind awakening for Ingrid. A single parent at the time she and May met, a graduate student and instructor in literature at UCLA, she was a person of great intellectual curiosity as well as emotional intensity caught up in a new sense of freedom. She enrolled in an interdisciplinary master's program at Teachers College that mixed the humanities, social work, and psychology, and participated in various therapy and women's groups. She also brought the feminist revolution home to Rollo in just about every way possible. The Mays settled into a New York apartment in the fall of 1971, and soon their home hummed with activity, as did the summer home in Holderness. Ingrid's feminist commitments, especially her turning over to Rollo basic housekeeping and cooking duties, didn't clash with her enjoyment of entertaining. Fearless, intelligent, and beautiful, for a few years she pulled May out of loneliness and regret and encouraged him to enter the social whirl of the New York intelligentsia. According to May, she "would go up to anybody, the King of England, and invite them for dinner." Her estimable cooking skills and provocative conversation enlivened dinners and cocktail parties whose guests ranged from the popular philosopher Max Lerner and May's Yale friends Bob and Betty Jean Lifton and Bill Coffin to Kurt Vonnegut and his wife, Jill Krementz, whose photographic portraits of May graced his book covers. He and Ingrid regularly socialized with Joe Campbell (even though she often lit into Campbell for his political views) and his wife, the choreographer Jean Erdman. A widening circle of friendships included the poet Stanley Kunitz and painter Jules Olitski, whose appreciation of May's work gave him added confidence in writing about creativity.

Ingrid's lack of inhibition and European sensibility about sex blended well with the historical moment but led to much heartache for May, not only because of her various infidelities but also because she, not he, was in charge. These combined with May's fears of aging and simple jealousy wreaked havoc in the household. After little more than a year, doubts he had about having married Ingrid and new suspicions of her sexual life began to lead

286 PSYCHE AND SOUL IN AMERICA

their roller-coaster relationship down a steep slope. He suspected she was having affairs with one of her professors, as well as with women friends in New Jersey and Los Angeles. She commenced a lengthy affair as well with Harold Taylor, who was captivated by Ingrid's beauty and magnetism. By the time May found out, he professed that he no longer cared.

A more nuanced vision of Ingrid comes from Lisl Malkin, a young Austrian Jew who had emigrated to England as part of the *Kindertransport* just before the beginning of World War II. Malkin met Ingrid, six years her junior, while they were both students at Columbia in 1972. Each "gravitated" toward the other. Malkin was struck by her Nordic accent and looks—"tall, broad-shouldered, and beautiful"—as well as her outgoing warmth. Despite a frisson when she discovered Ingrid was German and not, as she had imagined, Scandinavian, they managed to forge a warm friendship. Malkin challenged Ingrid by revealing that she was Jewish but also realized that Ingrid was all of thirteen years old at the end of the war. Ingrid's free spirit reinforced Malkin's own emerging sense of self, one first given shape by reading Betty Friedan's *The Feminine Mystique* almost a decade before.[10]

Ingrid often invited Lisl to lunch at the May apartment and the Malkins as a couple to dinners. If Malkin's husband couldn't come on one or another evening, Ingrid urged her to come alone. When Ingrid and Lisl traveled to Massachusetts to attend a workshop led by Virginia Satir, one of the pioneers of family therapy, Malkin saw more of the liberated side of Ingrid. Ingrid decided to swim nude in the indoor swimming pool at the workshop hotel as Malkin sat by the pool fully clothed, a forty-something "chaperone" to her only slightly younger friend. Ingrid also invited her into a women's consciousness-raising group whose other members, including novelist Helen Yglesias and women of various ages and sexual preferences, discussed cultural and social oppression as well as personal issues with mates and authorities. The key rule was simply: "You could only talk about yourself, your own thoughts, even better, your own feelings—not what your husband, partner, or boyfriend thought." Malkin praised its effects on her own consciousness, and, despite some rockiness along the way, she credited her new assertiveness (combined with an inborn conservative nature) as ultimately beneficial for the marriage.

The same could not be said of Ingrid's marriage to Rollo. For Rollo, his years with Ingrid were, among many other things, an education in a wildly assertive variety of second-wave feminism. All that was happening in America seemed to merge with his personal experience to create a rich canvas for his next book.

By late 1970, when May began outlining a new work that would both extend the analysis of *Love and Will* and break new ground in response to the whirlwind of rebellion, reaction, and cultural battle abroad in the land, he focused on what he saw as some of the potent roots of social and personal violence. He never imagined that he had a "solution" to Vietnam, racial inequality, or the problems highlighted by successive uprisings among gays, women, Mexican Americans, Native Americans, and other oppressed groups in American society. Rather, May sought insight into the ongoing crisis brewing in American society by focusing on a what he saw as a troubling simplification of two terms—power and innocence—in the rhetoric of political and cultural debate. A hint of the broader argument he was working on came during the question-and-answer period at a lecture on *Love and Will*. When asked how he would end the student rebellion then sweeping college campuses across the nation, he answered simply: "Give the protesters more power."[11]

Behind this terse response lay the basic point of *Power and Innocence: A Search for the Sources of Violence*, published in November 1972. May argued that a major cause of civil unrest and violence was the desperate quest for self-affirmation among individuals and groups of human beings trapped in situations that rendered them helpless and insignificant. His was essentially the same existential formulation that Betty Friedan found so convincing in the late 1950s. Yet in at least two ways *Power and Innocence* advanced significantly beyond May's prior formulations. First, though in the past he had theorized about apathy ultimately leading to violence, apathy as the symptom of impotence had been the focus. Now, in an age of violent unrest, violence became the phenomenon to explain. Second, in prior work he addressed human beings in universal terms, making few distinctions of gender or ethnicity in his description of the human costs of mass society. Now he differentiated the powerful from the powerless along lines of race and gender. Wide-ranging in its references, rich in case histories as well as literary and historical example, *Power and Innocence*, like *Love and Will*, sought to reimagine what May saw as overly simplistic keywords used freely in contemporary culture in favor of a more complicated understanding of both.

May explained the book's deep origins in a preface that linked personal reminiscence to his view of the world of the early 1970s. "As a young man," he began, "I held innocence in high esteem. I disliked power, both in theory and practice, and abhorred violence." May repurposed the story of his time at the Trudeau Sanatorium. At first, he had passively followed a routine dictated by doctors and nurses, an "innocence" born of helplessness. Only when he developed a sense of "power"—a spirit of "fight," an assertion of his "own will to live"—did he put himself on the road to recovery. The problems of various patients who "felt or were powerless" in relation to dominating institutions or persons or passive "while others (like the t.b. bacilli in my analogy) did significant violence to them" allowed him to formulate an approach to power rooted in his own and their experiences. The cure was power, he argued, that derived from "self-affirmation and self-assertion" rather than the military or corporation or state.

Then came a paragraph that was awkward in presentation and at first glance a non sequitur, yet somehow bracingly relevant:

> I had, then, to confront my own relationship to power. No longer could I conceal behind my own innocence my envy of those who had power. This, I found, only follows the general procedure in our culture: power is widely coveted and rarely admitted. Generally, those who have power repress their awareness of this fact. And it is the dispossessed in our society, represented by such movements as "women's power" and "black power," who, when they are able, force a direct confrontation with the issue.

Here, one could argue, was May's admission of his own blindness to the privilege automatically accorded him as a white male professional and a testimonial to all he had learned from the arguments and actions of the "dispossessed."[12]

It also obliquely revealed May's identification with those rebelling against the inequities of American society. Less visible were the class and cultural insecurities he had grappled with since his youth. His private narrative, constructed in diaries and interpretation of dreams as well as an incomplete autobiography he wrote in the 1980s, depicted a man disadvantaged by his upbringing and in combat with entrenched power and lesser minds, often holding back from fully asserting himself. May struggled with an inner voice tinctured with resentment and self-contempt, emotions not entirely erased by worldly success. It might well have given him a fictive sense of what damage powerlessness could wreak among the truly disempowered.

That is perhaps why May was particularly attracted to the work of the black psychologist Kenneth B. Clark, whose *Dark Ghetto* (1965) provided a socio-psychological analysis of urban unrest that confirmed May's sense that the angry reaction of young blacks to oppression had to do with a desperate assertion of their power and humanity. James Baldwin, rooted in his own embrace of existentialism, had made a similar point in *The Fire Next Time* (1963), a book May had read but did not cite. Baldwin excoriated the "innocent country" that had set blacks "down in a ghetto in which, in fact, it intended that [they] should perish." To Baldwin, perishing meant "never being allowed to go behind the white man's definitions, by never being allowed to spell your proper name."[13]

Power and Innocence highlighted the case of African Americans and saw theirs as the most extreme example of a far more widespread malady about which he had been writing for two decades—the fate of individuals who felt "insignificant to other people and, therefore, not worth much to ourselves." He interspersed definitional chapters and theory with illustrative examples from literature and history as well as from the cultural crisis of the 1960s and 1970s. May defined power in general as "the ability to cause or prevent change." Power to prevent change was all too obvious in society and could involve coercion of one person by another person or authority, whether through force, manipulation, exploitation, or simply unthinking tradition, the kinds of power that destroyed people, literally and spiritually. However, May concentrated on the power to effect change through creativity, self-affirmation, and self-assertion in the face of those who would deny one a sense of self-worth.

As for innocence, May celebrated the "authentic innocence" of the poet and the artist or the spiritual attitudes exemplified by Saint Francis or Jesus—the child's ability to see the world with "awe and wonder." "It is the preservation of childlike attitudes into maturity," he argued, "without sacrificing the realism of one's perception of evil."[14] May contrasted this ability to see the world in both darkness and light with a "conscious divesting" of power without the recognition of evil, a state of what he called "Pseudoinnocence"— "childishness instead of childlikeness." It is an innocence that leads us to "close our eyes to reality and persuade ourselves that we have escaped it." One recognized neither the power of evil in others nor the complicity with evil within ourselves. May highlighted Melville's Billy Budd, who clings to this innocence until the moment of his execution for a crime he did not commit, and the national innocence of an America that believes in providence or chosenness and chooses in fact to justify every evil deed done in its name, from the slaughter of Native Americans to the war in Vietnam.[15]

May decried another kind of pseudoinnocence, that displayed in Charles Reich's 1970 bestseller *The Greening of America*. Reich argued that American culture had passed through three stages of consciousness and that the last (Consciousness III), marked by a turn toward peace and love heralded by the Woodstock Festival, was rapidly spreading and soon would become the dominant force in society. May had little argument with Reich's analysis of the past but objected to the ways in which Reich wished away the evils of the present and future. According to Reich, Consciousness III was an embodied force that was impossible to stop. It would "not require violence to succeed, and it cannot be successfully resisted by violence." As May derisively quoted Reich: "The hard questions—if by that is meant political and economic organization—are insignificant, even irrelevant." To which May asked, "Are there really no enemies?" and proceeded to enumerate the signs of "creeping fascism" already confronting America.[16]

Juxtaposed to these chapters were case histories that supported the general theory, highlighted by "Black and Impotent: The Life of Mercedes." Mercedes was a thirty-two-year-old black woman whose eight-year marriage to a white professional was teetering on the brink of dissolution because of their lack of success in having a child. Two prior therapists labeled her as "untreatable," but May took up the challenge of bringing her to full consciousness of her own humanity. In fact, he chose as the chapter's epigraph a passage from Kenneth Clark's *Dark Ghetto*: "The real tragedy for the Negro is that he has not taken himself seriously because no one else has. The hope for the Negro is that now he is asserting that he really is a human being, and is demanding the rights due to a human being."[17]

It was an especially difficult task. Mercedes had been exploited sexually as a child and taught to be submissive within her family, but she nonetheless possessed a strong will and intelligence and sought a college education and then nursing school. She entered therapy, however, because of vague feelings of depression and apathy, especially regarding her marriage. Indeed, when May was able to elicit Mercedes's goals in therapy, she answered: "Let me have a child, let me be a good wife, let me enjoy sex, let me *feel* something." She eventually did get pregnant, but her early sessions reflected a sense of helplessness not only from the legacy of sexual abuse at home but also, as symbolized in a dream of a police officer shooting her dog and carrying him off, from "members of the Establishment highhandedly discharging the 'white man's burden,'" demonstrating "no respect whatever" for "her feelings or her rights."[18]

She also displayed ominous symptoms of a possible miscarriage, one that May related to her bottled-up emotions—she could allow herself neither to feel nor to express a liberating anger toward her parents or much else. He decided, "not wholly consciously, to express *my* rage in place of hers," and attacked her mother and stepfather for how they had treated her. "I was allying myself with that faint autonomous element which we must assume is in every human being," he explained, "although in Mercedes it was practically nonexistent to start with." It was hardly standard therapeutic practice at the time, but the episodes of bleeding stopped, and within a few months Mercedes began to express that anger herself, both in dreams and in therapy. In later dreams, helplessness turned to fearlessness before the threats of mother and father. The baby boy had a normal birth, and the couple celebrated by giving him a Promethean name, in keeping with the event's momentousness in their lives and, in May's mind, the birth of "a new race of men."[19]

Case histories often have a storybook quality, raising and resolving problems stripped of much of the messiness of life's details. Mercedes's history comports with this pattern, a complicated and long treatment shaped to fit a particular lesson. However, May's rendering of the case revealed striking aspects of his conception of therapy and of the place of violence in society. He made sure to explain his decision to get angry for Mercedes, already noting that it was only a partially conscious decision. "I was not assuming a role," he emphasized; "I genuinely *felt* angry toward her mother and stepfather. . . . I was also not merely 'training' Mercedes to establish 'habit patterns' by which she herself could become angry. No, we were playing for keeps—to keep a fetus alive in her womb." It was a particularly intense expression of what he had come to believe about empathy and the therapeutic relationship, that a genuine encounter was possible that could not be written off by simply calling it transference or countertransference.

The ideal, he argued, was to encourage clients to assert repressed anger and aggression in the clinical setting so that its roots could be analyzed and understood, and actions in the world could be taken with a full, controllable sense of one's feelings. May titled the last section of Mercedes' case "Violence as Life-Destroying and Life-Giving," pointing out that "it was obviously present, and in abundance" in dreams and waking life, and it expressed itself without control, in self-defense but also against herself and those she loved. "In her fights at school or on the street she had become wild," he noted, "not knowing what she was doing." In her dreams, she lashed out not only at her mother and stepfather but also at her son and her beloved grandmother and had "hysterical fights" with her husband. These targets, according to May, were "all persons to whom she ha[d] subordinated herself" and "should be fought for the sake of her own autonomy. In this list, of course, he included himself, for the client "must fight the therapist . . . precisely *for* the reason that he is trying to help." After all, by coming to therapy they surrendered some of their autonomy.[20]

May found in Mercedes's "wild striking in all directions" another meaning. "Here lies an important part of the explanation of the ghetto riots," he argued, "the burning, looting, killing, which may turn out, paradoxically, to be against those closest and dearest to the rioters." Furthermore:

> There is thus a self-affirmation precisely in self-destructive violence. Ultimately the affirmation is expressed in the person's demonstration of his right to die by his own hand if he chooses. . . . For the self-respecting human being, violence is always an ultimate possibility—and it will be resorted to less if admitted than if suppressed. For the free man it remains in imagination an ultimate exit when all other avenues are denied by unbearable tyranny or dictatorship over the spirit as well as the body.[21]

The chapters that followed Mercedes's case history expanded upon the roles of power, innocence, aggression, and violence, the roots of which were in May's older idea of the daimonic. Violence and the ecstasy inspired by the daimonic could move an artist to deconstruct or purify old forms and create them anew, or for the powerful and those in search of power to destroy lives and social order without a vision of renewal. He offered a kaleidoscopic selection of examples, whether in the art of Mondrian, the monstrous violence of a stickup turned to murder, or, on a larger scale, the comradeship and meaning generated by soldiers in combat by violence and threat of violence that caused untold destruction. Only facing the fact of the human capacity for aggression and violence allowed one to choose how to use and control it. Pseudoinnocence provided no escape. Curiously, he illustrated the point with Allison Krause, one of the students killed at Kent State, who a day before her death had placed a flower down a guardsman's rifle barrel. While May greatly admired her action, he also argued that by upsetting the standing order of things from of the National Guard's point of view, she naïvely put herself in the line of fire by repressing her fear of their guns.[22]

In two final chapters, "The Humanity of the Rebel" and "Toward New Community," May moved from a stress on paradox and duality to more guardedly hopeful themes. They also broadened May's frame of reference to pinpoint at least one key source for social change—the individual rebel who seeks to reform social consciousness. He begins with an example from François Truffaut's *L'Enfant Sauvage* (*The Wild Child* in its American release), in which Victor, a young boy who has been rescued from an animal-like existence in the forest, is being trained in the ways of civilization by a doctor. Victor has learned to accept punishment for mistakes, but what if the doctor punishes him even when he behaves correctly? Victor angrily resists, which his trainer marks as a success. He acts like a real human being. May characterizes the boy's action as "the capacity to sense injustice and take a stand against it" as if his life depended on it. What made him human was "the capacity to rebel."[23]

Having lauded the rebellious instinct as among the most human of characteristics, May felt it necessary to distinguish between the "rebel" and the "revolutionary." Whereas the revolutionary sought to overthrow the existing order or government and often imposed on society a tyrannical system of their own making, the rebel fought a different sort of battle. He or she simply "oppose[d] authority or restraint" and "b[roke] with established custom or tradition." May expanded on these dictionary definitions with a description of the rebel that comported with his own self-image. The rebel suffered from a "perpetual restlessness" that sought "internal change" in himself and others, thought little of outward success, and instead focused on a new "vision of life and society." He used his personal power not to collect more power for himself but rather to share and inspire self-affirming power in others. Referring again to Prometheus, who stole fire from the gods and gave it to humanity, May compared the Titan's tortures to that of the "agony of the creative individual," whether artist or social rebel, who risked all in creating and recreating civilization. He culled a list of exemplary rebels from ancient Greece to contemporary America: Socrates, Jesus, William Blake, Buddha, and Krishna, as well as Daniel and Phillip Berrigan, radical antiwar Catholic priests, and Daniel Ellsberg, who leaked the Pentagon Papers. Nor did he ignore the rebellions of Van Gogh, Cézanne, Picasso, Jackson Pollock, and Mark Rothko against the artistic mainstream. He even put in a good word for the rebelliousness of the "dropouts" or "hippies" of the era who felt estranged from society as they knew it.[24]

May contrasted his emphasis on the role of the rebel in altering beliefs and aesthetic meaning to those writers (he named Erich Fromm and Wilhelm Reich as examples) who stressed the necessity for change on the structural level and who assumed that society rather than prophets were all-important in molding consciousness. May took what one might call a Freudian approach to the problem, one that posited that all societies, no matter their stated ideals or humane structure, posed limits on behavior and thought that rankled the rebel, inspired the gadfly, and drove others to myriad forms of neurosis. He felt most comfortable, however, quoting Albert Camus: "We all carry within us our places of exile, our crimes and our ravages. But our task is not to unleash them on the world; it is to fight them in ourselves and in others. Rebellion, the secular will not to surrender . . . is still at the basis of the struggle."[25]

The final chapter of *Power and Innocence*, "Toward New Community," summarized the book in sermonic tones, calling for individualistic, pseudoinnocent America to wake up to its own daimonic essence, its capacity for evil as well as good. It could then rejoin humanity through new-found capacities for compassion and an ethic of "intention," where "each man is responsible for the *effects* of his own actions" as they affected the broader community of humankind. "The future lies," he argued, "with the man or woman who can live as an individual, conscious *within* the solidarity of the human race. He then uses the tension between individuality and solidarity as the source of his ethical creativity."[26]

In making this argument, May attacked the individualistic emphasis on character rather than compassion in American Protestantism, which produced "the curious situation of the man of impeccable character directing a factory that unconscionably exploited its thousands of employees." Nor did much of the human potential movement fare better, in both its singular focus on the individual and its implication that one could achieve unlimited "growth." Both much of modern Christianity and humanistic psychology's "ethics of growth" ignored the permanence of the daimonic struggle and lacked "an authentic empathy with others, an identification with the woes and joys of those bereft of power—the blacks, the convicts, the poor." This was something very different than "tithing" or helping the "less fortunate." It was communicating empathically with all in an inclusive community, consciously balancing the needs of the individual with those of society.[27]

The reception of *Power and Innocence* reflected its seamless mix of psychology, philosophy, current affairs, and religious inspiration and criticism. Reviewers found it difficult to take in the entire work, so they generally chose to highlight one theme or another as they tried to fit it into the spate of books attempting to diagnose and suggest cures for the cultural crisis of the 1970s. Anatole Broyard, writing in the *New York Times*, responded viscerally to May's "gift for gut truths," recalling the reactions of the congregation to a black preacher to whom he would listen on the radio.

> When [May] says "powerlessness corrupts," I want to shout, "That's right!" When he says, 'I cannot recall a time during the last four decades when there was so much talk about the individual's capacities and potentialities and so little actual confidence" in them, I want to cry, "I know it's the truth!" . . . He says a hundred things I've been unconsciously hoping to hear from someone who could assert them with authority. He takes the vague, generalized anxieties of American life and dissects them into clear, concrete particulars.

The *Times* thought *Power and Innocence* important enough to review in the Sunday Book Review as well, but this time the reaction was strikingly different. Paul Robinson, a Stanford intellectual historian who had written about Freud and his followers, covered most of the same ground as Broyard, appreciated some of May's argument, but thought *Power and Innocence* generally lacked intellectual rigor. Furthermore, he took offense at what he called May's "bloated philosophical language" and faulted his lack of expertise when discussing American foreign policy. Robinson found unoriginal the very insights that caused Broyard to cheer, and the "gut truths" to which May gave voice for the first reviewer Robinson dismissed as "popular psychology" that "ma[de] no pretense to theoretical or empirical rigor."[28]

Reviews in religious periodicals concentrated on the implication of May's views of Christianity and the Christian concept of innocence and, predictably, were equally split in their opinions. "The only possible purpose this book can achieve," wrote Ronald Sampson in the liberal Catholic journal *Commonweal*, "is to sow the widest possible moral confusion." In fact, he called the book "morally twisted." William Hamilton, the radical theologian who helped pioneer the "death of God" concept in modern Christianity and shared Union Theological Seminary as an alma mater, agreed that May posed a threat to the status quo and thought that was all for the good. "My point is this," wrote Hamilton in the *Christian Century*; "the attack on innocence, if we allow Melville's Billy Budd to set the terms of the attack, is really an attack on Christ and Christian character as shaped in the West. . . . At the bottom of this wise, humane and admirable book rest two quite terrifying questions: Is America possible? Is Christianity possible?"[29]

These were two very good questions.

24

Looking Backward, Moving Forward

When Rollo May looked out the windows of his penthouse office in the Master Building at Riverside Drive and 103rd Street, he could literally see the sites of his forty-year life in Manhattan—Union Theological Seminary, Columbia University, the various dorms and apartments in which he had lived to the north, the William Alanson White Institute to the south, and, just beyond the treetops and meadows of Central Park, his and Ingrid's apartment to the east. He might have even imagined his church in Verona, New Jersey, twenty-five miles across the Hudson River. May had married and raised a family, built a career, and forged lifelong friendships in a city he had come to love. Yet by the 1970s the city had come to look very different than in its postwar glory days. Whatever the serene view from his office, the Upper West Side had succumbed to rising violent crime and a burgeoning drug culture. New York City itself was creeping toward fiscal disaster.

These difficulties were the backdrop to the anxiety and confusion May felt in his own life. Though the White Institute had been his professional base since the late 1940s, he increasingly found himself estranged from his colleagues, the price of personal jealousies on their part and May's neglect of his teaching and supervision duties at the institute. Finally, his marriage to Ingrid was becoming well-nigh intolerable, in no small part because of their differences in age and generation and the strain of liberties each took with the other. Ingrid challenged and exasperated him, and, though ultimately a failure, life with her shook up his sense of women, revealing to him a layer of anger and aspiration about which he had once seemed blissfully unaware. This awakening certainly helped to inspire *Power and Innocence*, a debt reflected in its dedication to Ingrid. Yet as their marriage sank more deeply into a morass of conflict, jealousy, and exasperation, a general alienation from key aspects of his New York life set in. May sought to reclaim himself by revisiting the most profoundly important aspects of his inner life. He was, after all, in his early sixties and had already experienced the loss of close friends and colleagues that signaled one's own coming mortality. It was time to return to his roots, to shore up his view of human purpose and commitment.

At the center, of course, was the influence of Paul Tillich. Hannah Tillich began pressing May to write a biography of his mentor soon after her husband's death in 1965. He found the idea attractive but impossible to consider immediately, since he was in the final stages of writing *Love and Will*. Besides, as he added in a letter to her, "one can never 'decide' point blank to write a book—one has to grow into it—it's harder even than marriage, for in marriage you can get divorced, but once you commit your mind and spirit to a book, the daemon gives you no peace." He would want to plunge deeply into the soul of Paulus, May wrote, not just skim the surface of his life and popular ideas. Crucial to May was Tillich's "relation to evil." He was the one thinker "who faced evil and the demonic, and the void and abyss of nothingness, directly and head-on, and was not afraid." May continued for over two single-space pages to grapple with the implications of this characteristic, comparing Tillich favorably to Reinhold Niebuhr and Fromm. A "white-washing" would do Tillich's memory no service, nor would a strictly psychological biography do, for "the spirit was decisive for his greatness." He worried that, in fact, "in our super-technical, adjusted, psychological age . . . [Tillich] may be the last of Faustian characters until a new age is born."[1]

The challenge of envisioning Tillich as a modern Faust proved seductive enough to overcome May's initial caution, and he came to believe that only he could do justice to Tillich's full genius. After all, René, the Tillichs' son, called Rollo the "spiritual son of Paul in a way I have chosen not to be."[2] May saw writing such a book as a heroic gesture. "Can I live with courage? In a disintegrating time?" he wrote in his diary as he wondered whether he was equal to the task. Yet May signed the book with Harper and Row in 1967 and by early 1969 had scaled the project down from a comprehensive biography to something at once less grandiose and more compelling—a portrait drawn from personal observation and conversation during their close relationship of thirty years. It was, as he noted in the preface, "the only area in which I could hope to do some justice." May began to write in 1972, after *Power and Innocence* was in press. The book appeared as *Paulus: Reminiscences of a Friendship* in October 1973. At 113 pages, it was a loving and at times strikingly subtle rendering of a complex and contradictory life.[3]

May began by recounting their first meeting in 1934 and underlined Tillich's German background, his staunch opposition to Hitler, and his escape from the Nazis in 1934. In the short chapter that followed, "Ecstatic Reason," he accounted for his own early attraction to him as mentor and human being. Having already imbibed the tragic richness of classical Greek culture at

Oberlin and in Greece itself, May saw in Tillich the modern reincarnation of an intellectual line that began with Aeschylus and Sophocles: "Each seemed to me intensely vital; each lived with a seriousness that was not sober. . . . Each burned with the gemlike flame that comes from the knowledge that we are on this crust of earth for our little moment to build our machines or think and speak our thoughts or sing our poems." Tillich believed most of all "in the value as well as the pleasure, at times even ecstasy, of sheer thinking."[4]

Tillich's capacity for both logic and ecstasy combined to create an authenticity that colored his very presence in the world, May asserted, whether satisfying deep needs of contemplative aloneness or even stronger urges to engage with others. May described a typical public lecture, noting that "Tillich's face changed expression with everything he said—showing sometimes agony, sometimes wonder, sometimes joy, but in any case, mirroring his inner, personal commitment to what he was saying." In personal relationships, his directness, caring, and inability to "hide his embarrassment or blushing or discomfort" invited honesty from friends or new acquaintances. Yet at times he could be oblivious to others. May remembered that once, while he was staying with the Tillichs in New York, Paulus passed him by in a hallway "as though he had not seen me."[5]

May related these two sides of Paulus to a creative grappling with *kairos* and void—to a combination of innate genius, the rich if stormily contradictory culture of Germany, a distant, authoritarian father, and a mutually worshipful and sensual love between mother and son cut short by her painful death. In a sense, his life's journey, whether expressed in theology or in everyday life, became the embrace of darkness and light, joy and fear, provisional peace and terrifying anxiety. As May noted, Tillich himself described a "constant and tense contest between these paternal and maternal influences" and a life lived "in the midst of struggle and fate," of "two principles wrestling with each other." He emphasized that these inner battles bred in Tillich a heroic if volatile creativity, a mind and soul honestly grappling with questions of good and evil, joy and despair.[6]

Only one topic proved awkward, Tillich's attraction to and extramarital pursuit of women. The issue temporarily ruptured May's relationship with Hannah when she announced that she would be writing a book of her own, a spiritual and sexual autobiography that inevitably dealt extensively with her marriage. Hannah's reasons for writing what became *From Time to Time* were many, not least of which was to tell her own fascinating story. It was one dominated by a tantric mysticism she expressed inwardly and mostly in private during Paul's lifetime because of her need to keep up appearances as a prominent theologian's wife. She worried that May would downplay Paul's "horrible shortcomings" as a husband in favor of pleasing "all the little girls, who felt he was hers [and] all the intelligent men, who struggled with his thoughts." It was not simply a question of infidelity (Hannah herself had dabbled with other men) or her own jealousies, though clearly they were at play. Rather, she saw Tillich's wanderings and his sexual inadequacies as she experienced them as part of a broader theory of intellectual aspiration. "Spirituality or 'intellectual genius' means, holding the physiological biological thirst back," she explained. "This has consequences." That is, "he will be a lousy lover." The fact that Tillich like some other geniuses "ejaculate[d] into the cosmos" made "his life miserable his love untrue, his passion falsificated [*sic*] . . . he ha[d] no heart."[7]

Hannah asked May to peruse her manuscript in the summer of 1972. It was a pastiche of older prose and poetry she had written over decades of her life, as well as newer chapters about her life before Paul, with him, and after his death. May reluctantly gave it a read and promptly urged her not to publish it. Other friends offered the same advice, and various presses turned it down before she signed with Stein and Day in early 1973. May felt "sick about the whole thing" and decided to include a chapter in his own book to counter what he saw as the bitterness and inaccuracy of Hannah's account. He emphasized that Tillich's sensuality and love of women more often than not featured a spiritual intimacy that fit no easy moralism. Furthermore, he doubted that many of his encounters with other women ended up in bed. Indeed, he celebrated this aspect of Tillich's personality as "the clearest demonstration of Eros in action I have ever seen. His relationships were always a pull toward a higher state, an allure of new forms, new potentialities, new nuances of meaning, in promise if not in actuality. . . . Thus, the beloved woman is the way to God, playing a role not unlike Mary in Roman Catholicism." At the same time, he admitted that Hannah Tillich (or any woman married to such a man) might not see it that way.[8]

For May it was not only a question of whether Tillich's intimacies with other women were "sensual" or "sexual," or even what one might say about these needs in relation to his theological radicalism. His disgust with Hannah's depiction had to do with a more general sense of cultural corrosion and the cheapening of relationships. In a revealing interview for *Christian Century* published six months after the release of *Paulus* and *From Time to Time*, he decried the increasing tendency to disregard greatness in human endeavor, to emphasize the sameness of all individuals and bring down heroes and geniuses to a common level. He complained that Hannah's account said "almost nothing about [Tillich's] intellectual greatness." Instead, she gave the unsuspecting reader a portrait of "another dirty old man."[9]

He had good reason for concern. The two books were published virtually simultaneously and more often than not reviewed together. In the books' most widely circulated review, *Time* magazine titled its seven-hundred-word dual evaluation "Paul Tillich, Lover," and led with Hannah's blunt account of Paul's seductive behavior at parties. *From Time to Time*, the reviewer noted, "barely mentions the theologian's pioneering work in existential theology," instead noting that life with him "was something like *Cabaret* played out in a seminary drawing room—or bedroom." Predictably, in turning to *Paulus*, the review focused entirely on May's less sensational appraisal of Tillich's sexual mores and ignored entirely his account of their relationship and elucidation of Tillich's thought and its place in Christian and modern culture. Numerous other reviewers followed suit.[10]

Most interesting, however, were the reactions of some theologians, for the 1960s and 1970s witnessed multiple radical innovations in liberal Protestantism, many deriving from Tillich's insights. Such American theologians as Paul Van Buren, Thomas Altizer, William Hamilton, and Gabriel Vahanian, each in their own way, sought a revitalized and more meaningful Christianity through the engagement of religious experience outside the churches. One of the most celebrated of the group was Harvey Cox, a professor at Harvard Divinity School, whose bestselling *The Secular City* (1965) and *The Feast of Fools* (1969) turned the concept of secularization on its head by asserting that God's presence lay in engagement with and celebration of everyday life. Cox gave both books majestic treatment in the Sunday *New York Times*. Cox began with *From Time to Time*, noting that Hannah Tillich was "immeasurably more" than Paul Tillich's wife, rather in her own right "a poet, a witch, a lover and a mystic." Cox, himself a former Tillich student but not as close to him as May, concluded that "after reading this unadorned account of what it was like to try to live with him, I now know and respect him more than ever."[11]

Cox praised *Paulus* as "a personal portrait which is as honest as Hannah's but sounds less abrasive, more benign, affectionate but detached." While mildly critical of May's psychoanalytic musings, Cox paid May an extraordinary compliment: "He knows theology well enough to have written as good an expliqué as I've ever read of Tillich's famous 'God beyond God,' described in the last chapter of *The Courage to Be*. And May skillfully answers those who blithely labeled Tillich an 'atheist.'" Nor did Cox scoff (as some others did) at May's comparison of Plato's account of Socrates's death to Tillich's last moments, finding that by the end of *Paulus* the comparison did "not seem strained," that he was "of all the men of his time whom I have known, the wisest, and justest, and the best." He was "grateful" to both authors for reminding him of "Tillich's amazing 'presence,' and his capacity to invest a simple word with whole universes of meaning."[12]

Other prominent liberal Christians, those with more traditional senses of church and sexuality, reacted cautiously but still admiringly to May's vision of Paul Tillich. Martin Marty contrasted *From Time to Time*—an "angry, wounded, acontextual, and psychoanalystically blurry version [that], frankly, I wish had not been published"—with May's account, which displayed "philosophic depth."[13] As for Tillich's infidelities, Marty noted that he was merely joining a long list of imperfect men who had been great moral leaders: King David, Martin Luther ("I was pretty well shaped by beery old Martin Luther"), Martin Luther King, Jr., and John F. Kennedy, among others. He feared that May's and Hannah Tillich's books would be most usable by Tillich's enemies. "Tillich's kind of theology," he imagined them shouting, "was produced by *that* kind of man!"[14]

Soon after publishing *Paulus*, May turned to the topic of creativity and questions that had "haunted" him for as long as he could remember. Creativity had become for him a watchword defining at first a healthy Christian psyche and later an aspect of the authentic existential life. In the 1950s, May had engaged the topic of creativity in earnest—lecturing, contributing articles to professional journals, and participating in panels and conference proceedings. However, it wasn't until about 1973 that he decided to link the articles and lectures together in a short book, *The Courage to Create*, which was published in 1975.[15]

May eschewed the time-worn psychoanalytic explanations of creativity as "compensatory" or "regression in the service of the ego." While not denying the applicability of these concepts to some artists, he saw them as reductionist and epiphenomenal, not at the core of creativity itself. Rather, he embraced the romantic vision of the creator as prophet, applying familiar existential themes and rhetorical strategies (including a highly Tillichian title) to the creative process and the role of the artist in society. The first chapter began with one of his favorite nostrums, that we were "living at a time when one age is dying and the new age is not born," and artists might provide the much-needed voice to move humanity toward solid ground. The courage to create involved, he argued, "the discovering of new forms, new symbols, new patterns on which a new society can be built." To May, artists of all types who were most profoundly in touch with the culture challenged the status quo and vexed those in power. He traced this phenomenon back as far as Genesis (Adam, Eve, and the Tree of Knowledge) to Greek mythology (Zeus's anger provoked by Prometheus's theft of fire from the gods and his granting it to human beings). Adam and Eve's expulsion from Eden and the binding of Prometheus on Mount Caucasus served as metaphors for the liberationist consciousness and its shadow, creativity's "yearning for immortality" in the face of death's punishing inevitability.[16]

May's framing of the creative drama moved far beyond academic psychology or psychoanalysis to poetic truths and the struggle for an authentic spiritual life. He quoted his friend Stanley Kunitz's feeling that "the poet writes his poems out of his rage," his passionate protest against the tragedies and unfairness of life and ultimately against the final injustice of death. More vivid still, May recalled the angry voice of Dylan Thomas facing his father's death—"Do not go gentle into that good night." May noted how frequently condemned rebels against accepted faiths and philosophies—Socrates, Jesus, Joan of Arc—were recognized after death as saints and cornerstones of civilization: "They rebelled, as Paul Tillich has so beautifully stated, against God in the name of the God beyond God." Theirs was "the mark of creative courage in the religious sphere." The chapter's final flourish, a clarion call to the creativity in all human beings, consisted of a democratically paraphrased version of the penultimate sentence of Joyce's *Portrait of the Artist as a Young Man*. May recognized the "profound joy" of "creative courage, however minor or fortuitous our creations may be," and rallied his readers to "go for the millionth time to forge in the smithy of our souls the uncreated conscience of the race."[17]

He did propose one caveat, that truly authentic creativity involved "encounter" with and "absorption" in the subject of their endeavors. Both were necessary to ensure truly original work. These phenomena, sometimes expressed as the Dionysian and Apollonian characteristics of creativity, were at their most powerful when combined in a state of ecstasy—that is, the supranatural state in which the line between subject and object is dissolved. Having invoked the passions of encounter, absorption, and even ecstasy, however, May reminded the reader of the role of life's inevitable and tragic limits, as well as the necessity of "form" in the pursuit of the creative moment. He argued that psychotherapy might help unleash the creative spirit but also aid in understanding the boundaries of symbolic and experiential authority and the facing of that ultimate limit—death. Nor did he confine the exploration of such understandings to psychotherapy. Indeed, in a chapter titled "The Delphic Oracle as Therapist" that originally appeared as part of a memorial volume for Kurt Goldstein, he noted the essential role of "symbol and myth" implicit not only in the ancient Greek wisdom seeking at Delphi but also in the proper use of such psychological tools as the Rorschach and Thematic Apperception Tests. All such symbolic structures, including religion, might inspire and put guiding frameworks around the ecstasy of creativity.

The reviews of *The Courage to Create* were in some ways surprisingly similar. They mostly agreed that May's sense of the artist as prophet overly defined creativity, yet they applauded the book's heartening and even inspiring tone. The ebullient Anatole Broyard described May as "a romantic psychoanalyst, a 'good father' in contrast to those forbidding Freudians" who threw cold water on life's pleasures. Broyard didn't so much object to May's basic take on creativity, as he found it, compared to *Power and Innocence*, "kindly, avuncular, almost plummy," and "sentimental." Similarly, Howard Gruber, a psychologist at Rutgers University, found May's vision of the emotional side of creativity "compelling" but criticized him for emphasizing its socially transformative possibilities. Still, Gruber concluded by noting the book left him "wondering," and that "there is no pleasure greater than wonder, and no wonder greater than human creativity, and this, after all, is just what May is trying to tell us." Irving Markowitz, himself an interpreter of creativity, remarked perceptively that *The Courage to Create* was more about courage than creativity and worried that May's approach was "more theologic than scientific."[18]

These critiques were reasonable but in one sense missed the point. May's implicit agenda for *The Courage to Create* echoed especially the concerns of *Love and Will* and its sweeping use of the Western tradition. Having posited that his readers were living at a time on the precipice between eras, it was as if he were saying: true, you feel lost in the world, but look at the wisdom that philosophers, writers, artists, and others have provided since the ancient Greeks to guide your vision of self and society. For those motivated by the spirit of creativity in any medium or field, he formulated an analysis to inspire, honor, and quicken such efforts. *The Courage to Create* technically had no "theologic" message, as Markowitz labeled it, but ultimately a spiritualized one built upon a symbolic and mythic groundwork revelatory to the creative imagination. May saw its historic roots in religion but its merger of the Apollonian and Dionysian expressed in many nonreligious ways of thinking. In short, "Aeschylus and Sophocles and the other dramatists could write great tragedies because of the religious dimensions of the myths, which gave a structural undergirding to their belief in the dignity of the race and the meaning of its destiny." In many ways, then, *The Courage to Create* returned May not only to the question of creativity but also to the importance of symbol and myth. He saw it as the key to community renewal in an age when even when humanistic psychology, the movement with which he most identified, seemed fixed on the individual, leaving the question of social cohesion and meaning as an afterthought at best.[19]

Meanwhile, as he felt increasingly alienated in his New York life and began to draw new meaning from longstanding concerns, May's attention increasingly turned to the West. Though he had lived for four decades as a Manhattanite, he may well have found the Bay Area as enticing for its reminders of his meanderings in nature along the St. John River as for its headlong thrust into an alternative future. Though May remained wedded to a tragic view of the world at odds with its bright, futuristic sheen, in the early 1970s he increasingly saw California as the plausible incubator of a new society imagined and hoped for in *Love and Will*.

He was not alone among his humanistic psychology colleagues in gravitating toward California. Indeed, other key voices in humanistic psychology had already moved there. In 1963, the young Irvin Yalom, who May had inspired to embrace existential attitudes in psychiatry, began a long career at Stanford Medical School. A year later, Carl Rogers left the University of Wisconsin to create his own research institute in San Diego. In 1968, Abraham Maslow abandoned Brandeis University for Menlo Park near Stanford. Up and down the coast, a network of psychologists, psychiatrists, and psychologically inclined humanists began to create a new epicenter of existential and humanistic psychology.

May's westward gaze began to take on more concrete shape when the historian Page Smith, an important educational innovator at the University of California's newest campus at Santa Cruz, invited him to be the visiting Regents Professor for the spring quarter of 1973. All augured well. The campus itself bordered on the paradisiacal. Its Great Meadow overlooked the small city and the Pacific Ocean beyond; its residences and classrooms were scattered among a forest of douglas firs and redwood groves. The northern portion of campus was preserved as a pristine forest, and the thick woods of state parks ringed most of the rest. The coastal highways took one to San Francisco in less than two hours and Big Sur in about an hour and a half. The Mays lived in comfort, house-sitting for Norman O. Brown, one of the leading lights of the university's experimental History of Consciousness program.

May's experience hardly measured up to Santa Cruz's Edenic surroundings. He found his teaching situation disappointing, and perhaps the class did as well. He recalled later that three or four weeks into the course one student even remarked to another, "I hate Rollo May." May had expected a small class with the opportunity for discussion of ideas. Instead, he was assigned a large lecture class in which students sat passively, treating him like a celebrity. "People were sitting on the window sill," he recalled, and "standing outside listening. It was as though I were a TV performer." Nor was May at his physical best. He often felt weak, his tachycardia returned, and his marriage tested both his mind and body. Ingrid frequently took the five-hour drive to stay with friends in Los Angeles. When in Santa Cruz, she pushed May to attend parties and seek adventures that, whether because of health or personality, exhausted him. She even gave him unsolicited (and unwelcome) advice about his teaching. As he noted later, "At that time we were very estranged." By the end of their stay, he told Ingrid that he wanted a divorce.[20]

Nonetheless, thoughts about a move to California soon became a plan. That decision was made in part because, despite his reservations about humanistic psychology, he came to see it as the one psychological movement capable of forging a synthesis of science and humanism. Instead of breaking ties with the AHP, May played the familiar role of gadfly. A signal moment came even before his time at Santa Cruz, when he wrote a blistering jeremiad concerning the 1971 annual meeting to Fred Massarik, president of AHP; John Levy, its executive officer, and Melanie Allen, program coordinator for the 1972 annual meeting. May's message fell on sympathetic ears and was published as the front-page story of the January 1972 issue of the *AHP Newsletter*. He made it clear that the future of psychology was theirs if they took themselves seriously, that it was "the New Underground." However, he worried that AHP might "kill" its potential leadership role because of the anti-intellectual and "huckster at a circus" tone of much activity at the last national meeting. Titles like "Childbirth for the Joy of It," "Risking My Craziness: Letting Go," and "Should a Therapist Go to Bed with His Patient?" became grist for the mill of articles in the *New York Times* and across the country. Furthermore, many sessions amounted to "fancy ways of advertising a particular encounter group site" or some other form of self-promotion. "There is a danger," he argued, "of AHP becoming identified with the various groups of nude, marathon, touchy, feely and other kinds of therapy."[21]

These were only symptoms, however, of a larger problem, which were ironically the "anti-humanistic" tendencies of the movement. He reminded the membership of the organization's early years and founders, and especially the high level of thinking at the Old Saybrook conference. Soon, however, AHP was "taken over" by those who invested everything in feeling rather than thinking, "representatives from Esalen, Perls, and all the other encounter groups." They need not be cast out but simply be given their "proportionate place." He quoted another member with a similar critique: "Indeed, wisdom, joy, understanding, compassion, love have all gotten progressively cheapened—and no really new psychology has emerged, but only scattered fragments for such a possibility that are then oversold before they are first carefully cultivated and nourished." May asked whether a "relatively large group" in the membership harbored similar feelings, specifically whether they were in favor of developing "the kind of psychology that speaks out of the being of man, rather than out of all kinds of techniques."[22]

The response was heartening. The June 1973 issue of the newsletter featured a front-page banner, "AHP's Year of Reappraisal," and an enthusiastic response to May's article by Kalen Hammann. Hammann recalled that as a psychology graduate student he had been excited by the new emphasis on encounter but also "somewhat dismayed by the 'let's all FEEL together—to hell with the mind' attitude a good many students" displayed. He hoped AHP would stress the need to integrate the "newly-recovered feelings-in-the-now" with the intellect-minded "old selves."[23] Such responses and discussions with other leaders at AHP led May to forcefully reinject himself into the organization. He agreed to chair a new "Theory Committee" tasked with "the development and clarification of the theoretical bases of humanistic psychology." It would work with the "Research Committee," of which May was also a member, to apply those "theoretical bases" in scientific experiments appropriate to the humanistic enterprise.[24]

Meanwhile, women in the movement also felt the urge toward more critical investigation, albeit from a feminist perspective. As Tom Greening, editor of the *JHP*, noted by way of introduction to one article in the spring 1973 issue, Carolyn Morell's "*Love and Will*: A Feminist Critique," "Women of the world are shaking off their chains, and sometimes they clash down on the heads of our great white fathers." Originally written as a term paper for a course at the Institute of Human-Potential Psychology in Palo Alto, Morell's piece acknowledged her great debt to May but probed May's conscious and unconscious visions of gender and found them sorely wanting. Her discomfort with *Love and Will* focused on "May's theories and assumptions about men and women, and the implication of these assumptions for the relationship between the sexes." She attacked his overreliance on the outdated concept of "anatomy as destiny" as applied to ideas of sexual difference and its implications for social role and power. May thereby more or less ignored the inequality that stemmed from such an approach, Morell argued, and "impose[d] mutually exclusive, complimentary [*sic*], and polar qualities on the categories 'masculine' and 'feminine.' "[25]

Most important, Morell observed that although May paid lip service to gender equality, equality meant little given the political and personal implications of traditional notions of sexual difference that remained unquestioned. "May has identified failings in loving and willing and proposes a way for the future," she concluded. "That future would rely on relationships based on care-relationships leading to a new consciousness. But the development of caring relationships involves a greater change than May foresees; it requires changes in the very stereotypes and analyses that May himself employs."[26]

In a response published alongside Morell's article, May embraced the spirit of her critique, admitted to having struggled with *Love and Will*'s "unintentional sex prejudices," and declared that Morell's piece "ha[d] been of considerable help in this awareness." He did wonder whether she had mistakenly asserted as fact positions on some issues not yet settled (e.g., the question of essential differences between the sexes) but noted that feminism was a revolutionary movement whose boldest and most useful advocacies might be modified later without doing harm to the cause. He also pointed to *Power and Innocence*, which Morell had apparently not read before finishing her article, as his "endeavor to illuminate the deeper issues underlying the exploitation of women, blacks, and other groups."[27]

Recognition of the problem did not guarantee amelioration. Most psychological theory did not lend itself to nuanced considerations of "nature" or "nurture" in the making of strongly gendered roles and hierarchies. In the mid-1970s, of course, few humanistic psychologists could see the profound effect nascent feminist theory would have on future answers to just this question. In fact, after Fred Massarik and May secured NEH funding to hold an AHP Theory Conference in April 1975, they proceeded to invite mostly male major luminaries whose presentations were almost entirely free of gender consciousness. In fact, the major impact of the feminist movement, one that had already affected many women who were members of AHP, was for the planners to make sure that at least some women were among those present (there were five of twenty-four). Little survived of their contribution, however, when the conference's transcript was rendered.

May opened with a keynote that reiterated his fear that an anti-intellectual emphasis on the emotions and the body would guarantee the movement's "demise." The purpose of the conference, he added, was to create a theory, what in the 1950s he hoped would be a "science of man," that might "be adequate to both the principles of science on the one hand, and to the problems of living human beings on the other." As Jonas Salk, the pioneering scientific researcher and one of the participants in the conference, had written to May as he perused the meeting's agenda: "We will be engaged in a hybridization of each other."[28]

The major participants—May, Salk, Carl Rogers, Gregory Bateson, Floyd Matson, Tony Athos, and others—declared positions and engaged in dialogues that illuminated common approaches or teased out differences on such key concepts as choice, decision, the nature of mind, and other abstractions and theories of human nature. For example, Salk presented a complicated theory of mind based in sociobiology, while Rogers talked about the role of therapy in moving an individual progressively toward better choices and more realistic senses of the world. May and Rogers crossed swords over the nature of evil, and Gregory Bateson sought an entirely new sense of mind, choice, and decision-making grounded in the convergence of consciousnesses from within and outside the individual. Some, like Stanley Grof and his wife, Joan Halifax Grof, spoke of transcendent consciousnesses beyond the everyday, while others objected to the near-theological bent of some speakers. Of all these attempts to grapple with human nature, May found Bateson's approach most congenial to his own thought, and he even contributed a sophisticated appreciation of Bateson's work to the *Journal of Humanistic Psychology*.[29]

In late August 1975, the theoretical seriousness of the Tucson conference gave way to the more sensually freewheeling annual gathering of the AHP in Estes Park, Colorado, 7,500 feet above sea level in the Rocky Mountains. The location must have inspired nostalgia for May, who had attended YMCA meetings there in the 1930s, and was 120 miles north of Palmer Lake, where in 1936 he had declared his goal of revolutionizing religion for the world.

Mike Moore, a reporter and editor of the Colorado's *Mountain Gazette*, wrote a vivid account of that meeting and May's role as both gadfly within the movement and champion of socially embracing myths. The conclave offered lectures and hands-on workshops, all in search of individual "growth" and inner peace—even as, at sea level, defeat in Vietnam, urban riots, and a pervasive culture war gnawed at the sinews of American society. Moore arrived "hell-bent on writing a frolicsome satire," fantasized about being "touched, felt or laid," but also feared that he might be seduced by the "gaggle of massage persons, transcendentalists, Rogerians (they don't even talk), Frommists, Zen Buddhists, nudists, sexual acrobats, Sufi dancers, acid heads, Jungians and existentialists, lesbians, pederasts and feminists, brainwave synchronizers, Rolfers, seers and magicians."[30]

Moore passed up more sensually promising events, however, to hear a discourse by May, a Jeremiah who insisted that the individualistic goals of psychotherapy, meditation, and other rituals of inwardness were symptoms of the very condition they sought to cure—a thirst for personal meaning and connection in a world where a once shared system of values and accepted wisdom had been destroyed. May mixed references to familiar American virtues and vices with plainspoken renderings of Kierkegaard, Spengler, and Jung and made them "come alive and dance." He called for a vision of humanity that bound human beings in common cause even as it embraced individual freedom, and he etched his words in dark warning but always with a sliver of hope. He sought to remind those present of the myths that had made life comprehensible but had been lost in the whirlwind of change. May talked about the *Oresteia* and made a case for Fitzgerald's *Great Gatsby* as the controlling myth of American life. To know the past, its wisdom and especially its myths, he argued, was the first step toward creating the future. This "dinosaur of the human potential movement" left Moore "in the lofty regions" for the rest of the week. "That I spent the entire week of the convention untouched, unfelt and unloved would appear to be my own fault," Moore mused. "But I would rather blame it on Rollo May." A prophet of the tragic at odds with so many of the cultural innocents at Estes Park had blessed the journalist with a bracing spiritual equivalent of naked encounter.[31]

Meanwhile, May, having made the decision to move to the Bay Area, was already based in California. He informed patients and advisees of his plans and tried to place them with appropriate colleagues. He and Ingrid moved together but with the understanding that once in the West she would search for a home of her own. May's hunt for a new place in the Bay Area echoed many aspects of his personality. He sought a perch like his Manhattan office, sweeping in its views and distant from the ordinary sounds of life yet close to the excitement of San Francisco. He could not have chosen better. An agent showed him a house in Tiburon on Sugarloaf Drive, high atop the peninsula and with panoramic views of San Francisco Bay that on clear days stretched north toward Napa, east toward Berkeley, south toward San Jose, and southwest to San Francisco. Most days the only sounds were the whispers of gentle breezes and fog horns from the boats below. In such a setting, he hoped to regroup and begin a new and final chapter of his life. It was as if he had found a spot that combined some of New York's vigor with the solitude and the beauty of Holderness.

25

"I Don't Have Time to Die"

The breathtaking beauty surrounding his Tiburon home and the air of freedom and experimentation in Northern California of the late 1970s and early 1980s proved seductive for someone used to life in Manhattan. Even May's view from the penthouse of the Master Building could not compare to the sweeping vistas and quiet he experienced every day in Tiburon. He did miss the cultural intensity of New York and the proximity to decades-old friends, though he retained his home in Holderness and had some access to the city during the summer. At the same time, the Bay Area's expanding and increasingly influential psychotherapeutic community embraced him as something of a prophet, and he gladly continued in the role of Jeremiah to his chosen people—the humanistic psychologists.

Contrast that role to the petty conflicts and mutual suspicions at the White Institute—jealousies, competitiveness, and splits over internal issues. In March 1977 he returned to the institute to give a lecture, and, as he wrote to Jack Schimel, the editor of WAWI's *Report* (its newsletter), "I felt the competitive feelings so strongly as to make it practically impossible for me to continue speaking." "It was good to meet you at that fiasco at the White Institute," he wrote to his protégé Bob Akeret soon after the disastrous lecture. "I haven't had such an unhappy experience in years." May also complained that the newsletter had ignored his recent "serious" publications (two articles in professional journals and a speech at the recent APA meetings) in favor of mentioning among his recent accomplishments a fluff piece in *Harper's Bazaar* based on a phone interview. The newsletter also referred to a reprint of *The Art of Counseling* as a "new book," though May noted it had been written in 1938 and was "as naïve as such a young person's first book [was] bound to be." Nor did May understand why the *Report*, in summarizing reviews of *Love and Will*, chose to highlight a "terrible review" it had received in a predictably hostile psychiatric journal.[1]

More affirmative signs soon appeared. Clement Reeves, a recent PhD of the University of Ottawa, published his dissertation in 1977 as *The Psychology of Rollo May*. It offered a detailed, serious study of May's developing vision of human consciousness from the 1930s through *The Courage to Create*. May was so impressed with Reeves's manuscript that he accepted an invitation to write a detailed and mostly appreciative afterword, "Reflections and Commentary," as part of the book.[2] Furthermore, May's integration into the Bay Area's world of therapy proceeded smoothly, not only because of his fame but also because of the connections he had already made over the years. He helped bolster the reputation of the fledgling Humanistic Psychology Institute (HPI). In addition to HPI (which would become Saybrook Institute), he taught at the California School of Professional Psychology (CSPP) and Langley Porter Institute of the University of California, San Francisco.

Though May preferred teaching the occasional seminar to a regular faculty appointment, it was not for lack of interest in mentorship. Stephen A. Diamond, a practicing psychotherapist in Los Angeles, had an initial contact with May in 1980, one that led to an important mentorship and mutuality of interest. Diamond had read some of May's writings, wanted to investigate the question of anger in psychotherapy, and took the brave step of phoning him. May greeted the call with interest and soon invited him to become part of a clinical seminar at his home. Diamond eventually published his doctoral dissertation as *Anger, Madness, and the Daimonic*—with a foreword by May. Another future psychotherapist, Ed Mendelowitz, encountered May at the Berkeley campus of CSPP while pursuing an MA and PhD. He was his teaching assistant for one course and saw him as a model as to how a therapist might enrich the lives of his clients by integrating philosophy, music, and art into a broad approach to treatment. Philip Keddy met May in a seminar at the San Francisco campus of CSPP as well, having read some of his work as an undergraduate in Toronto. Keddy joined a small study group at May's home and also initiated a five-year analysis with him, learning much that he utilized in his own practice.[3]

If in many ways he made a smooth transition from New York to California in his professional life, private realms remained a problem. He was lonely. He had been married for forty of his almost seventy years of life and had only recently separated from Ingrid. He had affairs even before their separation, as well as after, but none that made him lay down the shield protecting him from hurt and disappointment After the day's work and evenings seeing friends, he watched the beautiful view of the bay from his home alone.

Then, in February 1976, less than a year after he had moved to Tiburon, May felt strongly drawn to another woman. S. was attractive, intelligent, an MSW with a bent toward feminism, and about forty years younger than

314 PSYCHE AND SOUL IN AMERICA

Rollo. Like Ingrid, she was in awe of May's fame and deeply flattered by his attraction to her. They met at one of his campus talks and exchanged letters, and S. moved to the Bay Area while Rollo was in Holderness. In late September they had lunch, and the following weekend they went bike riding on Angel Island. May invited her to his home for dinner, and they just talked, mostly about how each was recovering from a bad relationship and nervous about being rejected. He was in any case too busy with teaching, writing, and seeing clients.

It wasn't until December that they saw each other again and edged closer. In late January 1977 they overcame hesitancies and for the first time slept together. That evening began a whirlwind of intimacy, travel, and declarations of love. A trip by S. to Holderness in July 1977 seemed to cement things. Then came gnawing doubts on her part about other women in Rollo's life and her need to tell him that she had slept with another man while he was still in New Hampshire. May was crushed. "I feel I've been had," he confessed to his journal, "all this good time this summer, 'love you the most I've ever loved' . . . 'Best sex ever,' then suddenly this change." "I live alone, am alone, feel alone . . . many friends around, but I still live in my own solitary house, my own emptiness, my own long day." And two weeks later: "God damn S!!!!! . . . I sleep on sleeping pills and I live on valium."[4]

May began seeing a Jungian analyst, and S. saw a therapist. He also consulted his friends in both New York and California. Ellie Roberts flew out to meet S. and advised May not to marry her. Norma Lyman recommended the same. May himself began to move beyond hurt and rage to some understanding of S.'s situation as a single mother whose children needed a father for a longer time than May might live.[5] Still, he raged against her in his journal but found it difficult to get angry at her in person. Instead, he wrote off her actions as those of "a mixed-up, impulsive, undeveloped woman," a formulation he now saw that he had used to tolerate his mother and sister. "I always make woman I love seen as crazy . . mother, Ruth," he realized. "God damn it, if I could only get mad," he exclaimed to his journal. "I'm mad as hell!"[6]

In New York, he found few outlets for his anger or for even talking through his anxieties except in therapy. In California, for the first time in his life, he had a room full of male friends with whom he could share moments of anger, joy, self-doubt, and frustration. He had helped to found a "men's group," fashioned along the lines of the popular "consciousness raising" women's groups of the late 1960s and beyond. Members included Sam Keen, well-known for books that mixed theological, philosophical, and psychological reflections on life; Bill Jersey, an award-winning documentary filmmaker; Ron Garrigues, a distinguished Bay Area sculptor; Robert Gumpertz, a Marin artist; Clifford Janoff, a local environmentalist; Dick Galland, a wilderness guide; and other souls concerned about the inner lives of men at a moment of cultural revolution. The group functioned as a respite from their careers, a psychic space in which they could talk about themselves—their fears, failings, joys, and vulnerabilities. It created something like the male companionship for which he yearned in New York, where almost all of his confidantes were women. The men's group's opinions of S. comprised variations on a theme. In May's paraphrasing, Sam Keen saw her as a "self-seeking woman" who was after a father figure. Other men chimed in, Dick Farson exclaiming, "Don't let this second-class woman (block, harm, kill?) our Rollo." Visiting from New York, Harold Taylor took a slightly different tack, noting that May was entering "the most creative period of [his] life" and that it would be "a shame" if S. "ruin[ed]" even part of it." They all expressed rage for May, much as May had become angry for Mercedes in *Power and Innocence*.[7]

Less obviously "intimate" but supportive in its own way was his membership in a self-created Philosophers Club, another small group of men bent on exploring the complexity of human nature and social systems. Closest to May's background was Huston Smith, a famous scholar of religion who had retired to the Bay Area and taught as a visitor at Berkeley. Don Michael, professor emeritus of planning and public policy at the University of Michigan, lent a very different if complementary point of view. Contributing still another dimension was Peter Koestenbaum, who had trained in philosophy, physics, and music and taught philosophy for thirty-four years at San Jose State University before becoming a consultant and theorist on the intersection of business and philosophy. Jay Ogilvy, somewhat younger than the others, was another philosopher and business visionary.[8]

May also counted Irvin Yalom among his new friends. Yalom, a professor of psychiatry at Stanford, had already published the key professional text on group psychotherapy and, in 1974, *Every Day Gets a Little Closer*, an innovative and accessible book for a general audience. Such professional success, however, did not allay deep anxiety about death. It turned him again toward existentialism (even as May's *Existence* had directed him toward a career in psychotherapy decades before) and to lead therapy groups with terminally ill patients. However, the groups only increased his anxiety. When Yalom heard of May's move to Tiburon, he sought him out and began a helpful course of therapy made successful by May's unflinching willingness to deal with the question of dying. Unusually for therapist and client, after a few years the two became close friends.[9]

Yalom, the men's group, and others, however, were perhaps less aware of a profound drama unfolding in May's life—the death of Ruth May. Rollo and S. visited her in March 1979, in Placerville, about a two-and-a-half-hour drive from Tiburon. He wrote an account of the visit a few days later and described a macabre scene, "the smell of death all about. . . . Her face ashen, her legs very thin, her stomach distended." Ruth lay on a sofa, her face turned away from the door, her sallow skin wrapped around a wasted body but with eyes as alive as ever and only an occasional profanity cursing her excruciating pain. S. sat beside her until it was too much to face. Rollo then took the chair and put his hand on Ruth's arm. "It was a heavy, very heavy hour," he wrote soon after in his journal. "I felt her lack of vitality . . only a little bit of it . . dragged down to a little circle . . where her life still was." Ruth died the next day.[10]

With Ruth's death Rollo experienced an exorcism of guilt and mourning. Even as he wrote out the narrative of his trip to Placerville, he experienced an attack of neuropathy, "the most severe yet." He continued to write despite physical distress, which he viewed as transferred from Ruth's body to his: "My pain . . the throat comes at me when I least expect it." The pain became too intense for him to write: "I writhe on the floor . . There is something about it that I feel is justified . . I lie on the floor, how much more can I take." S. called and the neuritis again floored him. Guilt and anger were building into an emotional whirlwind that broke open his life. Ruth's death and the debacle of his relationship to S. marked the beginning of a subtle but significant refocusing. At first, one could hardly notice it in his public presence. He continued to lecture publicly and continued to agitate within humanistic psychology for social and political advocacy and formulating major writing projects in a form similar to his past successes.[11]

Ruth's death as well as the "destructive and devilish effect" of his affair with S. drove May into therapy, and, not surprisingly, therapy helped to dictate the shape of his next major work, *Freedom and Destiny* (1981). Like a number of his earlier books, it mixed hidden autobiography with a discourse on the qualities, possibilities, and limits of authentic freedom. He distinguished the various forms of freedom and deemed some more authentic than others. Destiny referred to the limits placed upon individuals by the circumstances of life and the historical moment into which they were born. In simple terms, human beings played out their lives with the cards they were dealt. May argued that human freedom could only find meaning within these limits as well as by facing the omnipresence of evil and ultimately the tragic certainty of death. Equally important, authentic freedom came from the vital confrontation of these realities in thought and action. May concluded a multidimensional exploration of this theme with a contrast of life goals:

> Happiness is the absence of discord; joy is the welcoming of discord as the basis of higher harmonies. . . . The good life, obviously, includes both joy and happiness at different times. What I am emphasizing is the joy that follows rightly confronted despair. Joy is the experience of possibility, the consciousness of one's freedom as one confronts one's destiny. In this sense despair, when it is directly faced, can lead to joy. After despair, the one thing left is possibility.[12]

As before, May illustrated his point by relating a case history in which he was both therapist and Philip, an imagined patient. He retold fictionalized versions of his childhood, his time in Greece, and the psycho-religious experiences that transformed his life. Like May, Philip was trying to make sense of a painful romantic breakup and his history of unsatisfactory relationships with women. May the therapist led him back to the tortured relationships with his now dead mother and sister and encouraged him to imagine and act out both sides of confrontations with each of them. First, Philip raged against his hysterical and mean-spirited mother. He then took her part, assuring the son that she was always proud of him and loved him and that he was her "favorite child." "I used to lie awake nights regretting my blow-ups and making resolutions to stop them," Philip had his mother admit, but she couldn't change. Philip moved to the empty chair of his imagined mother and admitted that he always knew he was the favored one but found it more convenient to play "the misunderstood genius, nobody to help me, and so on."[13] As he played this role, he began to see that Nicole, the fictive equivalent of S., became for him the best and worst of his mother—sometimes loving and passionate, other times distant and cruel.

May also asked Philip to contemplate a photograph of himself as a "little boy" and one with his sister Maude that he had brought to an early session, to imagine a chat with "Little Philip" from this most "walled off" part of his memory. "Little Philip" described "how frightening it was" to be in the same house with "two hysterical zombies," his mother and his "schizophrenic" older sister. "It was constant inconstancy, unpredictability, insecurity," Little Philip added, "and especially loneliness." As Philip listened to himself speak the part, the once anxious boy became more relaxed. The two Philips almost seemed to merge. "He [Little Philip] now sat in the Lotus position," May wrote, "appearing like a little Buddha, wise beyond his years."

Philip's therapeutic journey was not yet complete. As he began to confront and express rage at his mother and sister, Philip personified his anger as "a green-blue lad . . . of indeterminate age but somewhere in his late teens." May informed him that green and blue symbolized anger and fear in Chinese culture but also observed that Philip's "green-blue lad" was paradoxically "completely open and honest and full of energy" and "the stimulator of Philip's sense of humor." Later, Philip revealed the full significance of his new imaginary companion in his diary: "There is no such thing as defeat for me, for the issue is within me. . . . The green-blue lad and I know only the word *can*; we know only possibilities. There is no such word as *impossible* for the green-blue fellow and me when we stand together."[14]

Philip's last session revealed even more autobiographical inspiration. May the therapist listened as his "patient" used the words "loneliness" and "honesty" to describe the ironic desolation of losing his mother and sister despite their legacy in his life. He told May of his "nervous breakdown" while teaching at "Robert College" in Istanbul, where he hid his sense of isolation by "thr[owing] himself into his work with ever greater zeal" and exhausting himself to the point of collapse. Emerging from that crisis, Philip found a new and freer life. He took up drawing and experienced the world without a plan or direction. He joined a group of traveling artists and fell in love and "lost [his] virginity with the greatest of joy." Philip's story vividly summarized May's working through his checkered relationships with women in the shadow of Matie and Ruth, one that was slowly lifting as he widened his sense of connection with the world.[15]

No matter its possible value to May's own psychological well-being, *Freedom and Destiny*'s awkward merging of Philip's story and its more philosophical and psychological pages made it a difficult work to review. The reception was decidedly more muted than those of *Love and Will* or *The Courage to Create*, and most reviewers more or less ignored the narrative of Philip's journey from psychological dependence to freedom in favor of more familiar terrain. To some it seemed too familiar. *New York Times* critic Anatole Broyard, an enthusiastic fan of May's earlier work, deemed it "an attempt at consolidation rather than a Kierkegaardian leap." He thought the book too often sounded like the "wail" of a Salvation Army "trombone" rather than the "thunderclap" more often evident in *Power and Innocence*. "There's no question that his heart is in the right place," Broyard noted. "It is his rhetoric that's getting tired. He needs a new vocabulary, for even truth needs a change of clothes now and then." Some greeted the book with more enthusiasm. Norman Cousins noted its distillation of a lifetime of ideas and called it "a feast for the mind." Ed Mendelowitz recommended it as the best introduction to May's work. Canadian philosopher Michael Fox, in a piece entitled "Whatever Happened to Existentialism?," went one step further, recommending *Freedom and Destiny* as a reminder of "how a human life is to be actualized, played out, constructed by oneself as a middle path between the conflicting pulls of freedom and necessity." The book "unfold[ed] as a profound commentary upon the human condition," Fox continued, "and upon the prospects for achieving in the modern world the delicate balance between these polarities which constitute a healthy psyche." Yet May deemed it "a failure." Some years later, he remarked to Mendelowitz that "*Freedom and Destiny* [was] a plagiarism of myself."[16]

Meanwhile, May remained deeply concerned that the AHP was avoiding engagement with the vital social and political issues of the day: civil rights, gender equality, ending poverty, minimizing the threat of nuclear war, and saving the environment. He worried that too many members were afraid to confront the problem of power in the world—the fact that changes in individual consciousness must be related to a robust understanding of society's structures of power in order to move toward a more just and humane future. "We cover over our powerlessness," he declared in a talk at 1979 meetings of the AHP, with the notion that individuals were responsible for all that happened to them, that "self-actualization" or "human potential" could be cures for all that ailed the planet. It enabled many in the movement to act "like spoiled children, sit[ting] tight in our innocence."[17]

May's longstanding critique of humanistic psychology found reinforcement in the broader appraisals of American society that began to appear in the mid-1970s. Popular writers castigated the socially destructive results of therapy in general in such widely read articles as Peter Marin's "The New Narcissism" (1975) and Tom Wolfe's "The Me Decade: Reports on America's New Great Awakening" (1976). The more comprehensive indictment offered by Christopher Lasch's *The Culture of Narcissism* became a bestseller. Lasch's dismal vision of a psychocultural wasteland of narcissists become part of the background reading for Jimmy Carter's speechwriters when they penned his famous "crisis of confidence" (often wrongly labeled "malaise") speech. It focused on energy policy but along the way lambasted selfishness, acquisitiveness, and other narcissistic qualities that according to Lasch more and more characterized American life and sacrificed the common interests of the nation.[18] May agreed with these characterizations of therapeutic culture but was bothered that Lasch had not credited him with pointing out the "narcissistic" aspects of modern American society in *Man's Search for Himself* almost thirty years before.[19]

May's discomfort with the AHP's general lack of a tragic vision merged with his general feelings about California. In the notes for a 1981 address to an AHP gathering, he applauded the organization's success at posing an alternative to behaviorism and orthodox Freudian psychoanalysis. However, he declared the next crucial agenda: "Can we be genuinely realistic about the future? Is this what our community [was] for? Or are we to be escapist?" He worried that escapism was indeed still a strong theme in the movement, that "California [was] full of illusions." He mocked the illusory romance of quick fixes through Eastern religion: "Heretofore it has not been possible to gain *satoris* (in Buddhism, an awakening to true self-knowledge) easily but follow such and such a Guru you can now get *satoris* over the week-end."[20]

May's criticisms were aimed at an American culture of the late 1970s caught in a vortex of anxiety and exhaustion provoked by successive public traumas: the Watergate break-in and Richard Nixon's resignation from the presidency; the Arab oil embargo of 1973; and between 1973 and 1975 the defeat of US forces in Vietnam and the ultimate unification of the country under Communist rule. Such crucial domestic problems as civil rights, the environment, and nuclear danger had hardly disappeared, but remedies were held in check by a certain public exhaustion. A fitting finale to the late 1970s occurred in 1979 with the nuclear plant disaster at Three Mile Island, Pennsylvania, in March and, in December, the taking of American hostages by the revolutionary government of Iran. May argued that humanistic psychology, at least in its more solipsistic forms, could not help supply the energy and direction needed to cure the ills of American society. Nor was he the only member of AHP to feel the pull toward social engagement.

One sign of this change appeared in the theme of the August 1978 general meeting of the AHP, "Between Dreams," and those inside the organization detected a significant shift toward public action. The October 1978 *AHP Newsletter* even featured a long article about the conference by Marilyn Ferguson, author of the bestselling *Aquarian Conspiracy*, entitled "AHP Goes

Public, Launches Era of Social Involvement." May was skeptical. He wondered openly how the lofty goal of instigating a "paradigm shift" could be accomplished and how many members would pay more than lip service to the effort. "We may be 'between snoozes,'" he warned. "There is that danger." Even Liz Campbell, member of the advisory committee to the executive board, admitted that "some did not identify with the theme and found the conference too serious; some wanted more parties and felt a lack of community."[21] Yet the October 1979 *AHP Newsletter* trumpeted on its cover "Executive Board Votes Nuclear Free Resolution" and featured essays by George Leonard, Theodore Roszak, and others that pointed to the need for integration of humanistic values into politics and social policy.[22]

Underlying the debate over politics was another, less visible fissure, one that pitted those who believed in inevitable progress toward a better spiritual and social world against those who possessed a more contingent and even tragic view of the future. The tension had been present from the founding days of humanistic psychology but became more explicit beginning in the late 1970s. One flare-up had its roots in the summer 1981 issue of *Perspectives*, a publication of the Humanistic Psychology Institute, which devoted itself entirely to a celebration of "Rollo May: Man and Philosopher." Among the many essays and interviews that attested to the substantive influence of his work, just one took serious issue with May's vision of the world, and only in one very long paragraph. Carl Rogers, one of the other great living founders of the movement, punctuated his deeply appreciative portrait of May with a caveat about evil. As opposed to May's positing of a daimonic (Rogers misnamed the concept "demonic") core of human nature that guaranteed a struggle between creative and destructive behavior in human beings, Rogers argued that culture—child rearing, inequality, a warped educational system, and "cultivated prejudices against individuals who are different"—"warp[ed] the human organism in directions which are antisocial." Rogers predicted a future in which a new and saner generation would correct these flaws and signal a progressive betterment of society.[23]

May responded to that short but essential caveat with an eleven-page piece, "The Problem of Evil: An Open Letter to Carl Rogers," published a year later in the *Journal of Humanistic Psychology*. He pointed out that Rogers had misunderstood the use of the word *daimonic* as a synonym for evil, whereas May meant the term to describe that primary "urge in every being to affirm itself, assert itself, perpetuate and increase itself." It acted on the "organized bundle of potentialities" that were the "source *both* of our constructive and destructive impulses." He reminded Rogers that society was not some entity created apart from humanity but rather a reflection of the creative and destructive elements of human personality writ large—human beings created society, and society in turn created humans. The driving force was the daimonic, an urge constantly at war with itself and likely to remain at the center of individual and social life.[24]

May fought a related battle against a growing interest in what came to be called "transpersonal psychology." Transpersonalism's roots in professional American psychology ranged as far back as the nineteenth century's Society for Psychical Research and William James's theories of "multiple universes" and the "reality of the unseen." James posited a scientific method based on "radical empiricism," one that included experiences of transcendence and other states beyond the norm as authentic dimensions of human consciousness. For most of the twentieth century, professional psychologists and psychiatrists ignored such notions in favor of a narrower reading of empiricism based on observable facts, carefully conceived experiments, and data-based theories and conclusions. Even psychoanalysts, while emphasizing the power of the unconscious as a powerful alternative reality, saw it as a strictly human phenomenon untouched by transcendent worlds.

A striking renewal of interest in the transcendent among psychologists began in the late 1950s and blossomed in the 1970s. Maslow's idea of self-actualization and peak experiences, drug-induced altered states of consciousness common to the era, and various adaptations of Eastern and indigenous religions—all contributed openings to a more positive view of alternative consciousnesses. Even Abraham Maslow, once a declared atheist and champion of traditional empiricism, became sympathetic to radical empiricism and joined with Willis Harman, Ken Wilber, Stanislav and Joan Halifax Grof, and Anthony Sutich, among others, in exploring transcendent states. By the late 1960s, they put such research in a more organized and comprehensive form, founding the *Journal of Transpersonal Psychology* in 1969 and the Association for Transpersonal Psychology a few years later.[25]

May declined Anthony Sutich's invitation to join in their efforts even though he was no stranger to altered states of consciousness, whether from LSD or transcendent moments of his youthful religious experiences. May saw similarities between transpersonalism and what James had called, with mild contempt, the "religion of healthy-mindedness." At heart May's problem with transpersonalist thinking involved what he saw as its unfortunate mixing of religion with psychology. His opposition may have been surprising to some, even those who were not fully aware of his prior career in the ministry and his relation to Paul Tillich. Readers of *Freedom and Destiny*, for example, might have noted his use of quotes from Thomas Aquinas, Augustine, the mystics Jacob Boehme and Meister Eckhart, Kierkegaard, and Tillich. He merged their wisdom with secular voices from Nietzsche and Freud to Gregory Bateson, as well as practitioners of Zen Buddhism and Taoism—not as definers of truth but rather as serious thinkers who understood elements of life's deepest challenges. Pondering the relationship between religion and psychology had been crucial to May's intellectual odyssey, and no better illustration of that evolving vision can be seen in May's changed definition of the term *destiny*. While still a minister, he had used "Freedom and Destiny" as a chapter title in *The Springs of Creative Living*. In this youthful work, he defined destiny as God's will. By 1981, May's use of the term had become an existential vision of human beings thrown willy-nilly into the world and left to find meaning within the finite circumstances of their lives.

He remained firmly committed to the separation of religion and psychology but rarely addressed the issue as such until an occasion came the early 1980s. Willis Harman, head of the Institute of Noetic Sciences and a major figure in transpersonal psychology, objected to an AHP statement crafted at its 1981 general meeting that attempted to define the "values" of the organization. Early in 1982, Harman wrote to Jacqueline Larcombe Doyle, president of the AHP executive board, that the term "values" suffered from "mushiness . . . because we all claim to hold more or less the same ones." "Beliefs" better defined the movement's distinctiveness, Harman argued, ones that focused on psychology's role in transforming individual lives and societies and an underlying faith that "all human beings are basically creative, that intentionality and values are basic determinants of human action, that the search for meaning reveals a need as basic as the need for food and oxygen." Like Rogers, Harman thought social change would come not from heated conflict but as the result of individual and cultural transformation, since each person was "ultimately free" to cast out "unwholesome beliefs" that were the true cause of "evil" in the world. Change based on love and compassion would follow.[26]

Doyle passed the letter on to May, who responded soon after with a respectful but unequivocal rejection of key elements of Harman's position. They highlighted for him the problem he had identified in *Freedom and Destiny*: a dangerous naïveté among many in humanistic psychology who ignored the cruel realities of power and evil in the world. Freedom for every human being was compromised by the threat of nuclear war, yet, May argued, Harman's views "le[d] to a quietism with respect to our efforts to halt nuclear stockpiling." Harman's views could be seen as a form of "Pietism."[27] May's assessment was in fact a bit skewed. Harman certainly counted on a transformation of consciousness to effect change, but, unlike many in the transpersonalist camp, he had rather strong and specific views of the world economy as the node of a coming crisis. He worried about unbridled industrialization and sought in consciousness studies a route for directing human energy and resources in more rational and humane ways. He hoped that humanistic studies and transcendence could work toward reforming the world of business. There can be no doubt that he had values *and* beliefs as well as a vision that looked toward social change, yet Harman exuded a cosmic optimism that May the existentialist eschewed.[28]

The case of Ken Wilber, guru extraordinaire, presented a different sort of problem. In his books and public appearances, Wilber created complicated road maps and connections that he claimed synthesized all realms of knowledge into an "Integral Theory," one that would guide individuals toward the goal of "the simple feeling of being." The authoritative (some would say authoritarian) tone of his prose as much as his grand design offended May, who saw Wilber's work as theology rather than psychology and a dubious theology at that. An encounter with Wilber at May's home in Tiburon added personal affront to intellectual disagreement. Apparently, a gathering of friends had gotten into a brisk but respectful dialogue about humanistic and transpersonal psychology, one in which May asserted the view that neither individual nor social progress was automatic but rather that human beings were in a constant state of internal struggle. Wilber objected and removed himself from the discussion. "He wouldn't listen," May remembered later, "implying that his ideas had reached some state of perfection and he shouldn't be questioned."[29]

This incident helped push May toward what to many of his friends was a shocking open letter in the *APA Monitor* opposing a petition asking the APA to grant division status to transpersonal psychology. The *Monitor* caught the tone of his argument in its heading for the declaration: "Transpersonal: Humanism leader says proposed division would confuse psychology and religion." May criticized Maslow's advocacy of a "fourth psychology" that was, in Maslow's own words, "transpersonal, transhuman, centered in the cosmos." As for Sutich's enthusiastic, utopian laundry list of humanity's transpersonal future, May had a concise reply: "But what about human suffering, sadness, guilt, anxiety, envy, jealousy, and the whole line of negative characteristics? . . . The problem with the term 'transpersonal' is its implication that we can 'leap across' the negative aspects of human behavior." He found it "inadequate as a philosophical doctrine, because the evil facts which it positively refuses to account for are a genuine portion of reality; and they may after all be the best key to life's significance, and possibly the only openers of our eyes to the deepest levels of truth."[30]

Joining him in battle was a young therapist, Kirk Schneider, whom he had met in December 1980 at an HPI function. Schneider was working at several clinics in the East. He and May kept in touch, and Schneider entered the debate over transpersonal psychology with pointed attacks on Wilber. The two crossed swords in the *Journal of Humanistic Psychology* between 1987 and 1989 in articles mixing theoretical and definitional questions about therapy and philosophy and, not incidentally, seasoned with a fair helping of ad hominem needling.[31]

Tom Greening, the editor of the *JHP*, sensed the need for an open debate. He solicited a number of articles for a special issue on the question of humanistic psychology's identity, especially in relation to the transpersonal challenge. It included a variety of perspectives, among which was a position paper by Ken Wilber that expressed his disappointment in May's *APA Monitor* piece. May's response in the same issue attacked Wilber's insistence that his work fit into the category of "psychology" at all. He saw the claims in his work as "beliefs" rather than "facts," which as such should properly be labeled religion. May had made this argument before but this time with pointed vigor.[32] In making his case for the separation of religion and psychology, May sought to prove his own qualifications for such a task by recounting prior experiences that certainly qualified as transpersonal. He also revealed his interest in parapsychology and in the realms that William James called the "fringe of consciousness." May noted his fascination with "the sacraments of primitive sects of Brazil" and also revealed his "two experiences with faith healers" while he had tuberculosis. "All of these I choose to call religion," he argued. "My objection to transpersonal psychology is that it blurs the distinction between the two."[33]

Despite the vigor of May's attack, the transpersonal feud did cause him moments of self-doubt. He realized that he and they had a common cause, if not a similar method. He wanted to save religion from psychological reduction—"I want to fight vs. secularization of everything." The transpersonal psychologists wanted to save the spiritual by merging it with

psychology. He didn't want to hurt them by his disapproval, especially because they probably thought they were "doing [his] program." "I was not
upset objectively," he wrote, "but sadness that I had hurt them—they sought
religion under a different heading."[34]

In October 1981, May received a long and extraordinarily frank letter
from Herman Reissig, with whom he had interned in his first year at Union
Theological Seminary. They had been confidants at key moments ever since
but had not been in touch much since, in part because of May's whirlwind life
but also because, after the death of Reissig's wife, his old friend had courted
and married Florence. However, each missed the other, and as Reissig entered
his eighties and May his seventies, they corresponded about reaching "old
age." The question inspired Reissig to reflect at length in a depressing piece,
"My Life at Eighty-Two," that he seemed to share only with May. It ended
with a searing critique of his own "egotism." Though a minister, he doubted
he ever truly loved God or another human being and blamed it in part on "an
undisciplined sexual life."[35]

May's answer does not survive, but Reissig's letter may have quickened
May's own need to reckon with his life. Despite the endemic self-doubt and
guilt expressed in his diaries, he certainly had a more positive view of his professional and personal contributions. Still, he worried about his legacy to future generations in a world that seemed more and more to fulfill some of his
direst predictions. Perhaps that is why he chose to reassert his role in bringing
existential psychotherapy to America by reprising his important existential writings in *The Discovery of Being* (1983). He included the introductory
chapters of *Existence* and presented slightly revised conference papers and
articles from decades before as well as a few new chapters with reworked if
mostly familiar themes. May explored not only the existential movement but
the paradox of its "affinity for our American character and thought" as personified in William James. He grappled with the hostility raised against it by
others in psychology who hewed more to psychoanalysis and the dominant
academic focus on behaviorism and experimental psychology. One reviewer
aptly noted that even skeptical professionals would "find *The Discovery of
Being* clear, accurate, and interesting. There is no better short introduction to
the existential approach to psychology."[36]

As for his inner life, May continued ruminating, accusing, questioning
himself as he had for fifty years of diary-keeping. He allowed his public persona few such revelations in his role of prophet and caring philosopher,
though the careful reader or listener might intuit it in his writings and public

appearances. Only in his fictive "case studies" in which he was both therapist and fictionalized client did he ponder his life in public. These case studies often became the centerpiece around which more general themes emerged. "Philip's" family and romantic life as recounted in *Freedom and Destiny* was perhaps the most intimate rendering of all. In the late 1970s, he contemplated writing an autobiography, to which he gave the working title of "Wounded Healer." However, he gave up after producing a few chapters, frustrated by the difficulties of relating the intimate details of his family life and the messier moments of his adult life, especially in relation to women. However, May did reveal a bit more of himself in the interviews Linda Conti conducted for HPI's special *Perspectives* issue, "Rollo May: Man and Philosopher." He also permitted the editors to feature full color examples of his paintings interspersed with pithy quotes from an interview that focused on art, beauty, creativity, and form. Until then, May's forays into art had remained more or less a private passion.[37]

As luck would have it, his life as an artist became a key subject of his next book. R. Patton (Pat) Howell from Dallas, Texas, a wealthy former journalist, financial consultant, and free spirit, found himself inspired by May and his art while earning a doctorate in psychophysiology from Saybrook Institute (formerly HPI). He encouraged May to write a book about beauty and art, *My Quest for Beauty* (1985). It wove together a selection of May's drawings and paintings, general ideas about the relation of beauty to the authentic life, and the previously disguised renderings of his time in Europe in the early 1930s.[38]

Whether within *Freedom and Destiny* or the public revelation of his art attendant to *My Quest for Beauty*, May was experiencing a slow opening up of his emotional life in the early 1980s. The search for a woman to love, especially one who expressed attraction not only to his fame but also to his vulnerability, led May to engage in multiple affairs. Yet the fear that one or another woman might engulf him cut short what at times seemed like promising (though sometimes situationally impossible) relationships. Most were not casual but rather encounters in which there seemed to be a mature mutuality. If the sexual encounter was short-lived, the connection often continued in friendship.[39]

These intimacies often began in classes May taught or in the socializing that often accompanied guest lectures. One such event in November 1978 took him to the Mann Ranch at the crest of the coastal mountain range near Ukiah. In the 1970s, the ranch hosted retreats and seminars featuring luminaries of therapeutic culture, Jungian psychology, and political dissent, as well as feminist and gay activism. Attendees listened to lectures, participated in small group workshops, ate meals together with the invited speakers, and in free periods enjoyed walks around the ranch's scenic grounds. Among the thirty-five attendees was Georgia Lee Johnson, a Jungian therapist who after a recent divorce had moved from the wealthy community of Woodside, south of San Francisco, to a basement apartment shared with other therapists in the city. Attractive, warm, with an ebullient laugh and strong will, she, like May, had grown up in the Midwest. Johnson trained in occupational therapy at Washington University's School of Medicine in her native St. Louis. She then studied psychology at the Menninger Institute in Kansas, where she later worked, and became deeply interested in Jungian therapy. Life and marriage eventually took her to Northern California. Building a practice in a profession dominated by men, raising a family, and suffering the disruptions of a failed marriage toughened her resolve to survive yet did not close down her faith in the possibility of intimacy.[40]

At such a liminal moment, she received an advertisement in the fall of 1978 for May's Mann Ranch workshop. She had heard of May but had never read any of his work and thought this would be an opportunity to expand her therapeutic horizons. The last thing she imagined was what in fact transpired. Georgia sat in the back row for May's first lecture and noticed that he seemed preoccupied, nervously telling jokes and reciting limericks to ease the tension and eventually moving the audience with his sense of the tragic and his unwillingness to settle for easy answers to the problems of life. Georgia was struck by his vibrant, handsome presence. She encountered him as she was returning to the ranch house, just as he had begun to take his own solitary tour of the grounds. "Come walk with me," he suggested, and on that walk something ignited between them. They talked about their divorces, problems with tachycardia, and culinary preferences, including a shared love of Greek food that inspired him to talk about his revelatory years in Greece. The walk over, they returned to the lecture hall for group discussions. Rollo realized that he hadn't gotten Georgia's phone number, so as he finished the question-and-answer period, he called out to her with that request. She was embarrassed by his jocular, almost innocent forwardness amidst an adoring audience but acceded to the request.

Of course, May was still in a protective mode and delayed calling her. Finally, Georgia invited him to her apartment for a Greek dinner. He was delighted, but on the day in question he called to say that his tachycardia was acting up and that he was afraid to drive. Georgia asked whether he had taken his tachycardia medicine, and when he said no, she ordered him to do just that and brought the Greek dinner to his house. Rollo told her that she was the kindest person he had ever met. He signed one of his books to her that evening, "To Georgia, who restores my faith in humanity." The following week he took her to an intimate French restaurant. She was a significantly different sort of woman compared to others he had known, but fears of womanly enslavement were at first as vivid as in the past. She invited commitment with kindness and warmth but also a keen sense of intellectual engagement and protective self-respect.

Gun-shy as he was from two failed marriages and the affair with S., May resisted being "in love." Georgia was equally protective as she recovered from her own divorce and began to build her practice. They saw each other intermittently for a few years as he continued a busy schedule of lectures, conferences, and intellectual debates within the community of humanistic psychology. Sometimes he attempted to make sense of his own life by theorizing (as did many at the time) on the nature and future of marriage. In one newspaper interview, he asserted that "everybody you meet has been divorced" and predicted that the future might lie in "serial marriage" in which a person marries for "children and sex" and after twenty years marries again for "companionship." As the journalist noted, "He extrapolates from his own experience."[41]

However, by 1983, Rollo and Georgia were moving toward a committed relationship. Even then, Georgia, who had set up a home and office across the bay in Emeryville, usually only spent weekends in Tiburon. And May's moods could turn on a dime. Occasionally she would arrive to find him grumpy, depressed, or openly hostile, but mostly he would greet her dressed in an ascot and smoking jacket, fireplace ablaze, and an uncorked bottle of wine on the coffee table. Georgia understood his moods and protected her autonomy. She intuited that Rollo was tired of always being the great man and at the same time afraid of giving up the mantle of authority and control. He was in need of simple human love and care. She calmed him, and he delighted her. They shared interests in art and literature and, most of all, were transported by similar music—the slow movements of Mahler's symphonies, the rich voice of Kiri Te Kanawa, the mature elegance of Mozart's late piano concerti, and the sheer joy of Haydn's Saint Cecelia Mass.

May allowed and indeed thrived on her companionship and abiding love, not to mention her transforming what had once been his spare, semi-"bachelor pad" in Tiburon into a comfortable and welcoming home. Its decor freely mixed their tastes and was enlivened by his paintings and those of others. Rollo and Georgia spent summers together in Holderness, traveled to Greece to revisit May's haunts of the early 1930s, and regularly entertained their circles of friends in Tiburon and New Hampshire. They threw dinner parties on special occasions and to bring their families and worlds of friends together.

Sometime in the early 1980s, Rollo had a gold ring made for Georgia and presented it to her in the company of a few close friends in Tiburon. In a warm, informal ceremony, he declared his commitment to her and noted that the shape of the ring symbolized "two existential freedoms forever joined and forever autonomous." In August 1988, at the Squam Lake boathouse of their friends Sidney and Jean Lanier, and in the presence of New Hampshire friends, among them Harold Taylor, the artist Jules Olitski and his wife, and Georgia's daughter, they confirmed their love in marriage. There were three ministers present (a client of Georgia's later remarked that they could have done the ceremony with just one rabbi). Olitski presented them with a picture created especially for the occasion that found a prominent place in their Tiburon home.[42]

Meanwhile, May also journeyed to Sweden in the mid-1980s to star in a documentary film, *Sagolandet* (called "Land of Dreams" in its American release), by the famous Swedish director Jan Troell. Troell thought of May as the perfect commentator on a Swedish society that, in the filmmaker's view, had achieved material splendor at the cost of its humanity and sense of meaning. There was some irony in the fact that a small-town son of the Midwest came to remind Scandinavians (albeit Swedes, not Danes) of Kierkegaard's existential imperatives.[43]

Such comforts as well as May's advancing years and the spiritually open space of California also may have encouraged him to reopen the question of his inner life and its relation to formal religion. Of course, he had been writing about meaning that did not exclude transcendence even after his own loss of Christian faith, most often in the language of existentialism and as part of a concern for guiding myths and symbols. However, not until the 1970s did he begin to refer regularly again to forms of transcendence in his meditations, diaries, and even conversation with others. At first, he might express it about art, as in *The Courage to Create* or when he wrote in the guest book of the Rothko Chapel in Houston that he had accepted a speaking engagement in the city just so he could visit for a third time this "spiritual place that moves me tremendously."[44]

May's dreams also began to reflect some regrets concerning his leaving the church. "I was supposed to take charge of a service (in a church?)," he recorded about one dream. "I didn't show up—so they had to [conduct] their own service. I was irresponsible." The word "God" frequently reentered his vocabulary. He saw guilt in a spiritual as well as psychological light, as when he experienced a sense of a resurgent competitiveness over the announcement of a film about his old friend Joseph Campbell titled *The Hero's Journey.* He felt "mean, un-Christian," saw it as "a sin," and prayed to "God" as well as the "Zen spirits" to help him rise above "the grossness of this competition." The following summer, deep in the writing of his next book, he vowed not only "to plan for writing" but to do so "under god." And, on July 4, 1987, he reported to his diary: "Today I had a very satisfactory meditation—talking to God—period. I thought how different it is from what I wrote yesterday, [that] I had a hard time reaching 'God.'"[45]

He even began to attend church again, though not in the spare Methodist tradition of his youth. Rather, he sought out the symbolically richer liturgy of St. Stephen's Episcopal Church in the neighboring community of Belvedere. May was especially taken with the sacrament of the Eucharist, its symbolic rendering of the body and blood of Christ in bread and wine, and most of all the mystery of Communion. May also developed a fascination for Tibetan Buddhism. He and Georgia learned of its tradition firsthand at retreats in the Napa Valley. Such curiosity about other spiritual visions, East and West, made his response to a reporter from the Oakland *Tribune* who had asked about his motivation in writing books a little less surprising: "You know, I never considered myself a writer. I consider myself first a clergyman, then a psychotherapist. . . . I think what I have done, in each book is to go a little deeper."[46]

Such a statement could not have been made lightly, and a dream from early 1990 highlights the swirl of religious and psychological reference that remained alive in his mind:

I was being tried for my life by psychologists. I had been too depressed. The whole profession was too moribund and they didn't think enough, didn't dare enough. What had I done? I thought too much. My depression—I would be condemned to death. . . . Perhaps I would make a break for it—to run for it. . . . I was guilty for not being happy. I was guilty for not being free from my depression. I was tried at the University of Michigan. . . . I felt the depression was to be gotten over—but can I do it without taking on a religion? What is the connection with my mother? Can I be a happy man? I put the question to them—so I wasn't convicted—I won out.[47]

Such turbulent dreams furthered his inner reassessment and bolstered his pursuit of a public life. He wrote, attended conferences, gave lectures, and traveled. The positive side was evident to others, even in the retelling of his life story. In one interview from 1990, May displayed equanimity about his parents, emphasizing their hardscrabble life without a word of anger. He most often emphasized his joys—painting, writing, the comfort of his life with Georgia, the company of friends, and the natural beauty of Tiburon or New Hampshire. As for facing death, he remarked: "I don't have time to die."[48]

Early that same year, as May struggled with the final chapters of *The Cry for Myth*, a book he almost certainly knew would be his major valedictory statement, he was offered a fall 1990 residency at the Rockefeller Foundation's Bellagio Center. He and Georgia were looking forward to a trip to Italy and Bellagio's enchanting view of Lake Como, as well as the peace to write and enjoy the intellectual life free of everyday responsibilities. However, in May, as Georgia drove him back to Tiburon from San Francisco Airport, a drunk driver lost control at high speed and hit them on Highway 280. Rollo's head struck the ceiling of the car, and in the days that followed he suffered from symptoms of a concussion. In August, he had a transitory mini-stroke as he was preparing for the trip to Bellagio. He was, according to Georgia, "totally incapable of packing." She and Harold Taylor quickly put some clothes together, and the Mays boarded the flight. Once in Italy, Rollo and Georgia made a special trip to Milan to buy the underwear he had forgotten to pack. It was a harbinger of worse things to come. May lived in the shadow of depression and physical stroke symptoms virtually his entire time at Bellagio, often acted erratically, sometimes swallowed only with difficulty, and suffered attacks of shooting pain in his facial nerves.[49]

Upon their return to California in February 1991, May underwent treatment for the damaged facial nerves. He had a serious stroke during the surgery and lay in the hospital for five and a half weeks in something close to a coma. Georgia stayed with him virtually every night, making sure the doctors and nurses tended to his needs. Royal Alsup, who had studied existential psychology and trained members of a Northern California Native American tribe in that tradition, brought six healers to the hospital to pray for him. They gathered in Rollo's room to perform traditional chants. As they finished May awoke from his sleep and saw, with double vision, twelve Indians chanting. He was sure it had helped him to awaken.[50]

May lived for another three and a half years, at first recovering remarkably well but in time fading into moments of disorientation, psychic travel to his past, and depression mixed with a twilight sense of peace. He would sense the presence of his father, mother, or sister Ruth and converse with them. He would settle scores or make amends, clearly realizing that these might be his last moments to reimagine and close the book on unfinished business. Once he stopped a dinner conversation, turned to an empty spot on his right, and addressed an imagined Ellie Roberts. "You know," he said, referring to her husband's suicide, "I wasn't the only one at fault."[51]

As age claimed more of May's consciousness, other incidents and expressions of a past life and basic character appeared. Once, as Georgia drove Rollo and a guest down the winding road to a restaurant at the ferry dock for a leisurely dinner, he urged her to hurry, sure he was late for a lecture in New York. Another time, Georgia and her son, Boyd, and Rollo bought some takeout from an Indian restaurant in Berkeley. Boyd wanted to spend a few minutes at a bookstore, and Rollo offered to hold the food. Georgia went to get the car, and when Boyd came out of the shop Rollo was gone. Boyd finally found him getting into a cab and asking the driver to take him to his old New York address. He had given away the food to a few homeless people. As often as not after such episodes, Rollo displayed a bemused smile and welcomed himself back into the moment he had momentarily left.[52]

By his eighty-fifth birthday in April 1994, he had grown noticeably frail, though strong enough to enjoy a party. Tom Greening, editor of the *Journal of Humanistic Psychology*, wrote:

> In spite of Angst he's learned to thrive
>> And reached the age of 85

He grew weaker, napping a good deal each day and less able to focus on any subject for an extended period of time. In late October, Georgia felt certain that the end was near. She invited their closest friends to visit him with the understanding that they were saying goodbye. They arrived on Saturday, October 22, and spent time together with Rollo on the deck overlooking the San Francisco Bay. By the end of the day, only Irv and Marilyn Yalom and Georgia remained. At one point Rollo told Georgia, "Dear, I'm going to paint," got up, and slowly made his way to the bedroom. He lay sitting up in bed, took a few breaths and closed his eyes. Irv Yalom, a medical doctor, officially pronounced him dead.

Georgia and Irv washed and dressed Rollo so that he might remain in the bedroom. The night of his passing, a Buddhist friend read from the Tibetan Book of the Dead. Georgia's grandson, not yet a year old, tried to climb up on the bed to be with him. Georgia stayed up with Rollo the whole night. The following day friends, family, patients, and colleagues paid their last respects. At five on the afternoon of October 23, in the last hour of sunlight, representatives of a local crematorium came to take his body. The next day they delivered his remains in an urn. On the forty-seventh through forty-ninth days after his death, two lamas from the Napa Valley monastery at which he had studied came to accompany May through the *bardo*, the intermediate state between death and rebirth, by reciting from the Bardo Thodol. The wisdom and prayer of the text was meant to guide the recently deceased through storms of dreams and nightmarish visions toward a state of calm wholeness:

> When the roarings of savage beasts are uttered,
> Let it come that they be changed into the sacred sounds of the Six
>   Syllables;
> When pursued by snow, rain, wind, and darkness,
> Let it come that I see with the celestial eyes of bright Wisdom.[53]

* * *

A warm celebration of May's life was held a week later at Grace Cathedral in San Francisco. His son Robert read Robert Frost's "Birches." Sam Keen and Don Michael spoke. Later, there was a reception at the Fairmont Hotel. Tom Greening, bard for every occasion, read one more poem in May's honor. It ended:

> Dear Rollo now is God's resource
> for channeling daimonic force
> to aid us sinners left behind,
> as Huxley urged, to be more kind.[54]

Georgia gave the May children half of Rollo's ashes, which they later spread over the Holderness property. She kept the other half in a simple cylindrical urn in her bedroom, and when she moved from Tiburon to Carmel, and later to Palo Alto, Rollo moved with her.

Epilogue

Life after Life

In the summer of 2018, as she approached her thirtieth birthday and recovered from a serious car accident, Alexis Brown, a bartender in Chicago, ventured alone to Tulum, Mexico, to relax on the beach and think about her future. She felt overworked and exhausted, too ready to say yes to the demands of others but with little time to think about what she herself wanted from life. Brown brought along a stack of books but came away "obsessed" with one, *The Courage to Create*. "It's not a bartending book or anything that talks about making cocktails," she joked to reporter Anna Archibald. "[It is] basically about seizing the courage necessary to preserve our sensitivity, our awareness." Brown returned to Chicago bent on rebalancing her life and especially improving the lot of those she worked with as well as focusing on work she had already begun, to open doors for minorities in the bar industry. May's words so inspired her that she purchased twenty copies of *The Courage to Create* to give to close friends.[1]

May would have been happily surprised at the staying power of his work across decades and generations as well as genders and ethnicities. It answered a nagging question of his final years. On visits during the last decade of his life, I noticed that at times periods of quiet depression punctuated his usually cheerful demeanor. Such darkness had less to do with the fear of death than worries about the fate of his life's work. How much longer would his books be read and his ideas discussed? Who would even know his name? His fears were certainly reasonable, but for a while it looked as if they might be unwarranted. Saybrook University continued to function as a hub for humanistic psychology. Such protégés as Kirk Schneider, Steven Diamond, Ed Mendelowitz, and others expanded on May's therapeutic style and love of philosophy, literature, and the arts even as they found their own particular voices. May's friend Irvin Yalom, for whom *Existence* meant so much, had become the most notable American proponent of existentially rooted therapy among psychiatrists and psychologists, and his books, both fiction and nonfiction, had already reached out to a broad audience.

Still, May was keenly aware that psychotherapy's once vaunted place in American culture had declined precipitously since its halcyon years between the 1950s and 1970s. Since the mid-1970s, it had faced withering attacks from experimental psychologists who questioned the effectiveness of psychoanalytically based treatment and from proponents of cognitive behavioral therapy who claimed statistical evidence of more immediate practical results. Some critics saw the "therapeutic" as both cause and symptom of an increasingly narcissistic "me"-focused society, while others took special aim at the more radical wing of humanistic psychology, accusing it of subverting traditional norms and mores.

Structural blows in the 1980s and 1990s sent the therapeutic profession into further disarray. The first came with the rise of the health maintenance organization (HMO) as a key organizing principle of medical care, one that in the late 1980s denied or drastically limited benefits for outpatient psychotherapy. At the same time, the FDA approved Prozac in late 1987, and its dramatic amelioration of depression sparked a revolution in treatment—it was quicker, cheaper, and vastly more effective than psychotherapy. By 1990, Prozac was the most widely prescribed medicine for depression, and the development of other similarly potent drugs for anxiety relief and other conditions soon followed. A durable treatment regimen eventually emerged in the world of the HMO. Clients would see a psychologist or clinical social worker for short-term counseling and to get a diagnosis that fit the predetermined guidelines of the *Diagnostic and Statistical Manual of Mental Disorders (DSM)*. They would then visit a psychiatrist, who would prescribe and monitor one of the new psychotropic drugs based on that diagnosis. The use of these drugs became almost universal for depression-related disorders, while, according to one study, extended psychotherapeutic treatment declined significantly between the years 1997 and 2007. There seemed little reason to expend the time and money for long and often searing self-examination when relief using the new wonder drugs was just a pill a day away. Long-term psychotherapy and psychoanalysis had been priced out of the market and, in any case, could not demonstrate symptom relief comparable to the astoundingly rapid results produced by the Prozac revolution.[2]

If one legacy that May worried about was the survival of in-depth psychotherapy, perhaps even more important was his fear about the fate of his books. Here the story was more complicated, playing out over several decades and involving new business practices and technologies. Transformations in the book trade gave every author and publisher a case of whiplash. The 1980s marked the rise of national bookstore chains—B. Dalton, Waldenbooks, Crown Books, Bookstop, and a newly expanded Barnes and Noble—which by discounting bestsellers and limiting the stock of less popular titles challenged the business model and very existence of small, independent bookstores. Rollo May's works survived on the shelves of many chains into the 1990s but soon after his death met the fate of others on the backlist. Increasingly even his most popular works were no longer regularly stocked, and his work became literally more and more invisible to new generations of readers.

Then came an even more disruptive event the very year of May's passing—Jeff Bezos's launch of Amazon.com, an online bookstore from which one could order virtually any book in print and have it shipped to one's home. By 2000, Amazon's success and pressure from the national chains resulted in the closure of an estimated 40 percent of independent bookstores. Soon the chains themselves succumbed to the increasingly sophisticated marketing of books on the internet. Some book retailers filed for bankruptcy, and others further limited stock and attempted to match Amazon's deep discounts and services.

However, the impact of the internet on the availability of books came as a palpable boon to May and other backlist authors and also a new chance for the circulation of their ideas. One could find used or new copies of every book May had written, from *The Art of Counseling* to *The Cry for Myth*, at very affordable prices. Especially with the rise of social media, the blogosphere, and sophisticated search engines like Google, his work underwent fresh appraisal and excited reactions from a new generation of readers. At this writing, on any given day, a Google search for "Rollo May" generally yields between four hundred and six hundred thousand hits. Some are rogue sites offering free copies of his books, while others mention his name only in passing. However, literally hundreds, if not thousands, of hits contribute to an explosion of commentary on his ideas that widens each year. Amazon's and other online reviews echo the transforming thrill many of May's readers had experienced in the 1960s and 1970s. "Rollo May's *Love and Will* is the most important book I've read—of any kind, at any time," exclaimed J. Winokur about his 2010 Amazon purchase. "Its importance to me is not because of some specific thesis May advances, but for an integrated set of ideas and values, and an understanding of human nature, that May presents."[3] Caitlin O'Neil put it this way: "It is incredible that a book could be written fully 18 years before

I was even born, and yet gives possibly the most precise diagnosis of the present relational ills of our culture that I've ever read."[4]

The internet is filled with more extensive references to May's books and ideas and from a variety of contributors—ministers, social activists, philosophers, dissertation writers, and, of course, clinical psychologists and social workers as well as counselors. One example is Maria Popova's extremely popular blog, *Brain Pickings—An Inventory of the Meaningful Life*. Each week since 2006, Popova has highlighted, by her own description, the "most interesting and inspiring articles across art, science, philosophy, creativity, children's books, and other strands of our search for truth, beauty, and meaning." Along the way, she has published long excerpts from *Freedom and Destiny* as well as *Love and Will*.[5]

May continues to have a powerful impact on its readers across time, gender, and culture not only through the internet but also through the increased circulation of physical books, new and used, that the internet helped spark. One example is a conversation with Maral Mohammadian, a key animation producer at the National Film Board of Canada, which appeared on the Animation World Network website in 2017. She was asked what book she valued most. Her answer: "*Man's Search for Himself*, by Rollo May." I was intrigued by her response, of course, and asked her in an email to expand on this experience. She said she noticed the book during a period of "transition and personal reflection, struggling with anxiety, ghosts from my past that I could not understand." She purchased it, hoping it would help her, and soon found its "directness refreshing. It was sharp, succinct, but without the tone of pulp philosophy or self-help books." "Poetic and imaginative" and "inspiring and beautiful" as well as "humanizing"—these were the words she used to describe May's prose. "It hit an emotional nerve for me—it was nourishing, validating," she continued, "and it was somehow kind (by which I mean accessible)." More recently, she had reread it and was "struck all over again by how deeply it resonated": "I read it twice (often in tears, if I may be blunt). It transmits a painful kind of belonging. I find it therapeutic, especially because it's not a new book. It distills certain universal human traits in a poetic way."[6]

Mohammadian's deeply personal and perceptive email was one answer to the question of how a book published in 1953, worlds away from contemporary assumptions about self and identity, can nonetheless so powerfully affect an individual. His works offer historical breadth to generations in which technological innovation more and more has taken center stage at the expense of millennia of wisdom about the human condition. In a world enamored of data, robotics, and artificial intelligence, May underscores the resources of individuals in shaping their own existences. Love, courage, autonomy, creativity—reading Rollo May's work today reminds us that these endangered aspirations are as important today to the crafting of a meaningful life as they were during May's own lifetime and for millennia past.

Notes

All diary, letter, and document entries without a specific archival source were discovered as I researched Rollo May's papers in his Tiburon study. Since then, his manuscripts have found an excellent home in the Special Collections, Humanistic Psychology Archive, University of California, Santa Barbara. See "Guide to the Rollo May Papers," http://pdf.oac.cdlib.org/pdf/ucsb/spcoll/may.pdf.

Citation of May's various diary and journal entries over the years are identified only by "Diary" unless they come from notebooks or sections with titles, something more common in his early years than later on.

Citations that begin "Interview with author" refer to taped interviews made by Robert Abzug with Rollo May over a period of years in Tiburon, California, and Holderness, New Hampshire.

Citations from May's books use the following acronyms and refer to original editions and sole authorship unless otherwise noted:

AOC:	*The Art of Counseling: How to Gain and Give Mental Health* (Nashville: Abingdon-Cokesbury Press, 1939).
CBC:	*Existential Psychotherapy: Rollo May / Six Talks for CBC Radio* (Toronto: CBC Publications, 1967).
CFM:	*The Cry for Myth* (New York: W. W. Norton, 1991).
CTC:	*The Courage to Create* (New York: W. W. Norton, 1975).
DAS:	with Leopold Caligor, *Dreams and Symbols: Man's Unconscious Language* (New York: Basic Books, 1968).
DOB:	*The Discovery of Being* (New York: W. W. Norton, 1983).
EXP:	ed., *Existential Psychology* (New York: Random House, 1960).
EXP2:	ed., *Existential Psychology*, 2nd ed. (New York: Random House, 1969).
EXS:	with Ernest Angel, Henri F. Ellenberger, eds., *Existence: A New Dimension in Psychiatry and Psychology* (New York: Basic Books, 1958).
FAD:	*Freedom and Destiny* (New York: W. W. Norton, 1981).
LAW:	*Love and Will* (New York: W. W. Norton, 1969).
MOA:	*The Meaning of Anxiety* (New York: Ronald, 1950).
MQB:	*My Quest for Beauty* (Dallas: Saybrook, 1985).

MSH:	*Man's Search for Himself* (New York: W. W. Norton, 1953).
PAI:	*Power and Innocence* (New York: W. W. Norton, 1972).
PAU:	*Paulus: Reminiscences of a Friendship* (New York: Harper & Row, 1973).
PAU2:	*Paulus: Tillich as Spiritual Teacher* rev. ed. (Dallas: Saybrook Publishers, 1988).
PHD:	*Psychology and the Human Dilemma* (New York: D. Van Nostrand, 1967).
POE:	with Kirk J. Schneider, *The Psychology Of Existence: An Integrative, Clinical Perspective* (New York: McGraw-Hill, 1994).
SCL:	*The Springs of Creative Living* (Nashville: Abingdon-Cokesbury, 1940).
SRL:	ed., *Symbolism in Religion and Literature* (New York: George Braziller, 1960).

Preface

1. The file drawers and folders I researched in his home office contained an incredibly large collection of yellowing, crumbling newspaper and magazine clippings dating from the mid-1930s through the 1960s, filled with possible stories for his writings.
2. Philip Rieff, *The Triumph Of The Therapeutic: Uses of Faith after Freud* (New York: Harper & Row, 1966).
3. *AOC*, 224.
4. *SOCL*, 7.
5. "The Delphic Oracle as Therapist," in *CFM*, 110–11.

Chapter 1

1. Diary, August 22, 1987. Still, with typical self-scrutiny, Rollo asked himself whether the "aim of my whole life" should be "to have people acknowledge that I have made a contribution."
2. *CFM*, 49.
3. Ibid.
4. Diary, August 31, 1987.
5. *PAU*, 2–3, 13. The book was later published as *PAU2*.
6. Edgar Lee Masters, *Spoon River Anthology* (Clayton, DE: Prestwick House, 2007), 137.
7. Earl Tuttle May, travel diary, entry for January 3, 1904. Other quotations below from various entries. Diary in the possession of the late Dr. Gerald May, Rollo's half-brother and son of E. T.'s second marriage, who made a copy of the diary for the author.
8. Ruth May to Rollo May, March 14, [1967].

9. The Rollo books were favorites of Henry James and T. S. Eliot and most plausibly the ones that Matie herself had read as a young girl.

10. Rollo May, "The Wounded Healer," manuscript autobiographical fragments.

11. Diary, [July 1937].

12. The reference to the meaning of treehouses is in a newspaper interview. See Carol Horner, "An Expert on Love Is Still Looking for Answers . . . ," *Philadelphia Inquirer*, July 22, 1981, 1D, 3D. These self-reflections on the meaning of his love of heights are from diary entries after an analytic session with Dr. Alberta Szalita, a colleague at the William Alanson White Institute from whom he had sought help at a difficult moment. Diary, June 2, 1966.

13. Ruth May to Rollo May, [early 1960s?].

14. Interview with the author, May 5, 1990, Tiburon, CA.

15. Diary entry, January 19, 1967. This entry was written while Rollo was in psychotherapy.

16. The starting point for any historical look at the YMCA is C. Howard Hopkins, *History of the YMCA in North America* (New York: Association Press, 1951). An interesting study is David I. Macleod, *Building Character in the American Boy: The Boy Scouts, YMCA, and Their Forerunners, 1870–1920* (Madison: University of Wisconsin Press, 1983). See also Elmer L. Johnson, *The History of YMCA Physical Education* (Chicago: Association Press, 1979). However, a comprehensive interpretive study worthy of the organization's importance has yet to be written.

17. Frank Ritchie, *The Community and the Y.M.C.A.* (New York: Association Press, 1919), 11. Ritchie was community secretary of the International Committee of the YMCA.

18. J. Quincy Ames, *Social Adjustment through the Young Men's Christian Associations*, Changing Young Men's Christian Association 5 (Chicago: Young Men's Christian Association College, 1927), 32–33, 68.

19. Ruth May to Rollo May, March 14, [1967].

20. Rollo May interview with Shirley Kessler, July 23, 1982 in Holderness, New Hampshire. Typescript of Kessler interview, SR2, 39. Kessler interviewed May in preparation for an as-yet-unreleased documentary. I use the transcript with Kessler's permission. Gerald May, Rollo's half-brother and himself a psychologist, told me similar stories.

21. Kessler interview, SR2, 27.

22. May's own sense was that he was a poor student compared to his capabilities. His high school transcript somewhat bears this out. It notes an IQ of 134 scored on the Otis test when he was thirteen years old. All grades and scores from "Oberlin College: Certificate of Applicant for Admission—Transcript of Record of Rollo Reese [*sic*] May in the Marine City High School of Marine City, Michigan," Oberlin College Archives.

23. Rollo May, "Oberlin College: Application for Admission to Advanced Standing in the College of Arts and Sciences of Oberlin College," September 15, 1928, Oberlin College Archives.

24. For this and ensuing paragraphs on the river, see Emeline Jenks Crampton, *History of the Saint Clair River* (St. Clair, MI: St. Clair Republican, 1921).

25. May literally said this to me in an interview, March 1994, Tiburon, CA. He knew that he "wanted to become somebody" in high school but as yet did not know who that somebody might be.

26. Sam Walter Foss, "The House by the Side of the Road," in Foss, *Dreams in Homespun* (Boston: Lothrop, Lee & Shepard, 1897), 11–12. The anthology he received at high school graduation might well have been Roy J. Cook, ed., *One Hundred and One Famous Poems* (Chicago: Reilly & Lee, 1926), which contains the Foss poem.

Chapter 2

1. Essay section of Rollo R. May, "Oberlin College: Application for Admission to Advanced Standing in the College of Arts and Sciences of Oberlin College," September 15, 1928, Oberlin College Archives; Record Sheet for Rollo Reese May, Oberlin College Archives.

2. See Helen Lefkowitz Horowitz, *Campus Life: Undergraduate Cultures from the End of the Eighteenth Century to the Present* (Chicago: University of Chicago Press, 1987), and Paula Fass, *The Damned and the Beautiful: American Youth in the 1920s* (New York: Oxford University Press, 1977).

3. Paul L. Dressel, *College to University: The Hannah Years at Michigan State, 1935–1969* (East Lansing: Michigan State University Press, 1987).

4. "Pilgrimage to Man," n.d. A short meditation on his life. Though the manuscript is undated, internal evidence suggests the early to mid-1930s. Direct quotations in the pursuant paragraphs from this source unless otherwise noted.

5. Diary, March 23, 1932.

6. A complete run of *The Student* can be found at the Archives of Michigan State University, East Lansing, Michigan.

7. Rollo May, "Roosevelt in College," *The Student*, January 17, 1928, 4, 7.

8. *The Student*, April 23, 1928, cover; Elbert Hubbard's story was originally published as "A Message to Garcia," *Philistine*, March 1, 1899, 109–16. It has been reprinted in various forms since, and also shown to be historical fabrication.

9. Rollo May, "Are We Slaves?," *The Student*, April 13, 1928, 3–4.

10. Roscoe Bloss, "After All," *The Student*, April 13, 1928, 5; Rollo May, in Open Forum section, *The Student*, May 1, 1928, 6.

11. "Pilgrimage to Man."

12. The best source for information on Bennett Weaver's early life is a small entry in the biographical section of William Stanley Braithwaite, *Anthology of Magazine Verse for 1926 and Yearbook of American Poetry (Sesqui-Centennial Edition)* (Boston: B. J. Brimmer, 1926), section 3, 40. A brief history of the church can be found at Kevin Forsyth's Brief History of East Lansing, Michigan website, http://kevinforsyth.net/ELMI/peoples.htm, accessed January 26, 2020.

13. Diary, January 11, 1932, and March 24, 1932.

14. James Harris Fairchild, *Educational Arrangements and College Life at Oberlin* (New York: Edward O. Jenkins, 1866), 11, as quoted in John Barnard, *From Evangelicalism to Progressivism at Oberlin College, 1866–1917* (Columbus: Ohio State University Press, 1969) 8, 115.

15. Henry Churchill King, *Rational Living: Some Practical Inferences from Modern Psychology* (New York: Macmillan, 1905).

16. Interview with the author, November 1987, Tiburon, CA.

17. Bennett Weaver to Dean of Admissions, Oberlin College, September 22, 1928, Oberlin College Archives; W. W. Johnston to Dean of Admissions, Oberlin College, September 20, 1928, Oberlin College Archives.

18. Rollo May, Application for Admission to Oberlin College, September 15, 1928, Oberlin College Archives. The narrative is based on an informal conversation with May, especially the final "you're in."

19. Tuition was $150 per semester. See Rollo May, "Oberlin College Application for Scholarship Aid," 1929–30, Oberlin College Archives.

20. George Eliot, *Poems* (New York: White, Stokes & Allen, 1885), 201.

21. Will Durant, *The Story of Philosophy: The Lives and Opinions of the Greater Philosophers* (New York: Pocket Books, 1927). The importance of Durant to the proliferation of interest in Nietzsche and his influence on American culture can be followed in Jennifer Ratner-Rosenhagen, *American Nietzsche: A History of an Icon and His Ideas* (Chicago: University of Chicago Press, 2012). The book is relevant not only to May's early exposure to Nietzsche but also to his later romance with existentialism.

22. Rollo R. May, "A Philosophy of Philosophies," June 10, 1929, 6–7.

23. May, "Philosophy of Philosophies," 6.

24. Confidential Records of Rollo May, Oberlin College, Oberlin College Archives.

25. Indeed, so "Christian" were his outlook and surroundings that May hardly recognized the existence of any other religion at all. Quite innocently, he tried to recruit a Jewish friend, Harry Serotkin, to join his church. Serotkin simply said nothing, for he in his own way had perhaps felt the impact of Oberlin's Christian atmosphere. Protestantism reigned as a benign but unquestioned authority over campus life. Interview with the author, November 12, 1987, Tiburon, CA.

26. The Reverend James Austin Richards to Dean Bosworth, Oberlin, June 25, 1929, in Oberlin College Archives.

27. Although one can see the concept in the works of Freud and Jung, the "inferiority complex" was most of all a key construct of Alfred Adler, who soon would have a powerful influence on May.

28. See Edwin Diller Starbuck, *The Psychology of Religion: An Empirical Study of the Growth of Religious Consciousness* (New York: C. Scribner's Sons, 1899); William James, *The Varieties of Religious Experience: A Study in Human Nature* (New York: Longmans, Green, 1902), as well as Edward Scribner Ames, *The Psychology of Religious Experience* (Boston: Houghton Mifflin, 1910); Peter Gardella, *Innocent Ecstasy: How Christianity Gave America an Ethic of Pleasure* (New York: Oxford University Press, 1985), 140–49; G. Stanley Hall, *Adolescence: Its Psychology and Its Relations to Physiology, Anthropology, Sociology, Sex, Crime,*

346 NOTES TO PAGES 25–33

Religion, and Education (New York: D. Appleton, 1904); G. Stanley Hall, *Jesus, the Christ, in the Light of Psychology*, vol. 2 (New York: Doubleday, 1917); for a good history of the Emmanuel Movement, see Eric Caplan, *Mind Games: American Culture and the Birth of Psychotherapy* (Berkeley: University of California Press, 1998).

29. In addition, Norman Thomas, the Socialist Party leader, spoke on social justice. Kirby Page, an important voice in the interwar Christian peace movement, made the case for a modified pacifism using the revisionist arguments of Sidney Fay's *The Origins of the World War* (New York: Macmillan, 1928), which painted the Great War as a pointless bloodbath caused by nationalism, militarism, greed, and yellow journalism. See Rollo May, small notebook with printed cover "Young Man's Christian Association College / Chicago Lake Geneva." The source for the next paragraphs, unless otherwise noted, is this notebook. For a superb study of conflicting attitudes toward sexual knowledge among Christians of an earlier era, see Helen Lefkowitz Horowitz, *Rereading Sex: Battles over Sexual Knowledge and Suppression in Nineteenth-Century America* (New York: Alfred A. Knopf, 2002).

30. The quote is a rough paraphrase from Wordsworth's "Tintern Abbey." See William Wordsworth, *The Complete Poetical Works of William Wordsworth*, ed. Henry Reed (Philadelphia: Troutman & Hayes, 1854), 194.

31. Rollo May, "Oberlin College: Application for Scholarship Aid," forms for 1928–29 and 1929–30, Oberlin Archives.

Chapter 3

1. Quotes from typescript "Leisure," written on board ship to Greece, 1930. May misquotes Arnold's "Self-Dependence," which reads "Feel my soul" instead of "Feel myself." See Matthew Arnold, *Poetical Works of Matthew Arnold* (London: Macmillan, 1913), 255–56. May's essay itself showed no great imagination. It had identifiable sources. Professor Richards's final lecture addressed the centrality of soulful repose, as did a workshop at the Y camp. It was a hot topic at Oberlin in his senior year. Rollo's unremarkable conclusion: schoolwork must be put in its proper place next to other elements of life.

2. Kessler interview, SR3, 49.

3. Lord Byron, *Don Juan* (London: Penguin, 2005), 178.

4. Mark Mazower, *Salonica, City of Ghosts: Christians, Muslims, and Jews, 1430–1950* (New York: Vintage, 2006). Unless otherwise noted, all material on the history of Salonica in this chapter comes from this source.

5. Everett Stephens and Mary Stephens, *Survival Against All Odds: The First 100 Years of Anatolia College* (New Rochelle, NY: Aristide D. Caratzas, 1986).

6. Rollo May to "Mother, Dad, and all," January 23, 1931; the activities of the Athletic Council are described in *The 1931 Anatolian* (Salonika, Greece: Anatolia College, 1931).

7. *MQB*, 6.

8. May continued to call it by its older name. Rollo May, letter to "Folks," May 5, 1931. All texts for the section on his voyage are from this letter.

9. Charles Wager to Rollo May, Florence, Italy, July 23 and August 9, 1931.

10. Charles Wager to Rollo May, April 30, 1933.

11. *MQB*, 7–8.

12. Small notebook paper, the original notes written in the village. The ideas and quotations that follow are from a small, unlabeled notebook, unless otherwise noted.

13. *MQB*, 10.

Chapter 4

1. Matthew Arnold, *The Poetical Works of Matthew Arnold* (London: Macmillan, 1913), 226–27.

2. Joseph Wood Krutch, *The Modern Temper: A Study and a Confession* (New York: Harvest, 1956), 11, 101, 115; Wassily Kandinsky, *Concerning the Spiritual in Art* (New York: Dover, 1914), 14. The thirst for personal revelation analyzed by Krutch found enthusiastic expression in such artistic manifestoes as Wassily Kandinsky's. Decrying the soullessness of the age and the impotence of traditional religion in the face of science and modernity, Kandinsky identified literature, music, and art as "the first and most sensitive spheres" in which a new "spiritual revolution" had presented itself. "They reflect the dark picture of the present time," he argued, "and show the importance of what at first was only a little point of light noticed by few" (14). Indeed, Krutch had found art inadequate and only a temporary hedge against the essential meaninglessness of human life.

3. Tradition had it that the Virgin Mary and John the Evangelist, on their way to Cyprus to visit Lazarus, were forced to seek shelter on the peninsula. Mary so loved its natural beauty that she asked God to give Athos to her. The Greek Orthodox Church still considers it "the Garden of the Virgin Mary," though of course soon Mary would have been forbidden entry to its wonders.

4. I also worked from a typescript of May's account, which was lightly edited, amended, and illustrated with drawings Rollo did at the time. A slightly different version of the story can be found in *MQB*, 39–63. A short introduction to the legend and history of Mount Athos can be found at the website Mount Athos: The Holy Mountain, http://www.macedonian-heritage.gr/Athos/General/History.html, accessed April 2020.

5. *MQB*, 11.

6. Rollo May to parents, Salonika, June 2, 1932.

7. The best account and my source for the factual material on Adler, unless otherwise noted, is Edward Hoffman, *The Drive for Self: Alfred Adler and the Founding of Individual Psychology* (Reading, MA: Addison-Wesley, 1994).

8. Unless otherwise noted, quotations are from notes in unnumbered pages of a small blue notebook labeled "Individual Psychology Summer School, Dr. Adler and assistants, Semmering, June '32 Rollo R. May."

9. Quotes from Leonhard Seif and Erwin Krausz are found in Rollo's notes, headed "Conference with Dr. Seif."

10. The most accessible overview, in Adler's own words, of individual psychology's approach to dreams and its critical view of Freud's constructs appears in Heinz L. Ansbacher and Rowena R. Ansbacher eds., *The Individual Psychology of Alfred Adler* (New York: Harper & Row, 1964), 350–65·

11. Adler and the director of the Yale Institute for Human Relations quoted in \ Hoffman, *The Drive for Self*, 308.

12. May's later idea of the "unconscious" more resembled Freud's than Adler's conception, one that involved repression rather than simply inchoate, unformulated emotion.

13. Diary, June 6, 1937.

14. Susan Griffin· *The Eros of Everyday Life* (New York: Doubleday, 1995), 149·

Chapter 5

1. Kessler interview, SR4, 58.

2. Indeed, she devoted the rest of her life to this mission, not just in Europe but in Latin America as well. The best comprehensive source for understanding Elma Pratt's work and the ISA is Nicole R. Cardassilaris, "Bringing Cultures Together: Elma Pratt, Her International School of Art, and Her Collection of International Folk Art at the Miami University Art Museum" (master's thesis, University of Cincinnati, 2008). Pratt quoted on p. 12.

3. Joseph Binder and Carla Binder, *Joseph Binder: An Artist and a Lifestyle: From the Joseph Binder Collection of Posters, Graphic and Fine Arts, Notes, and Records* (Vienna: A. Schroll, 1976). May is quoted on p. 42.

4. Rollo May, "Colors in Czechoslovakia," 1932.

5. Kessler interview, SR4, 61.

6. Rollo May, letter to "Mother, Dad, and all," September 12, 1932.

7. Kessler interview, SR4, 64, and author's interview with May, as well as letters from Isabella Hunner ("Bets") in the months after she returned home.

8. Kessler interview, SR4, 62.

9. Isabella Hunner to Rollo May, Athens, September 18, 1932.

10. "Idea Notebook," October 10, 1932.

11. "Idea Notebook," October 8, 1931,

12. Rollo May to "Mother, Dad, and all," September 20, 1932.

13. "Idea Notebook," October 2 and 10, 1932.

14. Isabella Hunner to Rollo May, November 25, 1932.

15. Alfred Adler to Rollo May, November 28, 1932.

16. Undated insert into "Idea Notebook," but from internal evidence written in early 1933.

17. Isabella Hunner to Rollo May, January 2, 1933.

18. Isabella Hunner, letter to Rollo May, January 8, 1933.

19. Charles Wager to Rollo May, Oberlin, February 19 and March 23, 1933,.

20. Charles Wager to Rollo May, April 30, 1933,.

21. "Idea Notebook," February 2, 1933.
22. "Idea Notebook," February 22, 1933.
23. "Idea Notebook," March 10, 1933.
24. "Idea Notebook," March 10 and 15, 1933.
25. "Idea Notebook," March 27, 1933.
26. "Idea Notebook," March 18, 1933; Bertrand Russell, *Principles of Social Reconstruction* (London: George Allen & Unwin, 1916). Russell's *Principles* was first published in the United States as *Why Men Fight: A Method of Abolishing the International Duel* (New York: Century, 1917).
27. May's ruminations on Albert Schweitzer, *Out of My Life and Thought: An Autobiography* (London: George Allen & Unwin, 1933), in "Idea Notebook," March 27, 1933.
28. "Idea Notebook," March 27, 1933.
29. Commission of Appraisal (William Ernest Hocking, Chairman), *Re-Thinking Missions: A Laymen's Inquiry after One Hundred Years* (New York: Harper & Brothers, 1932), 327.
30. "Idea Notebook," April 27, 1933.
31. "Idea Notebook," April 7, 1933; Commission of Appraisal, *Re-thinking Missions*, 292.
32. Rollo recorded these and the other observations of the Gypsies at Larissa on four business-card-size pieces of pink cardboard.
33. Diary entry, June 24, 1933.
34. Diary entry, June 26, 1933.
35. Diary entry, in undated material after June 27, 1933.
36. Diary entry, July 4, 1933.
37. Diary entries, July 10–14, 1933.
38. Diary entries, July 10–14, 1933; interview with the author, March 20, 1987, Tiburon, CA.
39. Diary entry, July 20, 1933.
40. Interview with author, November 7, 1987, Tiburon, CA.

Chapter 6

1. Diary entry, April 17, 1933.
2. "Thoughts in New York (just after returning from Europe)," undated entry in back pages of untitled diary whose first entry is Friday, June 23, [1933].
3. "Thoughts in New York."
4. "My Mind's Diary, Union Theological Seminary, October 25, 1933, Rollo R. May," October 25, [1933].
5. Grades in the records of Union Theological Seminary, released with permission of Rollo May.
6. Reinhold Niebuhr, *Does Civilization Need Religion? A Study in the Social Resources and Limitations of Religion in Modern Life* (New York: Macmillan, 1927).
7. For more on Fosdick, see Robert Moats Miller, *Harry Emerson Fosdick: Preacher, Pastor, Prophet* (New York: Oxford University Press, 1985).

8. Matthew S. Hedstrom, *The Rise of Liberal Religion: Book Culture and American Spirituality in the Twentieth Century* (New York: Oxford University Press, 2012). Fosdick's most notable work in the 1920s was *Adventurous Religion and Other Essays* (New York: Harper & Brothers, 1926). He published many more books and sermon collections in the following decades, including *The Hope of the World: Twenty-five Sermons on Christianity Today* (New York: Harper & Brothers, 1933); *The Secret of Victorious Living: Sermons on Christianity Today* (New York: Harper & Brothers, 1934); and *On Being a Real Person* (New York: Harper & Brothers, 1943).

9. Fosdick, *Adventurous Religion*, 247.

10. Diary, November 2, 1933.

11. Diary, February 19, 1934.

12. "Thoughts in New York."

13. For the political evolution of Niebuhr in the 1920s, see especially Richard Wightman Fox, *Reinhold Niebuhr. A Biography* (New York: Pantheon, 1985), 62–141.

14. Reinhold Niebuhr, *Moral Man and Immoral Society: A Study in Ethics and Politics* (New York: Charles Scribner's Sons, 1932).

15. David Nelson Duke, *In the Trenches with Jesus and Marx: Harry F. Ward and the Struggle for Social Justice* (Tuscaloosa: University of Alabama Press, 2003).

16. Unpublished and undated letter to the editor of the *Christian Century*, June 1934.

17. Norma Abrams, "Rich Women Fight Reds at Church," *New York Daily News*, December 4, 1933.

18. "My Mind's Diary, Union Theological Seminary," January 5 and February 9, [1934], and undated entry following February 19, [1934]. On Pioneer Youth, see Joshua Lieberman, *Creative Camping: A Coeducational Experiment in Personality Development and Social Living, Being the Record of Six Summers of the National Experimental Camp of Pioneer Youth in America* (New York: Association Press, 1931), and the pamphlet *Pioneer Youth, 1924–1939* (New York: Pioneer Youth of America, 1939), celebrating the organization's fifteenth anniversary.

19. "My Mind's Diary, Union Theological Seminary," December 10, [1933]. Reissig was interested in politics and social welfare (he eventually became head of one of the major support committees for Republican Spain and in the 1950s a key advocate of rights for homosexuals in the United Churches of Christ). In the early 1950s, he was named as a fellow traveler of the Communist Party by the House Un-American Activities Committee. At the time of his working with Rollo, however, Reissig represented a more personalized grappling with the everyday impact of big issues on the average parishioner, an approach that fit perfectly with his Y background and introduction to Adlerian psychotherapy.

20. See June Bingham, *Courage to Change: An Introduction to the Life and Thought of Reinhold Niebuhr* (New York: Charles Scribner's Sons, 1961).

21. Hubert T. Herring, "Union Seminary Routs Its Reds," *Christian Century*, June 13, 1934. Rollo May, manuscript letter to the editor of *The Christian Century*, [June 1934].

22. "My Mind's Diary, Union Theological Seminary," April 28, 1934.

Chapter 7

1. Interview with the author, March 23, 1987, Tiburon, CA; "Thoughts and Experiences, summer of '35," October 24, 1935; Kessler interview, SR5, 75–76.
2. Interview with the author, November 7, 1992, Tiburon, CA.
3. Draft of "Report to Board in Control of Student Work, Peoples Church," October 22, 1934.
4. *Michigan State News*, n.d. [1934], May scribbling on an indecipherable clipping.
5. Draft of "Report to Board of Control of Student Work," January 28, 1935.
6. "The Purposeless Student," unpublished typescript, ca. 1934–35.
7. "The Fundamentalist Students," unpublished typescript, ca. 1934–35.
8. Rollo R. May, "Portrait of Men Students: A Study of Their Attitudes Toward College Life and Religion through Personal Interviews at Michigan State College," *Christian Education* 19 (April and June 1936), 394–402.
9. "My Mind's Diary," vol. 3, June 18, 1934.
10. Diary, September 24, 1934.
11. Diary, October 17, 1934.
12. Diary, October 17, 1934.
13. Diary, October 28, 1934.
14. Diary, October 18, 1934.
15. Diary, December 1, 1934.
16. Diary, January 24, 1935 and passim.
17. Rollo R. May, "Make Your Recreation Creative!," *Recreation*, February 1936, 553, 568.
18. In May's first book, *AOC*, there are case histories that, at least in fictive form, refer to some of his counselees from Michigan State. However, there is good reason to believe that these cases are amalgams of real students and autobiographical reflections. In any case, by the time May wrote the book he had accumulated a vast amount of theoretical knowledge about Freudian, Jungian, Rankean, and Adlerian psychotherapies. This knowledge shaped his telling of the cases so as to make them virtually useless as reflections of his experience as a counselor in 1934–35. For May's general contemporary view of his role, see draft of "Report of Director of Men Students and Y.M.C.A. Secretary to Board in Control of Student Work in Peoples Church."
19. Draft of "Report of Director of Men Students and Y.M.C.A. Secretary to Board in Control of Student Work in Peoples Church." Remarks on students in diary, undated [early summer 1935].
20. Diary, undated [early summer 1935].

Chapter 8

1. "Thoughts and Experiences, summer of '35," front pages and entry for July 21, 1935. Jung's quote can be found in C. G. Jung, *Modern Man in Search of a Soul* (New York: Harvest, 1933), 225.

2. Rollo R. May, "Review of C. G. Jung's 'Modern man in Search of a Soul—AND— Observations on the Bearing of Contemporary Psychotherapy on Our concept of Religious Education, Paper for R.[eligious] E.[ducation] s217e," July 25, 1935.

3. Ibid.

4. Ibid.

5. Ibid.

6. Ibid.

7. Ibid. Quotations selected by May for use in his paper are from Jung, *Modern Man in Search of a Soul*, 166, 169, 166.

8. "Thoughts and Experiences, summer of '35," [July 22, 1935]. May dated this entry as January 22, but it falls between entries for July 21 and another entry for July; "Review of C .G. Jung."

9. "Thoughts and Experiences, summer of '35," July 21, 1935.

10. "Thoughts and Experiences, summer of '35," unnumbered and undated page following epigraphs and titled "Fantasies."

11. "Thoughts and Experiences, summer of '35," n.d.

12. "Thoughts and Experiences, summer of '35," entries from July 17, [July 22], July 23, August 7, and August 31, 1935, last dream dated August 7.

13. "Thoughts and Experiences, summer of '35," August 8, 1935.

14. "Thoughts and Experiences, summer of '35," September 1, 1935.

15. "Reading: Aug. 1935 to ___; Comments, choice statements, and a record of my mental growth," September 1 and 2, 1935.

16. "Thoughts and Experiences, summer of '35," October 16 and 27, 1935.

17. "Reading: Aug. 1935 to ___," October 16, 1935; James Joyce, *A Portrait of the Artist as a Young Man*, in Harry Levin, ed., *The Portable James Joyce*, rev. ed. (New York: Viking, 1966), 526.

18. "Thoughts and Experiences, summer of '35," October 27, November 4 and 11, 1935 (he continued to use his summer notebook in Lansing). Jung, *Modern Man in Search of a Soul*, 236.

19. Lectures, exams, outlines, etc. for Religion in Modern Life. Paragraphs following use quotations from these sources.

20. However, he would soon be won over by Hermann Reissig, Paul Tillich, and Reinhold Niebuhr—all who had given up the pacifist ideal when the threat of fascism in Europe became apparent.

21. Loose note, "Conclusions re Experiment in Pedagogy," [winter 1936].

22. "Ideas and Experiences, My Mind's Diary, Beginning Nov. 25, 1935," May 7, 1936.

23. "Ideas and Experiences," May 7, 1936.

24. "My Mind's Diary; a record of my ideas, emotions and mental experiences, July 1, 36 to [?]," July 1, 1936.

25. "My Mind's Diary; a record," July 7 and 15, 1936.

26. "Ideas and Experiences," May 7, 1936. Lecture, "Religion and Sex," from Religion and Modern Culture course, 1935.

27. Small spiral notebook, section marked "Interlude," datable from internal evidence as from June 1936.

28. "Interlude"; "Religion and Sex" lecture.

29. "Reflections on Upper Reservoir, Palmer Lake, Colo.," September 12, 1936.

Chapter 9

1. "My Mind's Diary, Autumn, 1936 (Beginning of Second Seminary Course)," September 23, 1936; "My Mind's Journal, A Record of My Thoughts, Impressions, and Special Adventures (Beginning Feb. 11, 1937)," February 15, 1937.

2. Rollo May, "The Art of Student Counseling," *Christian Education* 20 (1937): 267–68.

3. Grace Loucks Elliott and Harry Bone, *The Sex Life of Youth* (New York: Council of Christian Association, 1929). For more on the subject, see Paula Fass, *The Damned and the Beautiful: American Youth in the 1920s* (New York: Oxford University Press, 1977); Helen Lefkowitz Horowitz, *Rereading Sex: Battles Over Sexual Knowledge and Suppression in Nineteenth-Century America* (New York: Alfred A. Knopf, 1992); and Jeffrey P. Moran, *Teaching Sex: The Shaping of Adolescence in the 20th Century* (Cambridge, MA: Harvard University Press, 2000).

4. Elliott and Bone, *Sex Life of Youth*, 138. Their source for gender role history was Mathilde Vaerting and Matthias Vaerting, *The Dominant Sex: A Study in the Sociology of Sex Differentiation* (New York: George H. Doran Company, 1923).

5. Elliott and Bone, *Sex Life of Youth*, passim, and 135–38.

6. E. James Lieberman, *Acts of Will: The Life and Work of Otto Rank* (New York: Free Press, 1985).

7. Anaïs Nin, *Incest: From "A Journal of Love": The Unexpurgated Diary of Anaïs Nin, 1932–1934* (New York: Harcourt Brace Jovanovich, 1992), 354–55, 361.

8. Program for "The Resources of Religion: the First Spring Conference of the Columbia Student Christian Council," March 6, 1937; "35 Begin Study of Key to Happy Marriage: Young Men and Women in Y.W.C.A. Course Advised Not to Wed Just to Get Girl to Cook Meals or Man to Provide Support," *Wilmington Morning News*, November 9, 1937. Quotations in the next three paragraphs come from this source.

9. May thus does not follow some of *The Sex Life of Youth*, which used Vaerting and Vaerting, *The Dominant Sex* to establish a theory of matriarchy as the original form of domination.

10. "My Mind's Diary, Autumn, 1936," September 23, 1936.

11. "My Mind's Diary, Autumn, 1936," February 15, 1937.

12. "My Mind's Diary, Autumn, 1936," February 18, 1937.

13. "My Mind's Diary, Autumn, 1936," February 20, 1937.

14. From Florence's letter to Lou, February 18, 1937.

15. Ibid.

16. Included in a letter to Florence, 3-page typescript, no title, dated June 5, 1937.

17. "My Minds Journal," December 14, 1937.

18. Miscellaneous personal notes, December 30, 1937.

19. Miscellaneous personal notes, December 29, 1937.

20. "My Mind's Journal, January 1938–," January 18, 1938.

21. "My Mind's Journal, January 1938–," January 19, 1938.

22. "My Mind's Journal, January 1938–," January 30, 1938, February 12, 1938; "My Mind's Journal," February 11, 1938.

23. "My Mind's Journal, January 1938–," February 23, 1938.

24. Rollo May to Florence DeFrees, April 16, 1938; Rollo May to Florence DeFrees, April 17, 1938.
25. Florence DeFrees to Rollo May, ca. April 1938.

Chapter 10

1. May, *PAU*, 1.
2. May, *PAU*, 3–4.
3. Wilhelm Pauck and Marion Pauck, *Paul Tillich: His Life and Thought*, vol. 1: *Life* (New York: Harper & Row, 1976), 224.
4. Interview with author, March 21, 1987, Tiburon, CA; Kessler interview, SR9, 130.
5. Tillich quoted in "My Mind's Diary, Union Theological Seminary," March 24 and April 28, 1934.
6. Pauck and Pauck, 41.
7. Ibid., 49.
8. Tillich quoted in ibid., 51, 53–54.
9. Paul Tillich, *Die religiöse Lage der Gegenwart* (Berlin: Ullstein, 1926);translated into English by H. Richard Niebuhr as *The Religious Situation* (New York: Meridian, 1956), 55–101.
10. Ibid.
11. Ibid., 138.
12. For the most complete and dramatic account of this aspect of the Tillichs' lives, see Hannah Tillich, *From Time to Time* (New York: Stein & Day, 1973), passim.
13. Pauck and Pauck, *Paul Tillich*, 132–33.
14. Ibid., 133–39.
15. Rollo R. May, "Comparison of Modern Psychotherapy and Christian Theology in Respect to Doctrine of Man" (BD thesis, Union Theological Seminary, 1938).
16. May, "Comparison of Modern Psychotherapy and Christian Theology," 2.
17. Ibid., 3–14.
18. Ibid., 15–20. May's is not a particularly subtle view of Freud, for instance calling his theory "hedonistic" and "anti-society."
19. Adler, Jung, and Rank are analyzed in ibid., 21–42.
20. Ibid., 48–49, 54, 57, 89–92, and passim.
21. E. M. Fleming to Rollo May, n.d., but ca. September 1938, since internal evidence suggests that Fleming wrote it just before Rollo's wedding.
22. *PAU*, 50–51.

Chapter 11

1. "My Mind's Diary," December 14, 1937.
2. "The Role of the Minister in a Small Town," undated manuscript (internal evidence reveals its time of composition).
3. Interview with author, November 7, 1992 Tiburon, CA.

4. Ibid.

5. "Suburban Christians," manuscript sermon, preached in Verona, NJ, October 15, 1939.

6. "Unto the Least of These," sermons notes, preached in Verona, NJ, December 4, 1938; even his Thanksgiving sermon contrasted American life to the fate of the Jews in Germany. See "Can One Give Honest Thanks?" preached in Verona, CA, November 20, 1938.

7. "Hold Only Unity Can Preserve Democracy; Rev. Mr. May Warns Against Undemocratic Influences," newspaper clipping, undated and unidentified; November 7. 1992, interview.

8. AOC; The key works of these two pioneers in this regard are William James, The Varieties of Religious Experience (New York: Longmans, Green, 1902), and G. Stanley Hall, Jesus, the Christ, in the Light of Psychology (Garden City, NY: Doubleday, Page, 1917).

9. Susan E. Myers-Shirk, Helping the Good Shepherd: Pastoral Counselors in a Psychotherapeutic Culture, 1925–1975 (Baltimore: Johns Hopkins University Press, 2009), is the most recent and most useful study of the history of pastoral counseling in the twentieth century. It contains an especially helpful chapter on Anton Boisen. John Sutherland Bonnell, Pastoral Psychiatry (New York: Harper & Brothers, 1938), xi and passim.

10. He claimed inaccurately that his was the first book on counseling in our interviews and to others as well. See Norma P. Simon, "A Revisit Worth the Trip: The Art of Rollo May," Contemporary Psychology 36, no. 11 (1991): 925–27; Harrison Sacket Elliott and Grace Loucks Elliott, Solving Personal Problems: A Counseling Manual (New York: H. Holt, 1936).

11. In fact, May's encomium to counseling contrasted with Harry Bone's somewhat tepid introductory remarks, ones that indicated sub rosa competition as much as objective judgment. Introduction to AOC, vii–ix, 15–17.

12. Ibid., 21–23.

13. Ibid., 24.

14. Ibid., 27.

15. Ibid., 27, 40–41.

16. Ibid., 44–74.

17. Ibid., 45–51.

18. Ibid., 51–53, 55–59, 61–67.

19. Ibid., 69, 67–74.

20. Ibid,75–77.

21. Ibid, 77–91, 86–87.

22. Ibid., 131–43. Bronson's counseling is the main example used in this chapter, "Confession and Interpretation." In conversation with me, May confirmed the autobiographical origins of these details.

23. Ibid., 211–12.

24. Rollo May to Florence DeFrees, April 16 and April 17, 1938.

25. AOC, 179–85.

26. Ibid., 186–92.

27. Ibid., 194–206.

28. Contemporary flyer for AOC, with comments, quotes from May, and order blank; Boisen, in the text of his full-fledged review, waxed enthusiastic despite feeling that May focused "too much on the writings of the psychotherapists and . . . too little . . . to the insights of the theologians and of the social philosophers." Boisen review in *Chicago Theological Seminary Register*, November 1939, 23–24; Robert A. Preston, review, *Journal of Bible and Religion*, May 1939, 90–91.

Chapter 12

1. Unknown to Rollo May, September 14, 1939. Only the first page of the letter survives. May's reply, if any, is not extant.

2. Linda Conti, "Rollo May: A Personal Look," *Perspectives: Humanistic Psychology Institute* 2, no. 1 (Summer 1981): 18.

3. Nikolai Berdyaev quoted on title page of *SCL*.

4. Ibid., 7 and passim.

5. Of special importance on the topic of spiritual middlebrow culture is Matthew S. Hedstrom, *The Rise of Liberal Religion: Book Culture and American Spirituality in the Twentieth Century* (New York: Oxford University Press, 2012). See also Janice Radway, *A Feeling for Books: The Book-of-the-Month Club, Literary Taste, and Middle-Class Desire* (Chapel Hill: University of North Carolina Press, 1997), Joan Shelley Rubin, *The Making of Middlebrow Culture* (Chapel Hill: University of North Carolina Press, 1992), and Lawrence W. Levine, *Highbrow/Lowbrow: The Emergence of Cultural Hierarchy in America* (Cambridge, MA: Harvard University Press, 1988), for complementary though in many ways different approaches to the question of "middlebrow" culture.

6. SCL, 34–35.

7. Ibid., 36, 40.

8. Ibid., 20–26, 36–42. Italics in the original text. May created his own narrative of psychology's relation to religion. The early hostility of each toward the other was one of misunderstanding and defensive rivalry, he argued, with the "fierce attacks and counter-attacks" one might expect from "members of the same family." Since 1920 or so, however, "it was discovered that most psychological problems are intertwined with religious, and that religious problems have in most cases a very clear psychological aspect." Jung, Adler, Rank, and Menninger each in his own way recognized that "co-operation" between the two fields were necessary. Even Freud had moved away from strict biology to a more philosophical understanding of life as a struggle between life forces and death forces, of Eros and Thanatos.

9. Ibid., 19–20, 31, passim.

10. The story and quotations that follow appear in ibid., 43–55, 61–73.

11. May does not deal with the threat of war or the details of authoritarian oppression even though he more specifically condemned them in his sermons and public activities; the Parable of the Talents is from Matthew 25:15–28; Adler quote from

Alfred Adler, *Understanding Human Nature: A Key to Self-Knowledge* (Garden City, NY: Garden City Publishing, 1927), 255–56.

12. *SCL*, 53–60.

13. Ibid., 61–72.

14. Ibid., 76–79

15. Ibid., 80–102.

16. Ibid., 128. Degas and Mann quotes from Thomas Mann, *Freud, Goethe and Wagner* (New York: Alfred A. Knopf, 1937), 85.

17. *SCL*, 158, 227.

18. *Publishers Weekly*, March 1, 1941; *Christian Evangelist*, August 28, 1941; *Church Management*, February 1941; Charles T. Holman in *Christian Century*, January 1, 1941 (clippings of reviews from Rollo May Papers.)

19. Reinhold Niebuhr to Rollo May, New York, November 14, 1940; Lewis Mumford to Rollo May, Amenia, New York, December 22, 1940.

20. *SCL*, 47.

21. Informal unrecorded interview with author, Tiburon, CA.

22. *SCL*, 13.

23. Interview with author concerning manuscript of Robert H. Abzug, "The Deconversion of Rollo May," *Review of Existential Psychology and Psychiatry* 24 (1999): 59–70.

Chapter 13

1. *SCL*, 13–14.

2. "Alcohol and Personality," *Epworth Highroad*, September 1939, 6–7, 63. The periodical changed names to the *Pilgrim Highroad* in 1941 and simply the *Highroad* soon after.

3. Rollo May, "Understanding and Managing Ourselves: A Series of Nine Lessons," *Pilgrim Highroad*, July 1941, 39–42, August 1941, 40–45. Other *Highroad* pieces included, "Spending Yourself," November 1941, 7–8, 57; "If You Like People," December 1941, 15–16, 58; "Getting Along with Your Family," January 1942, 14–15, 57; "I Am Also Timid," February 1942, 9–10, 49; "From Friendship to Love," March, 1942, 13–14, 55; "A Grown-Up Religion," May, 1942, 14–15. May also wrote similar articles for another denominational magazine, *Children's Religion*, including "Growing Up—The Problem of Adults," August 1941, 2–3, and "Religion is Caught in the Home," February 1942, 19–21.

4. "From Friendship to Love," *Pilgrim Highroad*, March 1942, 13–14, 55 "What to Expect from Your Counselor," *Pilgrim Highroad*, n.d., ca. 1940–41, 3–4.

5. "Understanding and Managing Ourselves: What Is Personality?," *Pilgrim Highroad*, July 1941, 39–40.

6. "Reason and Emotion," *Christendom*, n.d.; For example, "Does the War Destroy Our Values?" *Pilgrim Highroad*, March 1943, 5–7, 55–56. "Wartime Jitters the Inside Enemy," *Stationer*, n.d. [1943?], 3–4, 9–10.

7. He mentioned this to me during an informal unrecorded chat as we walked along a hiking path in Tiburon.

8. Edith Hammond to Rollo May, Elizabeth, NJ, July 13, 1941.

9. Edith Hammond to Rollo May, Elizabeth, NJ, July 28, 1941.

10. Ibid.

11. Edith Hammond to Rollo May, Elizabeth, NJ, August 3, 1941.

12. Edith Hammond to Rollo May, Elizabeth, NJ, August 27, 1941.

13. Pauck and Pauck, *Paul Tillich*.

14. For background on Goldstein and a general approach to his life and contribution, I have relied heavily on a strikingly original and important work, Anne Harrington, *Reenchanted Science: Holism in German Culture from Wilhelm II to Hitler* (Princeton, NJ: Princeton University Press, 1996), especially chapter 5, "The Self-Actualizing Brain and the Biology of Existential Choice," 140–74. I also found much of value in Oliver Sack's touching foreword to Kurt Goldstein, *The Organism: A Holistic Approach to Biology Derived from the Pathological Data in Man* (1939; repr. New York: Zone, 1995), 7–14.

15. Harrington, *Reenchanted Science*, 140–74.

16. Ibid.; for an introduction to Scheler's relevant thought, see Max Scheler, *Man's Place in Nature* (New York: Noonday, 1962).

17. Geoffrey Cocks, *Psychotherapy in the Third Reich* (New York: Oxford University Press, 1985); Harrington, *Reenchanted Science*, 140–74; the literature on Heidegger's Nazi past is vast and varied. A recent study provides one place among many to begin an exploration of the topic. See Elliot R. Wolfson, *The Duplicity of Philosophy's Shadow: Heidegger, Nazism, and the Jewish Other* (New York: Columbia University Press, 2018).

18. Harrington, *Reenchanted Science*, 164–65.

19. Ibid., 164–70; Kurt Goldstein, *Der Aufbau des Organismus: Einführung in die Biologie unter besonderer Berücksichtigung der Erfahrungen am kranken Menschen* (The Hague: Martinus Nijhoff, 1934); translated into English as *The Organism* (New York: American Book Company, 1939); Goldstein, *Human Nature in the Light of Psychopathology* (1940; repr. Cambridge, MA: Harvard University Press, 1959).

20. Susan Quinn, *A Mind of Her Own: The Life of Karen Horney* (Reading, MA: Addison-Wesley 1987), 324–27. Quinn notes that Horney herself had a rather mixed view of the Jewish refugees. See also Bernard J. Paris, *Karen Horney: A Psychoanalyst's Search for Understanding* (New Haven, CT: Yale University Press, 1996).

21. The best and most comprehensive biography of Erich Fromm is Lawrence J. Friedman, *The Lives of Erich Fromm: Love's Prophet* (New York: Columbia University Press, 2012); Svante Lundgren, "The Jewishness of Erich Fromm," paper presented at the 6th Congress of the European Association for Jewish Studies in Toledo, July 19–23, 1998 available online at http://www.fromm-gesellschaft.eu/images/pdf-Dateien/Lundgren_S_1999.pdf; Gail A. Hornstein, *To Redeem One Person Is to Redeem the World: The Life of Frieda Fromm-Reichmann* (New York: Free Press, 2000), 59–71.

22. Quinn, *A Mind of Her Own*, 349; Helen Swick Perry, *Psychiatrist of America: The Life of Harry Stack Sullivan* (Cambridge, MA: Harvard University Press, 1982), 380–86.

23. See Edith Hammond to Rollo May, September 5, 1941. After a successful freeing of her psyche, she displayed a good deal of therapist love but saw it as a problem: "You

have so thoroughly accomplished my worship of my therapist," she wrote, "that I'm afraid you're going to have a proportionate task of transference to perform."

24. Anton T. Boisen, *The Exploration of the Inner World: A Study of Mental Disorder and Religious Experience* (New York: Harper Brothers, 1936). See E. Brooks Holifield, *A History of Pastoral Care in America: From Salvation to Self-Realization* (Nashville, TN: Abingdon, 1983). Of particular importance is Susan E. Myers-Shirk, *Helping the Good Shepherd: Pastoral Counselors in a Psychotherapeutic Culture* (Baltimore: Johns Hopkins University Press, 2009).

25. Terry D. Cooper, *Paul Tillich and Psychology: Historic and Contemporary Explorations in Theology, Psychotherapy, and Ethics* (Macon, GA: Mercer University Press, 2006). See also Allison Stokes, *Ministry after Freud* (New York: Pilgrim, 1985). In addition to Fromm, Hiltner, Tillich, and May, at one time or another the participants included Ruth Benedict, Thomas Bigham, Harry Bone, Gotthard Booth (analyst and Episcopal priest, treated Walker Percy, wrote about psycho-healing), Harrison and Grace Loucks Elliott, Greta Frankenstein, Ernest Schachtel (another émigré member of the Institut für Sozialforschung), Martha Glickman (Jungian analyst), Howard Howson (professor of religion at Vassar), Elined Prys Kotschnig (psychologist and Quaker activist), Violet de Laszlo (Jungian analyst and writer), Carl Rogers, Elizabeth Rohrbach, and Frances G. Wickes (Jungian child psychologist).

26. Minutes of the Psychology of Faith Group, January 9, February 6, and March 6, 1942 (mimeographed copies).

27. Minutes of the Psychology of Faith Group, April 10 and May 1 and 20, 1942.

Chapter 14

1. Rollo May to Florence May, Chicago, Wednesday evening, n.d., [July 1943].

2. May told me that in those years "the crowd" in which he traveled indulged in serial affairs regularly, if discreetly.

3. Sheila M. Rothman, *Living in the Shadow of Death: Tuberculosis and the Social Experience* (New York: Basic Books, 1994), 2 and passim. In addition to Rothman, I have found Barbara Bates, *Bargaining for Life: A Social History of Tuberculosis, 1876–1938* (Philadelphia: University of Pennsylvania Press, 1992), extremely useful. Interestingly, even as May underwent treatment, scientists were testing drugs that by 1945 would begin to make great inroads in the disease, so much so that the entire caregiving establishment created in the United States for a vast pool of patients would collapse.

4. Shirley Kessler, interview typescript, July 1982, SR6, p. 86, and my own informal talks with May.

5. An interesting sidelight on May's irrepressible energy was his launching of a research survey at City College during his short stint there as a counselor, one that made news in October 1943. See "College Failure Is Laid to Parents; Forcing Education on Youths is Cause of Misfits, Survey at City College Shows," *New York Times*, October 17, 1943. Meanwhile, his dissertation committee was distinguished, one that was officially chaired by P. M. Symonds and also included Tillich and George Counts.

6. Rollo May to Erich Fromm, Lynnhaven, VA, June 15, 1943, Erich Fromm Papers, New York Public Library; Rollo May to Erich Fromm, Edward Sanitorium, September 8, [1943], in ibid.; Erich Fromm to Rollo May, November 6, 1943, in ibid.

7. For basic information about the history of Inwood House, see the Inwood House website at http://www.inwoodhouse.com/about/about.html, and "Inwood House," *All Souls Quarterly* 7, no. 2 (Winter 2000–2001), available online at http://www.allsoulsnyc.org/publications/quarterly/quarterly/inwoodhouse.html.

8. Rollo May, case notes at Inwood House, second interview with Lulu Richards, April 21, 1943.

9. Rollo May to Florence May, Chicago, Wednesday evening, n.d. [July 1943].

10. Ibid.

11. Florence May to Rollo May, n.d. [Summer 1943].

12. Florence May to Rollo May, n.d. [Late Summer 1943]

13. Ibid.

14. Florence May to Rollo May, n.d. [August 1943].

15. Dr. Frank Seligson, Medical Superintendent, Edward Sanitorium, to Mrs. Dorothy C. Jones, RN, Executive Secretary, Anti-Tuberculosis League of Norfolk, Naperville, IL, December 4, 1943; Florence May to Rollo May, [probably September 1943].

16. Erich Fromm to Rollo May, November 6, 1943, Erich Fromm Papers, New York Public Library; Paul Tillich to Rollo May, [Fall 1943].

17. Shirley Kessler interview typescript, July 1982, SR6, p. 8, and my own informal talks with May.

18. Professor Percival M. Symonds to May, Teachers College, New York, October 8, 1943; R. W. Frank to May, McCormick Theological Seminary, Chicago, December 27, 1943; John C. Millian to May, Baltimore, April 12, 1944.

Chapter 15

1. Philip L. Gallos, *Cure Cottages of Saranac Lake: Architecture and History of a Pioneer Health Resort* (Saranac Lake, NY: Historic Saranac Lake, 1985), 3–5. I am indebted to this book not only for its concise rendering of Trudeau's early career but also for the illuminating study of the origins and function of the cottages at Saranac.

2. Ibid. The cottages were renamed for Trudeau following his death in 1915.

3. Ibid., 16–17.

4. Two book reviews by Jean Mason that illuminate the Saranac experience are "Two Women Chronicle the White Plague: A 'Herstory' of America's Magic Mountain," *Journal of American Culture* 37 (June 2014): 2, and "Walker Percy's *The Gramercy Winner*: A Memoir of the American Tuberculosis Experience," *Journal of American Culture* 33 (June 2010): 2.

5. Lawrason Brown, *Rules for Recovery from Pulmonary Tuberculosis: A Layman's Handbook of Treatment*, 3rd ed. (Philadelphia: Lea & Febiger), 67. For fascinating anecdotes and historical material concerning Trudeau Sanatorium and daily life for the patients, see Victoria Rinehart, *Portrait of Healing: Curing in the Woods* (Utica, NY: North Country, 2002), 72–89 and passim.

NOTES TO PAGES 147–153

6. Kessler, Interview typescript, July 1982, SR6, p. 91.

7. Ibid.

8. Ibid., 91–93.

9. See Robert Taylor, *Saranac: America's Magic Mountain* (Boston: Houghton Mifflin, 1986), passim, for a lively history of the town within which Trudeau Sanitarium became a central institution.

10. Obituary for Cyril Richardson, *New York Times*, November 17, 1976, available online at http://www.nytimes.com/1976/11/17/archives/rev-dr-cyril-richardson-scholar-of-early-church-history-67-dead.html.

11. Jon M. Walton, "WORTHY," sermon preached on February 1, 2004, First Presbyterian Church, New York, NY, available on the church's website, http://www.fpcnyc.org/sermons/2004/web/040201.html; Cyril Richardson, *The Doctrine of the Trinity* (Nashville, TN: Abingdon, 1958). See also Robert Wilken, "The Resurrection of the Jesus and the Doctrine of the Trinity," *Word and World* 2, no. 1 (1982): 17–28, for a useful theological contextualization of Richardson's view.

12. For information on Rufus Moseley within the context of Pentecostalism, I am indebted to William L. De Arteaga, "Glenn Clark's Camps Furthest Out: The Schoolhouse of the Charismatic Revival," *Pneuma: The Journal of the Society for Pentecostal Studies* 25, no. 2 (Fall 2003): 265–85, especially 279–81.

13. Cyril [C. Richardson] to Rollo May, Trudeau, September 16, 1944.

14. Though May rarely mentioned this experiment in faith healing, he did refer to those experiences much later when arguing against what he saw as the confusion of psychology and religion in transpersonal psychology and especially the work of Ken Wilber. May wrote: "I do believe in parapsychology and of William James' studies concerning the fringes of consciousness. . . . When I was ill with tuberculosis I had two experiences with faith healers. All of these I choose to call religion." He did not name the second healer. See "Answers to Ken Wilber and John Rowan," misc. mss. 1987, UCSB.

15. Ibid.

16. Cyril [C. Richardson] to Rollo May, 89 Park Ave. S[aranac] L[ake], October 25, 1944.

17. Cyril [C. Richardson] to Rollo May, November 14 [1944].

18. Cyril [C. Richardson] to Rollo May, 89 Park. S.L., November 28 [19]44.

19. Ibid. Richardson also recommended that Rollo seek out a local palm reader in order to see useful "projection" in action, but apparently May didn't discuss this less ecstatic practice or seek a palm reading. Cyril [C. Richardson] to Rollo May, 89 Park, December 12, [1944].

20. Karl R. Stolz, *The Church and Psychotherapy* (New York: Abingdon-Cokesbury, 1943). Stolz was a well-known writer in the field of pastoral psychology and taught at Hartford Theological Seminary until his death in 1943, less than a year before the publication of this book. Cyril [C. Richardson] to Rollo May, 89 Park—Saranac, Dec[ember] 5, '44.

21. Cyril [C. Richardson] to Rollo May, 89 Park, Sunday [no date].

22. Ibid.

23. Ibid.

24. Cyril [C. Richardson] to Rollo May, Sunday [no date]; Cyril [C. Richardson] to Rollo May, 89 Park Avenue [Saranac], October 24, 1944; Walter Lowrie, *A Short Life of Kierkegaard* (Princeton, NJ: Princeton University Press, 1942).

25. May in *Existential Inquiries* 1, no. 1 (September 1959): 2.

26. Cyril [C. Richardson] to Rollo May, Sunday [no date].

27. Alexander Dru, ed. and trans., *The Journals of Søren Kierkegaard: A Selection* (New York: Oxford University Press, 1938), 220.

28. Florence May to Rollo May, fragment of letter; there is an unreadable word after "her."

29. Florence May to Rollo May, Thursday, [Fall 1944].

30. Cyril Richardson to Rollo May, Sunday, [January 1945]; interview with Rollo May, Tiburon, CA, November 7, 1992.

31. Harry Bone to Rollo May, New York, January 25, 1970.

32. Rollo May to Florence May, [Fall 1943?].

33. Ibid.

Chapter 16

1. Spinoza quoted in *AOC*, 20.

2. Elver A. Barker to the author, Denver, February 28, 2003. Quoted with permission of Mr. Barker. Barker's reference to "Hirschfeld" was to German sexologist Magnus Hirschfeld, whose *Die Homosexualität des Mannes und Weibes* (1914) and various other works made him a central figure in early twentieth-century German cultural modernism and sexology. A Jew and sex radical, Hirschfeld witnessed his books being burned by the Nazis in 1933 and was forced into American exile. In the 1930s, Barker might have read any number of articles about his work.

3. May was certainly not the only therapist to honor homosexual choices and freedom. Yet Barker's experience with other therapists was not unusual.

4. "Memories of the Search for Help," anonymous manuscript, dated by Rollo May, August 28, 1970.

5. Ibid.

6. See George Cotkin, *Existential America* (Baltimore: Johns Hopkins University Press, 2005), 35–87, for a pathbreaking treatment of Kierkegaard's moment in American culture and, for that matter, the history of existential interest in the United States.

7. G. Berrios, "Anxiety Disorders: A Conceptual History," *Journal of Affective Disorders* 56 (1999): 84.

8. Sigmund Freud, *Introductory Lectures on Psychoanalysis*, trans. James Strachey (New York: Liveright, 1966, 393; Sigmund Freud, *The Problem of Anxiety*, trans. H. A. Bunker (New York: Psychoanalytic Quarterly Press, 1936), passim; quote from 92. This latter essay is the version that May used in the 1930s and 1940s. There is also a later translation, with the title *Inhibitions, Symptoms, and Anxiety*, trans. Alix Strachey (New York: W. W. Norton, 1959).

9. *SCL*, 17.

10. Erich Fromm, *Escape from Freedom* (New York: Rinehart, 1941), passim; quote from 134 and mention of Kierkegaard and others from 133.

11. Kurt Goldstein, *The Organism: A Holistic Approach to Biology Derived from Pathological Data in Man* (New York: American Book Co., 1939); Goldstein, *Human Nature in the Light of Psychopathology* (New York: Schocken, 1963).

12. Goldstein, *Human Nature in the Light of Psychopathology*, 91–92, 112–13, 85–119, and passim.

13. Percival M. Symonds, *The Dynamics of Human Adjustment* (New York: Appleton-Century-Crofts, 1949), 133–91.

14. See O. H. Mowrer, "A Stimulus-Response Analysis of Anxiety and Its Role as a Reinforcing Agent" (1939), "Preparatory Set (Expectancy)—Some Methods of Measurement" (1938), and "Anxiety Reduction and Learning" (1940), collected in O. Hobart Mowrer, *Learning Theory and Personality Dynamics: Selected Papers* (New York: Ronald, 1950), 15–27, 28–64, 65–83. Symonds also cited a mimeographed paper by Mowrer titled "Anxiety: Some Social and Psychological Implications" (New Haven, CT: Institute of Human Relations, Yale University, 1940).

15. *MOA*, 44–45. In a footnote to these pages, he also notes that Erich Fromm's emphasis on human freedom and isolation in modernity present "striking parallels" to Kierkegaard despite major differences in view: "Both Fromm and Kierkegaard are centrally concerned with the individual as an existential unity, and both devote themselves to the problems of individual freedom and the sense of isolation so profoundly experienced by modern man." *MOA*, 85n. Kierkegaard quote from Søren Kierkegaard, *The Concept of Dread* (Princeton, NJ: Princeton University Press, 1944), 139. This is the translation May read, and in May's use of this quote he substituted "anxiety" for "dread."

16. Ibid., 48–86.

17. Ibid., 103–8.

18. Ibid., 108–10.

19. Ibid., 111–12. May claimed Jung had little to say about the subject.

20. Ibid., 138–46. Quoted phrases are May's characterizations of Horney's theory.

21. Ibid., 146–50.

22. Ibid., 151–89, Horney quoted on 185.

23. Ibid., 186–89, quotes from 186, 189.

24. Ibid., 190–93, quotes from 190, 191, 193.

25. However, according to May, these positive effects needed to be differentiated from the symbolic fear of death that often masked "*other conflicts and problems* within the individual" that produced "neurotic anxiety." See MOA, 194–95.

26. Ibid., 240–41.

27. Ibid., 331–7.

28. Ibid., 337–43, 343n22; May noted that his own thoughts seemed confirmed by another researcher, whose conclusion was that "not being loved is better than the experience of pseudo-love for a child." Ernest Schachtel quoted from an unpublished paper, "Some Conditions of Love in Childhood," March 1943.

29. *MOA*, 350–53; 355–56.

30. Rudolf Ekstein, *Bulletin of the Menninger Clinic*, March 1951, n.p.; Joseph Zinkin, *Journal of Nervous and Mental Disease* 118, no. 3 (1953): 280–82; Sylvan Keiser,

Psychoanalytic Quarterly 20, no. 3 (1951): 466–67. Other writers echoed this last point, even when they appreciated the book as a whole. Milton L. Miller, writing in *Psychosomatic Medicine*, found the work "thought provoking" but a bit "premature" "to offer evidence that the proletarian class may be less subject to anxiety . . . on the basis of only four unmarried mothers." Writing in the *American Journal of Sociology*, S. Kirson Weinberg praised the book as "illuminating reading for social scientists and other students of human behavior." However, he noted that May dismissed "somewhat lightly objective parental rejection," which could produce "acting-out, antisocial types in extreme cases and very emotionally cold in less extreme cases unless they cultivate other relationships in which they are accepted." See Milton L. Miller, *Psychosomatic Medicine* 14, no. 3 (May–June 1952): 237–38; S. Kirson Weinberg, *American Journal of Sociology* 56, no. 4 (January 1951): 381–83.

31. George F. J. Lehner, *Scientific Monthly* 71, no. 2 (August 1950): 130; E. T. Hall, Jr., *American Anthropologist I* 54, no. 2 (April–June 1952): 263–64; *Pulpit Digest*, July 1951; *Religion in Life*, date unknown, 139–41.

32. O. Hobart Mowrer, *Abnormal Reactions or Actions? (An Autobiographical Answer)*, vol. 2 of Jack Vernon, ed., *Introduction to Psychology: A Self-Selection Textbook* (Dubuque, IA: Wm. C. Brown, 1966), 13–20 and passim; Mowrer, *Learning Theory and Personality Dynamics: Selected Papers* (New York: Ronald, 1950), 531–61, quotes from 553–56. May's article "Historical and Philosophical Presuppositions for Understanding Therapy" is in Mowrer et al., *Psychotherapy, Theory and Research* (New York: Ronald, 1953), 9–43.

33. Interview with author, Tiburon, CA, November 7, 1992.

34. Interview with author, Holderness, NH, August 2, 1988. May noted that his staying away from the funeral infuriated Hannah Tillich.

35. Indeed, so strong was the theologian's continuing importance that Tillich's son, René, once wrote to his mother that Rollo was the "spiritual son of Paul in a way I have chosen not to be." René Tillich to Hannah Tillich, September 29, 1972.

Chapter 17

1. See Ellen Herman, *The Romance of American Psychology: Political Culture in the Age of Experts* (Berkeley: University of California Press, 1996), and Katherine Boone, "Peace of Mind: Military Psychiatry in World War II and the Creation of Combat Stress" (MA thesis, University of Texas at Austin, 2008).

2. John M. Reisman, *A History of Clinical Psychology* (New York: Irvington, 1976), 299, and, more broadly, 261–302.

3. In a published interview from late 1973, May summed up his analyses without naming names or dates, and certainly with much compression, merging of experience, and confusion. But the spirit of his remarks is clear: "I was in analysis for two years in New York, five and six times a week. It was the kind of analysis that did not take. Some take and some don't. . . . My analyst, who was a good man and an intelligent fellow, was from the Horney school. It just didn't do me much good." Howard

Martin, "A Famous Humanist Shares Some Personal Thoughts over a Picnic Lunch," *Human Behavior*, October 1973, n.p.

4. May to Clara Thompson, April 20, 1950, Archive of the William Alanson White Institute, hereafter referred to as WAWI.

5. Clara Thompson to May, May 22, 1951, May 25, 1951, December 31, 1951, WAWI.

6. *Bulletin of the New York State Psychological Association* 3, no. 3 (December 1950): 1; "A Certification Program for the New York State Psychological Association. Report of the Committee on Certification to the Board of Directors," New York State Psychological Association, mimeographed text of proposals distributed in preparation for an open meeting to discuss the proposals. For a brief history of these events, see Arthur W. Combs, "A Report of the 1951 Licensing Effort in New York State," *American Psychologist* 6, no. 10 (October 1951): 541–48.

7. "The Proceedings In Albany," *New York Times*, March 17, 1951, 21.

8. Soon after, May wrote to Fromm of their victory. Fromm wrote back on May 3: "I want to congratulate you personally for the victory of the Psychology Bill. I know that you put a great deal of effort behind it and I am sure it must be gratifying to you that the firm stand which you took proves to be the right policy." Erich Fromm to Rollo May, Mexico City, May 3, 1951; "Governor Dewey Vetoes Licensing Bill," *Newsletter of the Joint Council of New York State Psychologists on Legislation* 4, no. 1 (<<<YEAR>>>): 1; "Joint Council Plans," *Newsletter of the Joint Council of New York State Psychologists on Legislation* 4, no. 5, (June 8, 1951).

9. "Joint Council Seeks Agreement with Medical Group on Licensing Legislation," *Bulletin of the New York State Psychological Association* 4, no. 3 (December 1951): 3.

10. "Joint Council Leads Successful Fight against Restrictive Bill," *Bulletin of the New York State Psychological Association* 6, no. 1 (May 1953): 1, 6.

11. Roy Waldo Miner and Rollo May, eds., "Psychotherapy and Counseling," *Annals of the New York Academy of Sciences* 63 (November 7, 1955): 319–432, published also as a separate offprint with original page numbers.

12. Ibid., 344, 346–47.

13. Harry Bone to Clara [Thompson], New York, June 27, 1954; Janet MacKenzie Rioch, MD, to Clara Thompson, MD, New York, July 13, 1954, WAWI.

14. "A Resolution Addressed to the Council of Fellows of the William Alanson White Institute of Psychiatry, Psychoanalysis, and Psychology" (early 1956). WAWI

15. "Analysis and Report of the Fact-Finding Committee of the Harry Stack Sullivan Society of the 'Resolution Addressed to Council of Fellows of W. A. White Institute,'" March 26, 1956; "Fact-Finding Committee of the Harry Stack Sullivan Society," Final Report, September 14, 1956, members: Ben Brody, Alan Gray, Ed Levenson, Myer Mendelson, David Schechter, Hy Shatan, and Ben Wolstein at UCSB. Avram Ben-Avi, Harry Bone, Benjamin Brody, Edward M. L Burchard, Max Deutscher, Annette Herzman Gill, Anna Gourevitch, Rollo May, Ernest Schachtel, Erwin Singer, Joseph Steinert, Herbert Zucker to Institute members, [New York], April 2, 1956. WAWI.

16. Ibid.; "Fact-Finding Committee of the Harry Stack Sullivan Society," Final Report, September 14, 1956, WAWI; Earl G. Witenberg, MD, to the Fellows, New York, May 1956. WAWI.

17. "How to Backtrack and Get Ahead," *New York Times Book Review*, July 2, 1950; "The Ironic Prober" (Sullivan), *New York Times Book Review*, July 13, 1952; "What Are We Trying to Do?" (Adler), *New York Times Book Review*, August 19, 1951; "People Can Change" (Sullivan), *New York Times Book Review*, June 21, 1953; "With a Fresh, Keen Eye" (Fenichel), *New York Times Book Review*, January 31, 1954; "When Men Stand Alone" (Stanton and Perry, *Personality and Political Crisis*), *New York Times Book Review*, July 8, 1951.

18. Rejection Report, Manuscript Record for Personal Integration in a Disintegrating World, February 28, 1952, in Alfred A. Knopf Papers, Harry Ransom Center, Austin, Texas. May reported to Strauss that *The Art of Counseling* had so far sold twenty-five thousand copies and *The Springs of Creative Living* eleven thousand. *The Meaning of Anxiety*, according to May, had sold only a little more than three thousand copies by April 1951, a disappointing figure that May attributed to its publication on the Ronald Co. textbook list.

19. Ibid.

20. *MSH* ranked sixteenth on February 1 and fourteenth on February 15 on the *New York Times* bestseller list. *MSH*, passim, 13–19. Riesman's study, of course, does far more than establish these catchwords, and in any case uses "other-directed." See David Riesman, *The Lonely Crowd*, with Reuel Denney and Nathan Glazer (New Haven, CT: Yale University Press, 1950).

21. *MSH*, 15.

22. *MSH*, 22. The article was drawn from a series of articles in *Fortune* and appeared as "The Wife Problem," *Life Magazine*, January 7, 1952; *MSH*, 145–48, quotes from *Death of a Salesman* on 48–49.

23. *MSH*, 221.

24. *MSH*, 272.

25. Less apparent but implicit in some of its passages are the debts Tillich perhaps owed to May, especially concerning anxiety and in the use of contemporary American literature. Paul Tillich, *The Courage to Be* (New Haven, CT: Yale University Press, 1952), passim and 188–90.

26. Ibid.

27. *MSH*, 247–53.

28. *MSH*, 240–41.

29. *MSH*, 276.

30. Frances Witherspoon, "The Terrors of Emptiness," *New York Herald-Tribune Book Review*, January 11, 1953, 6; A. Powell Davies, "The Hollow People," *New York Times Book Review*, January 4, 1953, 3; Ann N. Hansen, "Analysis Valid but Solution Is Inadequate," *Columbus Dispatch*, February 15, 1953.

31. Seward Hiltner, "February Preview," *Pastoral Psychology Book Club*, n.d. [February 1953]; Gerald Van Ackeren, "Good Minds Missing Goals," *America*, March 21, 1953, 68.

32. David E. Roberts, review of *Man's Search for Himself*, *Union Seminary Quarterly Review*, 8:3 [March 1953], 48–50.

33. *MSH*, 276.

34. Erik Erikson to Rollo May, June 15, 1976, in Erik Erikson Papers, Houghton Library, Harvard University. May's letter does not seem to have survived, but he apparently wrote to Erikson after their first meeting in California. Erikson, who at the time was a major figure at Austen Riggs, replied: "I am glad you wrote since this issue has been on your mind all these years. I myself remember the Roberts case only vaguely. Such decisions as his visit home at Christmas time were made by the Medical Director after consultation with the staff, so I probably did not feel personally accused of misjudgment. I don't think I saw Dr. Knight's letter. But then, I may have 'repressed' the whole thing. At any rate, it was not on my mind when we met. I am glad we did!"

35. "David E. Roberts, Educator Here, 44: Religion Professor at Union Theological Seminary Dies—Author and Lecturer, *New York Times*, January 5, 1955, 23. See Paul Tillich, "The Sermons of David E. Roberts," introduction to David E. Roberts, *The Grandeur and Misery of Man* (New York: Oxford University Press, 1955), 12–13.

36. Ellie Roberts To Rollo May, Easton, Maryland, December 16, 1956.

37. Ellie Roberts To Rollo May, Easton, Maryland, February 7, 1957.

38. Ibid.

39. This happened in the presence of the author and May's widow, Georgia Johnson May, in the spring of 1994.

Chapter 18

1. Harold Taylor, interview with author, August 22, 1988, Holderness, New Hampshire. Later quotations of Taylor are from this interview.

2. May to Clara Thompson and Edward Tauber, January 8, 1957; Edward Tauber to May, June 19, 1957. May complained to Clara Thompson that a new brochure made the "double mistake" of trying to impress the medical profession while implicitly discouraging analytic training for lay therapeutic professionals. He thought the institute should "capitalize on the breadth of [its] viewpoint." When in early January 1957 the executive board of the institute made known its intention to hire new training analysts, May immediately suggested his own appointment and that of three other distinguished colleagues on the board of fellows: Ernest Schachtel, Milt Zaphiropolous, and Geneva Goodrich. WAWI. On NYU, see Bernard N. Kalinkowitz, revised by Spiros D. Orfanos, *History of the Postdoctoral Program*, https://as.nyu.edu/content/nyu-as/as/departments/postdocpsychoanalytic/training/history-of-the-program.html.

3. May to Lloyd Merrill, February 16, 1958; May to Clara Thompson, February 8, 1958; May to Edward Tauber, October 17, 1958; Edward Tauber to May, October 29, 1958, WAWI.

4. The best introduction to existentialism in American culture is George Cotkin, *Existential America* (Baltimore: Johns Hopkins University Press, 2003). I am indebted to Cotkin not only for the broad framework of his book but more specifically for its detailing of Kierkegaard's introduction to the United States. I also wish to thank him for his general encouragement over the years.

5. David E. Roberts, "Existentialism and Religious Belief," *Pastoral Psychology*, April 1957, 46. The article was published posthumously.

6. See Hazel Barnes, *The Story I Tell Myself: A Venture in Existentialist Autobiography* (Chicago: University of Chicago Press, 1997), 144 and passim.

7. *EXS*, viii.

8. Ibid., 3.

9. Rollo May, "The Art of Student Counseling," *Christian Education*, n.d., n.p.; *AOC*, 77, 82, 91.

10. *MOA*, 30, 30n35–36; Paul Tillich, "Existential Philosophy," *Journal of the History of Ideas* 5, no. 1 (1944): 44–70. It is unclear just how much of Sartre's work May had read at this point, when so little of it had actually been translated.

11. *MSH*, 16. Hazel Barnes had published a section of her translation of Sartre's *Being and Nothingness* as *Existential Psychoanalysis* in 1953, but there exists no reference to it in *Man's Search for Himself*, and I could find no reference at the time in his papers. In an interesting comment, May wondered aloud what would become of a movement built upon negations, noting that Gabriel Marcel, the most important of Catholic existentialists, "predict[ed] it will go Marxist." In Sartre's case that is exactly what happened. Later, in 1962, May wrote an introduction for a new edition of Barnes's translation of *Existential Psychoanalysis*, one more appreciative of Sartre's work, but noted that it was simply a philosophical prelude to analysis, an important but incomplete stage setting to escape what he and many others saw as the biological straitjacket of Freudian theory. *MSH*, 167; Jean-Paul Sartre, *Existential Psychoanalysis*, trans. Hazel E. Barnes, introduction by Rollo May (Chicago: Henry Regnery, 1962).

12. Immigration problems forced Ellenberger to seek another appointment at University of Montreal, where he moved in 1959. By the 1960s, he had become one of the most important historians of psychotherapy, especially known for his extraordinary survey and interpretation *The Discovery of the Unconscious: The History and Evolution of Dynamic Psychiatry* (New York: Basic Books, 1970).

13. *EXS*, vii–viii.

14. Paul Tillich, *The Courage to Be*, 136–39; *EXS*, 20.

15. *EXS*, 38–39. See Jean-Paul Sartre, *Being and Nothingness: An Essay on Phenomenological Ontology*, trans. Hazel Barnes (New York: Washington Square, 1956), 561.

16. *EXS*, 55.

17. Ibid., 38–41.

18. Ibid., 61.

19. Ibid., 79.

20. Fromm-Reichmann quotation in ibid., 81; Rogers quotation in ibid., 82.

21. Ibid., 80–91.

22. Edith Weigert to May, Chevy Chase, Maryland, June 12, 1957; Carl Rogers to May, Madison, Wisconsin, September 17, 1957; Erich Fromm to May, Zurich, April 4, 1958; Gordon W. Allport to May, Cambridge, Massachusetts, March 24, 1958, with attached "preview."

23. Carl R. Rogers, "The Way to Do Is to Be," *Contemporary Psychology* 4 no. 7 (July 1959): 196–97. This was not necessarily a surprising assessment, since, as the editors

of *Contemporary Psychology* pointed out, May had highlighted Rogers's work "as an independent American version of existential psychology." Henry Lowenfeld, review of *Existence* in *Psychoanalytic Quarterly* 28, no. 2 (1959): 258–61.

24. "Psychiatry and Being," *Time*, December 29, 1958, 26–27.

25. Ibid.

26. Ibid.

27. For Allport, see Ian A. M. Nicholson, *Inventing Personality: Gordon Allport and the Science of Selfhood* (Washington, DC: American Psychological Association, 2003), passim.

28. Carl Rogers to Rollo May, Madison, August 1, 1958.

29. Abraham Maslow to Rollo May, Cuernavaca, October 4, 1958.

30. Irvin D. Yalom, *Staring at the Sun: Overcoming the Terror of Death* (San Francisco: Jossey-Bass, 2009), 172–73. Yalom became one of the most distinguished writers and practitioners of his generation in the fields of existential psychotherapy and group psychotherapy. He noted that May's chapters were the source of inspiration, the chapters by other authors "less valuable."

31. May to Abraham Maslow, November 7, 1958.

32. Three years before, he created a short-lived study group to review the selections for *Existence*. Frieda Fromm-Reichmann to May, September 18, 1956, May Papers. Fromm-Reichmann's letter said she could not attend, but she suggested May contact Leslie Farber and Edith Weigert, both of whom eventually became active in existentialist activities. The group assembled in 1959 came from a fascinating mix of backgrounds. Thomas Hora (1914–1995) was a Hungarian émigré psychiatrist and psychoanalyst who sought to integrate spiritual and psychoanalytic realms and who won the Karen Horney Prize for the Advancement of Psychoanalysis in 1958; Henry Elkin (1914–1987) was an eminent psychoanalyst known for his work in child and adolescent psychology, creativity, and spiritual life. Antonia Wenkart (1896-1985) was a Polish émigré psychoanalyst whose interests turned to self-acceptance.

33. Organizing Committee to Dear Colleague (announcement of conference), February 10, 1959; Program of "Conference on Existential Psychotherapy, April 11 and 12 1959, Hotel Plaza, White and Gold Suite, Fifth Avenue and 59th St., New York City."

34. Mimeographed minutes, "Meeting—Saturday, May 9, 1959," and *Existential Inquiries: Journal of the American Association of Existential Psychology and Psychiatry* 1, no. 1 (September 1959). On the discussion of the name, see fragment of a circular letter, May to Drs. Benda, Colm, Elkin, Hora, Lefebre, Weigert, Wenkart (Council Members) and Mgr. Editor Van Dusen, Ashland, New Hampshire, June 24, 1959.

35. "Meeting * Saturday, September 26, 1959 at 2.30 PM," mimeographed minutes; EXP. May later published a revised edition with a more extensive list of readings. See EXP2. In 1967, May gave his own cogent summary of existentialism's relevance to psychotherapy in a series of lectures for the Canadian Broadcasting Corporation, see CBC. Feifel served as a psychologist in the Army Air Force during World War II and eventually found his calling working for the Veterans Administration in outpatient care. Feifel had organized a pioneering panel at APA on Psychology in 1956, "The Concept of Death and Its Relation to Behavior" and published the papers from that panel as

The Meaning of Death earlier in 1959. In 1960 he became the chief psychologist in charge of outpatient care for the Veterans Administration in Los Angeles.

36. "Meeting * Saturday, September 26, 1959 at 2.30 PM."

37. Typed documents, "Program Second Annual Conference on Existential Psychotherapy, Feb. 27–28" and typescript of minutes, "Business Meeting * Carnagie [sic] Endowment Center * February 28, 1960 * 4:00 P.M., Chairman: Rollo May; Van [Wilson Van Dusen] to Rollo and Toni [Antonia Wenkart], March 12 [1960]."

38. Andrew E. Curry, "Report on Existential Symposium," *Existential Inquiries* 1, no. 1 (September 1959): 32; programs, "Conference on Existential Psychology, Sunday December 13, 1959" and "Conference on Existential Psychology, Sunday, May 8, 1960," both sponsored by the Chicago Ontoanalytic Society.

39. Anthony Sutich to May, Palo Alto, April 22, 1960.

40. Jessica Grogan, *Encountering America: Humanistic Psychology, Sixties Culture, and the Shaping of the Modern Self* (New York: HarperCollins, 2013), 86–89.

41. Adrian van Kaam to May, April 9, 1960. The newly named journal also sported a much expanded editorial board including, among others, Rogers, Maslow, Allport, Straus, Tillich, Farber, and Frankel, as well as two other non-psychologists but major scholars of existentialism, Maurice Friedman and Michael Wyschogrod. See *Review of Existential Psychology and Psychiatry* 1, no. 3 (Fall 1961): 1.

Chapter 19

1. Rollo May, "Existential Analysis and the American Scene," in *Topical Problems of Psychotherapy III* (Basel: S. Karger, 1960), 57. This paper was reprinted virtually unchanged as "Existential Therapy and the American Scene" in *PHD*; quote on 134–35. It was originally delivered as a paper at the Fourth International Congress on Psychotherapy at Barcelona in 1958.

2. Tillich, "Existential Philosophy," passim. Indeed, only through Tillich's pioneering 1944 article "Existential Philosophy" did he become reacquainted with William James's relevance.

3. *EXS*, 9, 9n10–n11. He actually notes in passing a connection between James and existentialism, derived from the Tillich article, in *MOA*, 30n, but doesn't expand upon it.

4. "Existential Therapy and the American Scene," *PHD*, 129.

5. Ibid., 129–30.

6. Ibid., 130–31.

7. Ibid., 132–33. The key study of the origins and ongoing influences of these early 1950s critiques through the 1960s and 1970s is Daniel Horowitz, *The Anxieties of Affluence: Critiques of American Consumer Culture, 1939–1979* (Amherst: University of Massachusetts Press, 2005).

8. "Existential Therapy and the American Scene," *PHD*, 136.

9. Ibid., 136–37.

10. Henry A. Murray, "Vicissitudes of Creativity," in *Creativity and Its Cultivation: Addresses Presented at the Interdisciplinary Symposia on Creativity, Michigan State*

University, East Lansing, Michigan, ed. Harold H. Anderson (New York: Harper & Brothers, 1959), 98.

11. *MSH*, 139–42. This particular coupling of ecstatic moments might have had hidden autobiographical significance, since at one point Ellie rhapsodized to Rollo about a recent evening of listening to Brahms and making love.

12. Rollo May, "The Nature of Creativity," in Anderson, *Creativity and Its Cultivation*, 55–68, quotes on 57.

13. Ibid., 56

14. Quote most accessible in CTC, 54. I have quoted from the book rather than the original article because it is more easily obtained in its later form. May was referring to two major exhibitions at the Museum of Modern Art: *Picasso 75th Anniversary* [MoMA Exh. #619, May 4, 1957–August 25, 1957 (first floor and Auditorium), May 22, 1957–September 8, 1957 (third floor), MOMA website.

15. SRL.

16. Rollo May, "The Significance of Symbols," in ibid., 22, 29, and passim, 11–49.

17. Ibid., 45.

18. Rollo May, "The Man Who Was Put in a Cage," *Psychiatry: Journal for the Study of Interpersonal Relations* 15, no. 4 (November 1952), shortened and reworked in *MSH*, 145–48, and most easily accessed in *PHD*, 161–68.

19. *PHD*, 166.

20. Ibid, 166–67.

21. Manuscript in boxes 140–41, Rollo May Papers, Department of Special Collection, Davidson Library, University of California, Santa Barbara.

22. Rejection letter conquest of Apatheia, 1146.4 Knopf Edit Dept Rejection Sheets 1960–64 Ma, Alfred A. Knopf Papers, Harry Ransom Center, University of Texas at Austin.

23. Ibid, Alfred A. Knopf Papers, Harry Ransom Center, University of Texas at Austin.

24. Reader's report rejection, 2-25-1964, Alfred A. Knopf Papers, Harry Ransom Center, University of Texas at Austin.

25. Diary, August 6 [1959].

26. See Warren Goldstein, *William Sloane Coffin, Jr.: A Holy Impatience* (New Haven, CT: Yale University Press, 2004), passim, for a comprehensive account of Coffin's career.

27. Diary, July 20, [1959]. May was referring to a review by Philip Rieff, author of *Freud: Mind of the Moralist*, of an edition of Freud's collected papers that appeared in the book review of the *New York Times*, July 19, 1959, 1.

28. Diary, July 26, [1959].

29. Diary, July 3, [1959]

30. Diary, July 13, [1959].

31. A later dream reprised the earlier rescue of his sister from family strife, imagining that he was giving a girl—"like Yona?"—artificial resuscitation by remote control from Yankee Stadium. "I pushing buttons," he recalled the next morning, "then I count to do it more slowly; '1' '1000' . . then I try to get where girl is, do it directly, would work better." Diary, July 6, [1960], July 17, [1960].

Chapter 20

1. The panel consisted of Tillich; May; John C. Bennett, a church activist and soon to be Union's president; and the New School's Adolph Lowe, a Jewish émigré economist and dear friend of Tillich since the 1920s. My account of the "Theology of the Secular" conference is drawn exclusively from three compact discs (TT557777 82–84) available from the Union Presbyterian Seminary Library, Richmond, VA, as part of its Paul Tillich Collection of audio recordings. The recordings contain all or most of the conference dialogue. See the Union Presbyterian Seminary Library's website for the Tillich Collection, https://library.upsem.edu/research-resources/richmond-instructional-resource-center/digital-audio-collections/tillich-collection/,   last accessed December 2019.

2. Lowe in fact was not entirely happy with Kennedy but, since the alternative was Richard Nixon, voted for him. More positively, he compared Adlai Stevenson, with whom as an intellectual he felt much more comfortable, with Kennedy the pragmatist. Lowe was sure that what the world needed, in fact, was decisive, pragmatic leadership.

3. "The Anatomy of Angst," *Time Magazine*, March 31, 1961, 14, 44–51; Brock Brower, "Who's in Among the Analysts," *Esquire Magazine*. July 1, 1961.

4. Interview with the author, June 2002, New York.

5. *EXS*; for Strauss and phenomenology, see Rollo May, "Wish and Intentionality," in *Condicio Humana Erwin Straus on His 70th Birthday*, ed. Walter Ritter von Baeyer, (Berlin: Springer-Verlag, 1966), 233–40; Erwin Straus, *Phenomenological Psychology. The Selected Papers of Erwin Straus* (New York: Basic Books, 1966).

6. The best cultural history of humanistic psychology is Grogan, *Encountering America*. Grogan's account excels in placing the human dimensions of the leadership and the evolution of the movement as a whole within the broad and changing world of America from the 1950s onward.

7. Ibid.; see also Alan Petigny, *The Permissive Society: America, 1941–1965* (New York: Cambridge University Press, 2009), for a different perspective.

8. Interview with author, Holderness, NH, July 31, 1988.

9. Interview with author, Holderness, NH, July 31, 1988.

10. Interview with author, Tiburon, CA, October 21, 1987.

11. Interview with author, Holderness, NH, July 31, 1988.

12. May to Florence May, Friday (no date), handwritten single page note.

13. May to Florence May, March 27, 1962. Unless otherwise noted, the quotations in the next paragraphs are from this letter. I was not able to locate Florence May's letter to Alberta Szalita.

14. Interview with author, Holderness, NH, July 31, 1988.

15. Florence May to May, telegram, April 16, 1962.

16. Hannah Tillich to May, no date, but internal evidence suggests April 1962. May also marked these letters "'62."

17. Interview with author, Holderness, NH, July 31, 1988.

18. Interview with author, Holderness, NH, July 31, 1988.

19. Interview with author, Holderness, NH, July 31, 1988. Diary, November 9, 1964.

20. Here I rely on Jessica Grogan's account of the conference in *Encountering America*, 129–42.
21. Rollo May, "Intentionality: The Heart of Human Will," *Journal of Humanistic Psychology* 5, no. 2 (Fall 1965): 202–9.
22. Interview with author, Holderness, NH, July 31, 1988.
23. Ibid.
24. Ibid.
25. In 1966, he gave a series of six half-hour radio talks on existential psychotherapy for the Canadian Broadcasting Corporation that was published in Canada the following year. Rollo May, *Existential Psychotherapy* (Toronto: Canadian Broadcasting Corporation, 1967).
26. The society was an idea of Marvin Halverson, a Protestant theologian and activist who had a special interest in reconnecting modern artistic expression with religious issues. His own activities ranged from lecturing on church architecture to producing editions of plays with spiritual content that included the works of T. S. Eliot, Christopher Fry, and W. H. Auden. His interest in drama led to the production of such plays at the Phoenix Theater in New York and to his personal support of the Actors' Studio and its experimental dramatic endeavors. Halverson and Tillich became natural allies and friends in the 1950s, based on their belief that the most exciting religious art was being forged in the so-called secular realm.
27. "Imagination and Existence: Conference under the Auspices of the American Association of Existential Psychology and Psychiatry," program pamphlet.
28. Interview with author, Holderness, NH, August 1, 1988.
29. Robert S. Ellwood, *The Politics of Myth: A Study of C. G. Jung, Mircea Eliade, and Joseph Campbell* (Albany: State University of New York Press, 1999), 130–33. I find Ellwood's vision of Campbell fair and compelling. A summary of the opposing visions of Campbell as anti-Semite and racist can be followed in Richard Bernstein, "After Death, a Writer Is Accused of Anti-Semitism, *New York Times*, November 6, 1989, 51.
30. "Find No Rise in Evasion," *New York Times*, October 22, 1965.
31. Pauck and Pauck, *Paul Tillich*, 282–83; H. Tillich, *From Time to Time*, 219–24.
32. Diary, "Sept 20, [1965], Monday (after weekend at Tillich's)."
33. Diary, October 22, 1965.
34. Diary, "Nov. 15, 1965, After interment of Paul Tillich."
35. Rollo May, "Paul Tillich: In Memoriam," *Pastoral Psychology*, February 1968, 7–8.
36. Ibid., 8–9.
37. Ibid, 9–10.

Chapter 21

1. Max Frankel, "Demonstrators Decorous—3 White House Aides Meet with Leaders," *New York Times*, November 28, 1965, 1, 86.
2. See, for example, Todd Gitlin, *The Sixties: Years of Hope, Days of Rage*, rev. ed. (New York: Bantam, 1993), a standard work on radical student activism.

3. Aurobindo quoted in Michael Murphy, *The Future of the Body: Explorations into the Further Evolution of Human Nature* (Los Angeles: Jeremy P. Tarcher, 1992), 47.

4. The best short narrative account of Esalen's history is Walter Truett Anderson, *The Upstart Spring: Esalen and the American Awakening* (Reading, MA: Addison-Wesley, 1984), and I am indebted to Anderson's book for my rendering of Esalen's early history. Esalen intellectual life, more fascinating and profound than one would guess from its popular image, is told with great perception and detail in Jeffrey J. Kripal, *Esalen: America and the Religion of No Religion* (Chicago: University of Chicago Press, 2007).

5. Esalen Institute, Catalogue no. 9 W/S 1965.

6. Molly T. Day to May, Big Sur, April 2, 1965. Day was one of Michael Murphy's assistants and the daughter of a friend of May in Connecticut; "frontiers of human development," Esalen Catalog no. 11a, Fall 1965. The list of fall program leaders reads like a who's who at the intersection of religion, psychotherapy, and the arts: concerts by Ustad Ali Akbar Khan; a workshop led by Episcopal Bishop James A. Pike and Alan Watts on "Christianity in Revolution"; a harp concert; a seminar with Gardner Murphy; a program of Indian dance; seminars led by Carl Rogers and B. F. Skinner; "LSD and Human Potential," led by Sidney Cohen; Maurice Friedman on contemporary images of Man; Frank Barron on the "Psychology of Creativity"; George Brown on creativity; "The Family," led by Donald Jackson and Virginia Satir; a workshop by Virginia Satir, Sidney Jourard; parapsychology and J. B. Rhine; Clark Moustakas, S. I. Hayakawa, Robert Gerard and psychosynthesis; encounter group led by James Bugental and Fritz Perls.

7. May to Charles C. Dahlberg, New York, September 18, 1965.

8. Diary, October 28, 1965; November 17, 1965.

9. Diary, November 29, 1965.

10. Diary, March 25, 1966.

11. Diary, March 30, 1966; *The Daily Toreador* (Lubbock, TX), March 30, 1966, 1.

12. *DAS* and *PHD*.

13. "Mother" to "Rollo," Howell, Michigan, March 16, 1967, July 12, 1967, and September 8, 1967; Ruth May to "Rollo," September 18, 1967.

14. Hannah Tillich to May, n.d.; internal evidence suggests sometime in the first half of 1964; Pauck and Pauck, *Paul Tillich*, 280.

15. Diary, Monday, November 22, [1965].

16. Ibid.

17. Diary, April 27, 1966.

18. Mike Murphy to Rollo May, Big Sur, December 13, 1965.

19. Diary, April 27, 1966.

20. Diary, June 9 and 10, 1966. Here he refers to an early statement by George Leonard, a journalist and one of the founding fathers of Esalen, and Murphy, as to Esalen's vision for the good society.

21. Diary, June 10 and July 5, 1966.

22. Walt Whitman, "Facing West from California's Shores," in *Leaves of Grass* (New York: J. S. Redfield, 1871), 117. The poem was written in 1860 but not published until the late 1860s.

23. Diary, July 18 and 19, 1966.

24. Ibid.

25. Diary, July 29and 30, [1966].

26. Esalen Catalog for Summer 1966, August 5–12, 5–7 weekend seminar, 7–12 (five day workshop); Diary, August 18, 1966.

27. Diary, September 16, [1966].

28. Diary, January 8, 1967.

29. Diary, March [9 or 10], 1967 and for ensuing paragraphs describing LSD trip.

30. Diary, March 14, [1967]; Diary, April 13, [1967].

31. Diary, May 20, 1967, May 24, 1967.

32. Diary, July 4 and 5, [1967]. At the end of the summer, Rollo and Florence made a last desperate attempt at reconciliation on a trip to Europe. In response to May's writing her while in Europe with Florence, Ruth thanked him for his "lovely letter" describing their visit to the cave paintings in Lescaux, France, and offered, "Glad Florence was with you." Ruth [May] to Rollo [May], September 18, 1967.

33. Diary, July 7 and September 26–27, [1967].

34. Diary, January 25, [1965], January 2, 1967.

35. Diary, July 1, 8, 10, July 14, 1967.

36. Diary, July 8, [1967].

37. Diary, July 14, [1967].

38. Ibid.

39. Diary, July 11, November 13, November 15, [1967].

40. Diary, October 5 and 16, [1967].

41. Aldous Huxley, "Human Potentialities," *Psychology Today*, May 1967, 78.

42. Mary Harrington Hall, "Focus on Man," *Psychology Today*, September 1967, passim; Boring quote at 67.

43. Ibid., 28.

44. Ibid., 26.

45. Ibid., 29.

46. Diary, January 2, February 20 and 21, 1968; February 4 and 5, 1969; Rollo May, "The Daemonic: Love and Death," *Psychology Today*, February 1968, 16–25.

47. Diary, April 10, [1969].

Chapter 22

1. Diary, August 29, September 12, October 2, [1969]. John Lennon and Yoko Ono purchased the Ryan's apartment in 1973.

2. "The Message of History's Biggest Happening," *Time*, August 29, 1969, 32–33.

3. *LAW*, 9–10.

4. Ibid., 13–33.

5. Ibid., 45, 52.

6. Ibid., 53.

7. Ibid., 56.

8. Ibid., 105–6

9. Ibid., 325.

10. Anthony Storr, "A Psychoanalyst's Tract for Our Times," *Washington Post*, October 12, 1969.

11. John Leonard, review of *LAW*, *New York Times*, December 24 and 25, 1969.

12. May sold the paperback rights in 1970 for $500,000, and by 1976 *Love and Will* had sold half a million copies in the United States alone (and already had been translated into a dozen languages). These are rough figures drawn from Barbara Rowes, "'Love and Will'—You Need Them Both in This Age of Anxiety, Says Pioneering Psychoanalyst Rollo May," *People*, December 20, 1976.

13. "Yes Begins with a No," *Time*, June 22, 1970, 66–70, quote on 69.

14. V. to May, Montreal, August 2, 1973.

15. I have not footnoted this letter because the writer is still alive and I could not contact her. The original is in the May Papers.

16. Martha [Green?] to May, April 30, 1971, and May to Martha [Green?], June 1, 1971, in May papers.

17. William Douglas to May, August 30, 1971, May Papers.

18. The account of the trip to Death Valley comes entirely from one document, "With X in Death Valley." His account of the trip reads like a narrative expansion of his diary entries and a bit like his LSD trip.

19. Diary, January 6 and January 19, 1970.

20. Diary, n.d., ca. March 1, 1970.

21. Diary, March 6, 1970.

22. Diary, March 3 and 5, 1970.

23. Diary, April 29, 1970.

24. Diary, n.d., ca. May, 1970.

25. Diary, n.d., ca. March 1, April 13, August 27, and August 28, 1970.

26. Diary, October 16, 1970, and August 28, 1970.

27. Diary, November 2, 1970.

Chapter 23

1. William Butler Yeats, "The Second Coming," available online at https://poets.org/poem/second-coming. Significantly, Joan Didion's bestseller, *Slouching Toward Bethlehem* (New York: Farrar, Straus & Giroux, 1968), a wide-ranging collection of essays on contemporary society, drew its title from the same poem.

2. Marjorie Hunter, "Prominent Foes of War Arrested," *New York Times*, May 25, 1972. The complete text of the petition and the names of the signatories were published in Erna Acernigow, "Petition for Redress of Grievances," *New York Review of Books*, June 15, 1972, available online at http://www.nybooks.com/articles/1972/06/15/petition-for-redress-of-grievances/.

3. He did gain the notice of the Mississippi Sovereignty Commission, the state-funded anti-integration agency that secretly monitored civil rights activists, for contributing to the Poor People's Corporation, a support group for the Student Non-Violent Coordinating Committee's activities in that state during the Freedom

Summer of 1964. See "Poor People's Corporation" (pamphlet), in the papers of the Sovereignty Commission, Mississippi Department of Archives and History, Sovereignty Commission, available online at http://www.mdah.ms.gov/arrec/digital_archives/sovcom/result.php?image=images/png/cd07/049600.png&otherst uff=6|62|0|5|1|1|1|617|, accessed April 12, 2020.

4. National Advisory Commission on Civil Disorders, *Report of the National Advisory Commission on Civil Disorders: Summary of Report* (New York: A. Philip Randolph Institute, 1968).

5. Betty Friedan, *The Feminine Mystique* (New York: W. W. Norton, 2001), 429–31; *LAW*, 53. Of course, the roots of the crucial book in the history of feminism run wider and deeper than the question of personhood defined psychologically. See Daniel Horowitz, *Betty Friedan and the Making of "The Feminine Mystique": The American Left, the Cold War, and Modern Feminism* (Amherst: University of Massachusetts Press, 1998).

6. *LAW*, 53–54.

7. James R. Petersen, *The Century of Sex: Playboy's History of the Sexual Revolution, 1900–1999* (New York: Grove, 1999), 334–35. The next few paragraphs describing the show are from this source.

8. Ruth May to May, September 18, 1967, in May Papers; Ruth May to May, Placerville, CA, December 3, 1972, in May Papers.

9. David Dempsey, "Love and Will and Rollo May," *New York Times*, March 28, 1971, 26.

10. Lisl Malkin, *An Interrupted Life: A Holocaust Survivor's Journey to Independence* (Englewood Cliffs, NJ: Full Court Press, 2014), Chapters 35 and 36, Kindle edition.

11. Ibid.

12. *PAI*, 14.`

13. James Baldwin, *The Fire Next Time* (New York: Dial, 1963), 21.

14. *PAI*, 99, 48–49, and passim.

15. Ibid., 50–53.

16. Ibid., 54–55, quoting Charles A. Reich, *The Greening of America* (New York: Random House, 1970), 348.

17. *PAI*, 81, quoting Kenneth B. Clark, *Dark Ghetto: Dilemmas of Social Power* (New York: Harper & Row, 1965), 198.

18. *PAI*, 86.

19. Ibid., 87–88. It is simply a reference to the Greek Titan who forges man from clay, gives human beings fire, and is ultimately punished severely by Zeus.

20. Ibid., 93–96.

21. Ibid., 96–97.

22. Ibid., 208–9.

23. Ibid., 219–20.

24. Ibid., 221–22, 229, 233–34. May pointed out that though the rebel might eventually become accepted by the mainstream, it might have devastating effects on the artist, as in the suicides of Pollock and Rothko at the height of their fame.

25. Ibid., 238, quote from Albert Camus, *The Rebel: A Man in Revolt* (New York: Alfred A. Knopf, 1954), 301.

26. *PAI*, 253–54

27. Ibid., 241–60, especially 253–59.

28. Anatole Broyard, "Books of the Times," *New York Times*, November 2, 1972, 41; Paul A. Robinson, "An Innocent Defense of Power," *New York Times*, December 10, 1972.

29. Ronald Sampson, "An Opiate for Conscience," *Commonweal*, February 9, 1973, 427, 429; William Hamilton, "The Flaws of the Innocent," *Christian Century*, December 20, 1972, 1303–4.

Chapter 24

1. May to Hannah [Tillich], n.d., with note from May, "written in Autumn, 1966"]

2. René Tillich to Hannah Tillich, September 29, 1972. René continued: "My father, Paul, was a funny pot-bellied man who told me stories about mountain climbing and took me out in a row boat."

3. Diary, April 29, 1970; *PAU*, 1; for dates of contract and writing, see Elliott Wright, "Paul Tillich as Hero: An Interview with Rollo May," *Christian Century*, May 15, 1974, 530.

4. *PAU*, 1–24.

5. Ibid., 28–36.

6. Ibid., 45, quotations from Paul Tillich, *On the Boundary* (New York: Charles Scribner's Sons, 1966), 14.

7. Hannah Tillich, postcard and note enclosed in Hannah Tillich's personal stationery envelope and marked by Rollo May as "Crazy letter / May 5th", no year.

8. *PAU*, 52–53, 58.

9. Wright, "Paul Tillich as Hero," 530.

10. "Paul Tillich, Lover," *Time*, October 8, 1973, 79.

11. Harvey Cox, "The Wisest and the Justest and the Best," *New York Times*, Sunday Book Review, October 14, 1973.

12. Ibid. Plato quotation is from the *Phaedo*.

13. Martin E. Marty, "Eros and the Theologian," *Christian Century*, September 26, 1973, 959.

14. Ibid.

15. *CTC*.

16. Ibid., 12–35.

17. Ibid., 32–35.

18. Anatole Broyard, "From Oedipus to Prometheus," *New York Times*, November 10, 1975, 31; Irving Markowitz, *American Journal of Orthopsychiatry* 47, no. 2 (1977): 360–61.

19. *CTC*, 110–11.

20. Interview with author, August 1, 1988, Holderness, NH.

21. Liz Campbell, Reflections: Annual Meeting, *AHP Newsletter*, January 1972, 1–3.

22. Joe Brodbeck quoted in ibid., 2–3.

23. Kalen Hammann, letter to the editor, *AHP Newsletter*, May–June 1973, 1, 3.

24. "News," *AHP Newsletter*, January 1973, 4.

25. Carolyn Morell, "*Love and Will*: A Feminist Critique," *Journal of Humanistic Psychology* 13, no. 2 (Spring 1973): 35–39.

26. Ibid., 45 and passim.

27. Ibid., 45–47.

28. Rick Gilbert, ed., "Edited Theory Conference Transcript," Tucson, April 4–6, 1975. For a general account of the meeting, see Grogan, *Encountering America.*

29. Rollo May, "Gregory Bateson and Humanistic Psychology," *Journal of Humanistic Psychology* 16, no. 4 (Fall 1976): 33–51; the essay was later published in John Brockman, ed., *About Bateson: Essays on Gregory Bateson* (New York: E. P. Dutton, 1977), 75–99.

30. Mike Moore, "Breaking Free from the Human Potential Movement," *Mountain Gazette* 38 (October 1975): 17. A touching obituary for Moore can be found on the *Mountain Gazette* web page, http://www.mountaingazette.com/mountain-culture/ memorium-mike-moore/.

31. Moore, "Breaking Free from the Human Potential Movement,", 18, 23.

Chapter 25

1. May to Jack [John Schimel], 98 Sugarloaf, April 7, 1977. Schimel was the editor of the *Report.* The article to which May referred was probably "How to Cope with Rejection," *Harper's Bazaar,* July 1976; M to Robert Akeret, 98 Sugarloaf, March 28, 1977. Akeret made it clear in conversation with me that the event became the pretext for expressing longstanding tensions and jealousies that spilled over into this presumably valedictory event.

2. Clement Reeves, *The Psychology of Rollo May* (San Francisco: Jossey-Bass, 1977). May's response can be found on pages 295–309.

3. Stephen A. Diamond, "The Meaning of Mentors: Memories of Rollo May," *Psychology Today* (blog), June 16, 2012, https://www.psychologytoday.com/us/blog/evil-deeds/ 201206/the-meaning-mentors-memories-rollo-may; Diamond, *Anger, Madness, and the Daimonic: The Psychological Genesis of Violence, Evil, and Creativity,* Foreword by Rollo May (Albany: SUNY Press, 1996). Diamond was not the only recipient of such care. May had a more general impact on Ed Mendelowitz, now a Boston-area psychotherapist and explorer of the relationship of the arts, creativity, and the self. He was May's teaching assistant at the California School of Professional Psychology in 1982. For Keddy, see Philip Keddy, "My Experience With Psychotherapy, Existential Analysis, and Jungian Analysis: Rollo May and Beyond," *Journal of Clinic Psychology: In Session* 67, no. 8 (2011): 806–17. Keddy's account includes a reasonably detailed description of May's analytic technique, one quite similar to that described by Sabert Basescu, an analysand of May's in the 1950s and in his own right a major figure in New York's analytic world.

   Nor did one necessarily have to be a protégé to experience May's generosity in publicly supporting the work of others. Most poignant was his foreword to an extraordinary memoir, *Notes on an Emergency: A Journal of Recovery,* by Elizabeth Leonie Simpson. Simpson was a humanistic social psychologist who contracted tubercular meningitis, a disease that caused hallucinations and ultimately a coma, with attendant doctors pronouncing her terminally ill. He also wrote a foreword to Robert

Kramer's edition of lectures by Otto Rank, one that was published posthumously. See Rollo May, foreword to *Notes on an Emergency: A Journal of Recovery*, by Elizabeth Léonie Simpson (New York: W. W. Norton, 1982), xi–xiv; Rollo May, foreword to *A Psychology of Difference: The American Lectures Otto Rank*, ed. Robert Kramer (Princeton, NJ: Princeton University Press, 1996), xi–xii.

4. "Loneliness," typescript of private and unpublished self-analysis, September 10, [1977], and Diary, September 13, [1977].

5. May "To S_____," typescript.

6. Diary, September 26, [1977], and typescript, "S. on trip to Placerville; Norma", September 13 [1977].

7. Diary, September 26, [1977], and typescript, "S. on trip to Placerville

8. Both Don Michael and Peter Koestenbaum, in interviews with the author, talked much about May's naïveté when it came to the complexity of social and political questions.

9. Irvin Yalom, *Becoming Myself: A Psychiatrist's Memoir* (New York: Basic Books), 187–94.

10. Diary, March 19, [1979], "March 19—* Ruth *" above the entry.

11. Typescript of unpublished autobiography, "The Wounded Healer."

12. *FD*; quote from 282.

13. Ibid., 24–51, 88–91, 153–54, 234–35. May told me an interesting story about the autobiographical nature of the book: "The editor of Norton, I don't think he caught on to the fact that it was partly an autobiography. He said that when he first read it that it wouldn't work because the people I talked about were too unusual. I was 10 percent happy when he said that and 90 percent suspicious. We were having lunch together when he said that and I looked up at him to see if he was looking at me and to see if he even knew it was autobiographical. He just kept eating his lunch. I don't think he did know it ever." Interview with author, July 1, 1988, Holderness, NH.

14. *FD*, 45.

15. Ibid., 49–51.

16. Anatole Broyard, "Fashions in Madness," *New York Times*, November 21, 1981; *Kirkus Reviews*, October 21, 1981. Interview with author, March 23, 1987. For May's judgment, see Ed Mendelowitz, "Psychology and Paradox," PsycCRITIQUES 52, no.7, Article 17 (2007); Michael Fox, "The Editor's Column: Whatever Happened to Existentialism," *Queen's Quarterly* 90, no. 1 (Spring 1983): 284–88.

17. Notes for a talk at Princeton meetings of the AHP, August 27, 1979, May papers.

18. For a text and very useful interpretation of the Carter speech, see Daniel Horowitz, *Jimmy Carter and the Energy Crisis of the 1970s: The "Crisis of Confidence" Speech of July 15, 1979* (Boston: Bedford/St. Martins, 2004).

19. *MSH*, 234–36.

20. Notes for a speech, January 29, 1981; *FD*, passim.

21. Rollo May quoted in Liz Campbell, "Reflections: Annual Meeting," and Marilyn Ferguson, "AHP Goes Public, Launches Era of Social Involvement," *AHP Newsletter*, October 1978, 7, 8–11. May quote concerning "myths of the future" in text box, p. 15. See this issue for other assessments of the meeting.

22. *AHP Newsletter*, October 1979.

23. Carl Rogers, "Notes on Rollo May," in "Rollo May: Man and Philosopher," special issue, *Perspectives* 2, no. 1(Summer 1981): 16. The entire issue exemplified the supportive environment May enjoyed in California. Meanwhile, Rogers's rejection of what he called the "demonic" has had an important influence on the future "positive psychology" movement, though this new approach from the realm of academic psychology claimed that Rogers and other humanistic psychologists lacked the scientific evidence for much of their claims and that in any case humanistic psychology suffered from a tendency toward narcissism and worship of "self-esteem. See Daniel Horowitz, *Happier?: The History of a Cultural Movement That Aspired to Transform America* (New York: Oxford University Press, 2017), passim, and Jessica Grogan, *Encountering America*, 314–15.

24. May, "The Problem of Evil: An Open Letter to Carl Rogers," *Journal of Humanistic Psychology* 22, no. 3 (Summer 1982): 10–21. See also a more recent, historical reworking of the general idea of constant struggle in Jill Lepore, *This America: The Case for the Nation* (New York: Liveright, 2019), passim.

25. For a succinct view of the movement and its context within humanistic psychology, see Grogan, *Encountering America*, 250–51.

26. Willis Harman to Jacqueline Larcombe Doyle, February 10, 1982, May Papers.

27. Rollo May to Willis Harman, March 27, 1982.

28. Harman's work in the area of society was certainly optimistic in its hope for a new and more humane and creative paradigm for society. However, he shared May's concern that potentialities did not inevitably lead to progress. In fact, he concluded in a work of 1982: "[His view] should not be mistaken for optimism that industrial civilization will develop the requisite understanding, early enough, to enable it to navigate these troubled waters without nearly wrecking itself in the process." Harman became more and more interested in the relationship between consciousness and social change as the years went on but died in 1997, before the momentous impact of the internet and other aspects of the tech revolution, as well as the increasing disparities of wealth in the United States and more generally in the world, confirmed at least parts of this dire possibility but as yet little of his hoped-for change. See O. W. Markley and Willis W. Harman, eds., *Changing Images of Man* (Oxford: Pergamon, 1982, 198–99 and passim.

29. Wilber himself was reluctant to identify with the transpersonal movement, though it seems his was very much a minority opinion. May recounted the incident as part of a recorded discussion with Jackie Doyle and Stanley Krippner, published as Rollo May, Stanley Krippner, and Jacqueline Larcombe Doyle, "The Role of Transpersonal Psychology in Psychology as A Whole: A Discussion," *Humanistic Psychologist* 20 (Summer-Autumn 1992): 307–17.

30. Rollo May, "Transpersonal," *APA Monitor* 17, no. 5 (May 1986): 2. The issue of a separate division was part of an identity crisis in the movement that found many other participants besides May and Wilber, and at least the broader dimensions of this somewhat splintered debates found expression in the spring 1989 issue of *JHP*, where various authors attempted to define the essential characteristics of humanistic psychology, its various schools of thought and the issues that divided them, and ultimately what might hold them together.

31. Interview with Kirk Schneider, *Wise Counsel* (podcast), March 1, 2010, https://radiopublic.com/wise-counsel-podcasts-WP01Yj/ep/s1!2b675. Schneider began his direct connection to existential therapy at West Georgia College (presently the State University of West Georgia), where he did work with Don Rice, one of the early graduates of HPI. Rice was deeply influenced by the work of May and James Bugental, another distinguished humanistic psychologist in the Bay Area. Schneider took Rice's advice and transferred to HPI, chose Bugental as his mentor, and by the mid-1980s had struck up what turned out to be an ever-deepening personal and intellectual relationship. See also May to Kirk Schneider, Tiburon, January 20, 1985, letter supplied by Schneider to the author.

32. Rollo May, "Answers to Ken Wilber and John Rowan," *Journal of Humanistic Psychology* 29, no. 2 (Spring 1989): 244–48; These were not May's last words on the subject. As the hundredth anniversary celebrations of the founding of the American Psychological Association approached, May, Stanley Krippner, and Jackie Doyle met to discuss transpersonal ideas within the broader field of psychology. May, Krippner, and Doyle, "The Role of Transpersonal Psychology"; Mark A. Scholl, John Rowan, and Oliver Robinson, with comments by Angela Voss and Brad Adams, "Clearing Up Rollo May's Views of Transpersonal Psychology and Acknowledging May as an Early Supporter of Ecopsychology," *International Journal of Transpersonal Studies* 30, no. 1 (2011): 120–36.

33. May, "Answers to Ken Wilber and John Rowan," 244.

34. Diary, August 1, 1986.

35. Herman Reissig to May, Stamford, Connecticut, October 27, 1981.

36. DOB, passim; Peter Y. Gunter, "May Takes On Existentialism and Psychology, and Wins," *Dallas Morning News*, November 13, 1983, 4G.

37. "The Wounded Healer."

38. *MQB*, passim. Howell also reprinted *Paulus* and published articles mostly from the *JHP* and the *AHP Newsletter* that illustrated the kaleidoscopic vision and internal debates of the movement. See Rollo May, Carl Rogers, and Abraham Maslow, *Politics and Innocence: A Humanistic Debate* (Dallas: Saybrook, 1986).

39. Correspondence with various women in the May Papers. I have chosen not to quote or cite them in order to protect their privacy.

40. This and the following paragraphs recounting the relationship between Georgia Johnson and May derives from interviews with both Rollo and Georgia.

41. Carol Horner, "On A Lonely Mount With Rollo May," *Chicago Tribune*, September 7, 1981.

42. Georgia May interview with the author on various occasions, Tiburon and Carmel, CA.

43. See Jan Troell, dir., *Sagolandet* [Land of dreams], (Stockholm: Folkets Bio, 1988), 185 minutes.

44. Anne Mead to Chapel Board Members, "Re: Chapel Life," October 29, 1979, Rothko Chapel Library, Houston, Texas.

45. Diary, August 18 and 20, 1986; July 4, 1987; on *The Hero's Journey: The World of Joseph Campbell*, see the IMDb entry, http://www.imdb.com/title/tt0093183/?ref_=fn_

al_tt_3. This film is not to be confused with Bill Moyers's *The Power of Myth*, which appeared a year later on PBS.

46. Interview with Georgia May; interview with the author; Janet Silver Ghent, "For the Common Good: Doing's More Important Than Feeling, Says Psychologist," *Oakland Tribune*, clipping without date [1990].

47. Diary, January 28, 1990.

48. Marshall B. Stearn, *Portraits of Passion Aging: Defying the Myth* (Sausalito, CA: Park West, 1991), 100–103, quote on 103. The book contained thirty-two narratives of older intellectuals, artists, and others who continued to lead engaged lives into their seventies and eighties.

49. From unrecorded conversations with Georgia May in Tiburon and the late Diane Middlebrook in Austin. Middlebrook had been a fellow at Bellagio at the same time as May.

50. Georgia May's remembrance of May telling the story.

51. The author witnessed some of these incidents.

52. The author witnessed the drive to dinner. The story of the Berkeley trip was told to me by Georgia May.

53. "The Path Of Good Wishes Which Protecteth From Fear In The Bardo", Verse 7, Tibetan Book of the Dead, Part 21, https://buddhism.redzambala.com/tibetan-book-of-the-dead/tibetan-book-of-the-dead-part-21.html.

54. Georgia May interview; "Rollo May 1909–1994," in Tom Greening, "Poems for Rollo," photocopied collection of four poems distributed privately, n.d.

Epilogue

1. Anna Archibald, "Top Bartender Alexis Brown's Current Obsession: "The Courage to Create by Rollo May," *Daily Beast*, December 5, 2019, https://www.thedailybeast.com/bartender-alexis-browns-current-obsession-the-courage-to-create-by-rollo-may.

2. Peter D. Kramer, *Listening to Prozac* (New York: Viking, 1992), was the first widely read book on the drug, one that made the case for its use as a positive transformative experience. Scores of books on Prozac and other antidepressants have appeared since—memoirs, celebrations, and critiques of its use. HMOs and the new psychotropic treatment caused a significant shift in the training of psychiatrists toward the use of prescription drugs and less emphasis on "talk" therapy. See T. M. Luhrmann, Of Two Minds: An Anthropologist Looks at American Psychiatry (New York: Vintage, 2001), for an incisive study of this phenomenon. However, by the beginning of the twenty-first century, it began to become clear that these drugs, while often producing seemingly miraculous transformations, sometimes had serious side effects and in any case were most effective when combined with traditional psychotherapy.

3. J. Winokur, review of *Love and Will* on Amazon, https://www.amazon.com/gp/customer-reviews/RO7I1MLTF2QKS/ref=cm_cr_dp_d_rvw_ttl?ie=UTF8&ASIN=0393330052>, accessed January 6, 2020.

4. Caitlin O'Neil, review of *Love and Will* on Amazon, https://www.amazon.com/gp/customer-reviews/R1ZE7QU1IM4TDG/ref=cm_cr_dp_d_rvw_ttl?ie=UTF8&ASIN=B002KD2M74, accessed January 6, 2020.
5. See Maria Popova, "Existential Psychologist Rollo May on Freedom and the Significance of the Pause," *Brain Pickings* (blog), October 4, 2017, https://www.brainpickings.org/2017/10/04/rollo-may-freedom-destiny-pause/, accessed January 7, 2020.
6. Chris Robinson, "I Have a Question Maral Mohammadian," *Let's Go Eat the Factory!* (Animation World Network blog), August 2, 2017, https://www.awn.com/animationworld/i-have-question-maral-mohammadian, accessed April 5, 2020. Our email exchange occurred on August 6 and 13, 2017, text in possession of the author.

Index

For the benefit of digital users, indexed terms that span two pages (e.g., 52–53) may, on occasion, appear on only one of those pages.

The photo insert images are indexed as *p1, p2, p3*, etc.